Contents

Preface   5

PART I • THE INTERNAL ORGANS & THEIR Y-SCORES   7

  1   *The Chinese Theory of Internal Organs*   9

  2   *Y-Scores of the Internal Organs*   23

  3   *Identifying Your Own Signs and Symptoms*   31

  4   *Recording and Calculating the Y-Scores of Your Internal Organs*   52

PART II • THE SYNDROMES   77

  5   *Choosing Foods and Herbs to Boost the Lungs and Cure Applicable Symptoms and Diseases*   79

  6   *Choosing Foods and Herbs to Boost the Large Intestine and Cure Applicable Symptoms and Diseases*   97

  7   *Choosing Foods and Herbs to Boost the Spleen and Cure Applicable Symptoms and Diseases*   105

  8   *Choosing Foods and Herbs to Boost the Stomach and Cure Applicable Symptoms and Diseases*   125

  9   *Choosing Foods and Herbs to Boost the Liver and Cure Applicable Symptoms and Diseases*   137

  10   *Choosing Foods and Herbs to Boost the Gallbladder and Cure Applicable Symptoms and Diseases*   156

11 *Choosing Foods and Herbs to Boost the Kidneys
and Cure Applicable Symptoms and Diseases*   160

12 *Choosing Foods and Herbs to Boost the Bladder
and Cure Applicable Symptoms and Diseases*   174

13 *Choosing Foods and Herbs to Boost the Heart
and Cure Applicable Symptoms and Diseases*   179

14 *Choosing Foods and Herbs to Boost the Small Intestine
and Cure Applicable Symptoms and Diseases*   192

15 *Choosing Foods and Herbs to Boost Two
Internal Organs Simultaneously and Cure
Applicable Symptoms and Diseases*   197

PART III • CHINESE FOOD CURES   221

16 *An Overview of Chinese Food Cures*   223
17 *Six Classes of Foods and Their Effects*   246

GUIDE TO APPROXIMATE EQUIVALENTS   267

INDEX   268

CHINESE SYSTEM

SYSTEM

OF

FOODS

FOR

HEALTH

&

HEALING

Henry C. Lu, Ph.D.

Sterling Publishing Co., Inc.   New York

Library of Congress Cataloging-in-Publication Data

Edited by Laurel Ornitz

1   3   5   7   9   10   8   6   4   2

Published by Sterling Publishing Company, Inc.
387 Park Avenue South, New York, N.Y. 10016
© 2000 by Henry C. Lu
Distributed in Canada by Sterling Publishing
c/o Canadian Manda Group, One Atlantic Avenue, Suite 105
Toronto, Ontario, Canada M6K 3E7
Distributed in Great Britain and Europe by Cassell PLC
Wellington House, 125 Strand, London WC2R 0BB, England
Distributed in Australia by Capricorn Link (Australia) Pty Ltd.
P.O. Box 6651, Baulkham Hills, Business Centre, NSW 2153,
Australia

Sterling ISBN 0-8069-7065-0

Preface

Traditional Chinese medicine is based on the fundamental belief that ten vital internal organs in the human body play a crucial role in both health and illness. The ten organs have their respective duties, which need to be performed adequately and effectively. A Chinese medical classic published more than thirty centuries ago pointed out that the ten organs must be coordinated properly in order to maintain good health, and that at no time should they neglect or harm one another in any way. If you have nine strong, healthy organs working hard for you every day, but one organ that is failing you miserably, you would not be in good health—on the contrary, your very existence could be in jeopardy.

This book introduces two simple and yet very useful concepts— the y-scores of the internal organs and the organ y-scores of foods— which are the two key working concepts in traditional Chinese medicine for the promotion of good health. The y-scores of the internal organs have to do with identifying the yin-yang status of the internal organs; the y-score can range from 0 to -8 or +8, which indicates to what extent your internal organs are yin or yang. Having identified the y-scores of your internal organs, you need to know the organ y-scores of foods, so that you can choose the right foods not only to cure any diseases you may have but also to promote your health.

The organ y-scores of foods are used to determine what foods can help the internal organs increase or decrease their y-scores. If the organ y-score of a food is Liver -2, for example, this means that food is useful in bringing the y-score of your liver to -2. Assuming that the y-score of your liver is 4, food with Liver -2 would be beneficial for you, because it could help you bring down the y-score of your liver.

Health and illness are not two isolated states, but there exists a continuity between them. However, if you are in good health, you will still have different y-scores for the ten vital organs. Having gone through the steps for diagnosis, you may find that the y-score of your liver is 3, which is within the healthy range. This y-score can fluctuate up or down over time. If it goes down to 1 or -1, this indicates that your liver is becoming healthier. If it goes up to 8, you may start to display symptoms such as headaches, dizziness, or hypertension. When this occurs, you are no longer healthy.

When you are sick, the illness and the symptoms can be traced back to disorders of the internal organs, which are described in Chinese medicine as "syndromes." For example, if chronic bronchitis is due to the syndrome of Lungs Energy Deficiency, this syndrome should be treated in order to cure it. The same theory applies to virtually all diseases and conditions, and is the focus of this book. It is a far cry from the current Western understanding of diseases and their treatment in which illnesses and symptoms are treated as such directly. In traditional Chinese medicine, illnesses and symptoms are traced back to their respective syndromes, and the methods of treatment are directed toward the syndromes that are responsible for them.

This book is designed for you whether you are healthy or ill. If you are in good health, it will help you maintain your good health, because it will show you how to bring the y-score of your liver down to 1, 0, or -1, for example. If you are ill, this book will show you how to eat the right foods and take the right herbs to correct the illness.

Part I

THE INTERNAL ORGANS & THEIR Y-SCORES

1

The Chinese Theory of Internal Organs

FUNCTIONS OF THE TEN INTERNAL ORGANS

The Heart

In traditional Chinese medicine, the heart is the ruler or the monarch. When the ten internal organs are all assigned duties, the heart becomes the monarch from whom the spirits are derived. Therefore, the activities of all internal organs are under the control of the heart. The heart is also the master of the blood vessels, which means that blood can circulate in the blood vessels without a break and supply nutritive energy to various tissues of the human body only under the direction of the heart. Normal blood circulation will be impaired if the conditions of the heart are themselves impaired.

The heart also takes charge of the spirits, as mentioned above. The spirits are the state of mind, as the mind and the heart are regarded as identical. All the mental activities, including sensation, consciousness, thought, and emotion, are associated with the heart. You will display normal spirits as long as your heart continues to function normally. On the other hand, many symptoms of the mind can arise when there is a disorder of the heart.

The Lungs

The lungs are the master of energy. One of the most important functions of the lungs is to take charge of energy. Initially, the lungs take charge of air, which is the energy of space; this is done through respiration, with the lungs inhaling clear energy and exhaling turbid energy. In Chinese medicine, this phenomenon is called "exhaling the old and absorbing the new."

Later, after foods have been digested in the stomach and the spleen, the energy of grains is transported to the lungs. There, the energy of air and that of grains meet to combine with the pure energy of the kidneys for transformation into true energy, which is then distributed throughout the entire body for nourishment.

The Spleen

The stomach and the spleen are both regarded in Chinese medicine as officials in charge of food storage, but they serve different functions. After foods enter the stomach, the spleen spreads the energy of foods to other internal organs. In other words, the stomach receives foods and the spleen spreads them for nourishment.

The spleen controls the blood, so that blood will flow within the blood vessels regularly and constantly. The spleen can produce energy, and when the spleen is full of energy, blood circulates normally. But when spleen energy is deficient, blood can escape from blood vessels and cause various types of bleeding.

The Liver

The liver is the largest organ in the human body. It contains the largest quantity of blood among the internal organs, which is why it is considered the "sea of blood" in traditional Chinese medicine. As the liver stores the blood and as the blood stores the soul, it follows that the liver is not only capable of regulating the conditions of the blood but is also the source of strategies that direct our course of action.

The Kidneys

The kidneys are capable of steaming and regulating water, in order to spread it throughout the entire body to maintain the normal distribution of water in the body. The stomach receives water from the outside, the spleen moves it throughout the body, the lungs regulate it, and the bladder expels it through urination. This whole process depends on the energy transformation of the kidneys, because the kidneys control the bladder and keep it closed so that urine does not escape, and they open the bladder so that urination can take place.

The kidneys produce marrow to fill bones, and, as teeth are an extension of bones, it follows that the kidneys are also responsible for the health of teeth. The kidneys are in charge of the growth of bones, which is why in the treatment of fracture it is customary for Chinese physicians to tone the kidneys to speed up recovery. Marrow is inside bones, and the kidneys are capable of generating marrow; because the brain is full of marrow, it is said that "the brain is the sea of marrow." A Chinese classic states: "The kidneys are the roots of sealed storage, they are the residence of pure energy, their glory is manifest in the hair on the head, they fill up the bones."

The Small Intestine

The small intestine is the receiving official from whom pure substances are derived. This means that the small intestine distinguishes refined energy of foods from turbid energy; it assimilates refined energy and excretes waste matter. This process takes place in the following way. The small intestine receives decomposed and cooked foods from the stomach, digests these foods, and separates them into clear and turbid substances. The small intestine absorbs the clear substances for distribution through the entire body by way of the spleen; then it sends the turbid substances out as waste matter, moving water to the bladder for discharge as urine and residue to the large intestine as stools.

The Large Intestine

The large intestine primarily acts as the official of transportation, receiving waste matter from the small intestine, absorbing its water, and discharging the residue as stools. When the large intestine is too deficient and cold to absorb the water contained in waste matter from the small intestine, this will give rise to intestinal rumbling, abdominal pain, and diarrhea; on the other hand, if the large intestine has accumulated too much heat and absorbs too much water from waste matter, this will lead to dry stools and constipation.

The Stomach

Foods gathering in the stomach can be compared to water gathering in the ocean, which is why the stomach is regarded as the "sea of water and grains." The stomach is the grand source of nutrition for all the other organs.

The stomach is in charge of decomposing and cooking, as well as pushing down turbid substances. The term "turbid substances" refers to water and grains in the stomach. After preliminary digestion, the stomach must send the digested foods to the small intestine by pushing downward.

The Gallbladder

The gallbladder is the impartial judge from whom judgments are derived. The gallbladder performs the duty of passing good judgments in protecting the spirits, eliminating emotional disturbances, and directing other internal organs to take an adequate course of action. It also separates bravery from cowardice.

A Chinese classic says: "A brave person has deep eyes and high eye sockets, looking at objects so firmly that the eyeballs stay put without turning, eyebrows standing up, with rough stripes on the muscles and a straight heart and a big, hard liver; and, also, his gallbladder is full of bile almost overflowing on the sides. When this person is angry, he is full of energy with the chest expanded, his liver lifts up, and his gallbladder expands toward the sides, his eyes are wide open as if about to break, his hair stands up, and his face turns green. Such are the factors that account for bravery."

The Bladder

Among the ten internal organs, the bladder, located far from the other organs, is the district official in charge of storing urine. The symptoms of the bladder are primarily associated with urination and include difficult urination, blocked urination, discharge of urine containing blood, enuresis, and frequent urination.

FACTORS SHAPING THE CONDITIONS OF THE INTERNAL ORGANS

The internal organs are continually under adverse influences from both external and internal factors. Among the external factors are the six atmospheric energies: wind, cold, summer heat, dampness, dryness, and fire; among the internal factors are energy and blood, emotions, fatigue, and the foods we eat. Each factor can affect the internal organs differently. In order to stay in good health, it is important to constantly keep track of the conditions of the internal organs and then to eat the right foods to counteract any adverse influences.

The Six Atmospheric Energies

The ten internal organs are all subject to attack from the six atmospheric energies—wind, cold, summer heat, dampness, dryness, and fire—which can give rise to various syndromes. It is important to understand the nature of such an attack so that you can figure out the y-scores for different syndromes. Each of the five major internal organs is most susceptible to the attack of one specific atmospheric energy: The liver is most susceptible to the attack of wind, the kidneys are most susceptible to the attack of cold, the heart is most susceptible to the attack of summer heat, the spleen is most susceptible to the attack of dampness, and the lungs are most susceptible to the attack of dryness; all the internal organs are more or less susceptible to the attack of fire.

Wind (y-scores of 2 within the healthy range and 6 within the pathological range)

Wind affects the human body constantly, and it can also attack it from time to time. When wind merely affects the human body, the organs affected may display a y-score of 2, in which case no symptoms are observed and the organs remain in good health. On the other hand, when wind attacks the human body, the organs under attack may display a y-score of 6; in this case, certain symptoms are seen and the organs under attack have become sick. Among the internal organs, the liver is most frequently under the influence of wind. When wind affects the liver, the y-score of the liver is 2; when wind attacks the liver, the y-score of the liver is 6.

Wind is a yang energy, because it tends to move upward and stay high. Wind has a tendency to attack the upper regions of the human body, causing such symptoms as headache, sore throat, and cough, which are common symptoms of a bad cold. Wind moves fast and constantly undergoes rapid changes, which is why when we are under the attack of wind, the symptoms often move from one place to another and also undergo rapid changes. For example, when wind attacks the joints causing arthritis, this will affect the joints all over the body.

When wind attacks the liver, the liver may start to shake. Although we do not actually see the liver shake, we can observe the victim suffering from shaking symptoms, such as shaking of the head and the hands, twitching of muscles, wry eyes or wry mouth, and sudden fainting. The head, limbs, eyes, mouth, and muscles can be compared to the leaves and branches of a tree, and the tree can be compared to the liver. In Chinese medicine, the shaking symptoms are called the "symptoms of liver wind."

The Chinese believe that, in order to counteract liver wind, it is necessary to tone the blood and promote blood circulation so that the wind will stop. In Chinese medicine, this strategy is commonly put like this: "When the blood begins to circulate, wind will stop by itself." Blood deficiency is an important factor accounting for the attack of liver wind, which is why it is important to tone the blood and promote its circulation.

Cold (y-scores of -4 within the healthy range and -8 within the pathological range)

Cold affects the human body continually, but it can also attack it every now and then. When cold merely affects the human body, the organs affected may display a y-score of -4; in this case, no symptoms are apparent and the organs affected stay healthy. However, when cold attacks the human body, the organs under attack may display a y-score of -8, in which case certain symptoms are observed and the organs under attack are now sick. Of the ten internal organs, the kidneys are most frequently under the influence of cold. When cold affects the kidneys, the y-score of the kidneys is -4; when cold attacks the kidneys, the y-score of the kidneys is -8.

Cold is a yin pathogen, meaning that it can harm yang energy easily. When cold attacks the body, the first victim is yang energy. Under the attack of cold, yang energy causes shivering sensations initially. Gradually the pores are blocked by the invading cold energy, preventing perspiration. Once cold has defeated yang energy and victoriously penetrated the body further, the pores become almost completely shut off. The result is that body heat has nowhere to go and accumulates inside the body. The accumulated body heat will finally be forced to break open the blocked pores, which is why profuse perspiration begins at this stage.

Summer Heat (y-scores of 3 within the healthy range and 7 within the pathological range)

Summer heat affects the human body during summer, but it can attack it during summer as well. When summer heat merely affects the human body, the organs affected may display a y-score of 3, in which case no symptoms are observed and the organs affected remain in good health. Yet when summer heat attacks the human body, the organs under attack may display a y-score of 7; in this case, some symptoms are detected and the organs under attack have become sick.

Summer heat is a yang energy and the dominant atmospheric energy in summer. Because summer heat is a yang pathogen and a hot pathogen, when the body is under the attack of summer heat there will be high fever, thirst, and profuse perspiration, all of which are yang symptoms. Moreover, summer heat is especially harmful to body fluids, for it sucks moisture and water from the body. Therefore, a person under the attack of summer heat will feel extremely thirsty as well as very fatigued, have a dry mouth and dry lips, suffer from constipation due to a dry intestine, and discharge meager amounts of urine because of a shortage of water in the body. Among the internal organs, the heart is most susceptible to the attack of summer heat. When summer heat attacks the heart, this can cause an eye infection, thirst, nosebleed, vomiting of blood, and even a loss of consciousness in severe cases.

Dampness (y-scores of -1 within the healthy range and -5 within the pathological range)

Dampness affects the human body continuously and especially in late summer; it can also attack it from time to time. When dampness just affects the human body, the organs affected may display a y-score of -1; in this case, no symptoms are detected and the organs affected stay healthy. But when dampness attacks the human body, the organs under attack may display a y-score of -5, in which case some symptoms are seen and the organs under attack are sick. The spleen is especially sensitive to the influence of dampness. When dampness affects the spleen, the y-score of the spleen is -1; when it attacks the spleen, the y-score of the spleen is -5.

Dampness is the dominant atmospheric energy in late summer. It is a yin energy, which is why its y-score is either -1 or -5, both of which are yin scores. Because dampness is a yin energy, its nature is to move downward. Dampness is heavy and turbid and moves slowly, in contrast to cold, which is clear in nature and moves more freely. Dampness often causes a disease that takes a long time to heal as a result of its slow movement; in this respect, it is the opposite of wind, which moves fast.

When dampness causes pain, as with rheumatism and arthritis, the pain always stays in the same spot, and as time goes on swelling will occur due to an accumulation of dampness in the affected region. When dampness causes a headache, we feel dull pain in the head and sleepy as if the head were wrapped up in a wet towel; in Chinese medicine, this is called "muddy dampness surrounding the head."

Dampness is heavy with a tendency to move downward to attack the lower part of the body, as opposed to wind, which is light with a tendency to move upward to attack the upper part of the body. Because of the downward propensity of dampness, the person under attack often displays a swelling of the lower limbs, experiences the legs as too heavy for walking, and has a sense of the whole body sinking down. Dampness and heat often work together as a formidable team causing all sorts of symptoms, including discharge of yellowish urine, frequent and difficult urination, and vaginal discharge with an offensive smell in women. Such symptoms are called the "symptoms of damp heat" in Chinese medicine.

Because of its natural inclination to attack the lower part of the body, dampness frequently causes rheumatism and arthritis involving the lower limbs, eczema of the lower limbs, and wet beriberi, which is a type of vitamin-B1 deficiency disease that is characterized by swollen legs, numbness in feet, walking difficulty, difficult urination, and cold limbs.

Dryness (y-scores of 1 within the healthy range and 5 within the pathological range)

Dryness affects the human body constantly, but especially in autumn; it can also attack the human body from time to time. When dryness only affects the body, the organs affected may display a y-score of 1, in which case no symptoms are apparent and the organs affected remain healthy. On the other hand, when dryness attacks the body, the organs under attack may display a y-score of 5; in such instances, certain symptoms are observed and the organs under attack have become sick. Of all the internal organs, the lungs are most often under the influence of dryness. When dryness affects the lungs, the y-score of the lungs is 1; when dryness attacks the lungs, the y-score of the lungs is 5.

Dryness is a yang energy, unlike dampness, which is a yin energy. Dryness is the dominant energy in autumn, because there is low humidity in the atmosphere then. In autumn, we are more susceptible to the attack of dryness, with such symptoms as a dry cough, a sore throat with dryness, dry skin, a dry nose, thirst, meager urine, and constipation with dry stools. These are called the "symptoms of autumn dryness" in Chinese medicine, because they occur most frequently in autumn due to the dryness of the atmosphere.

Dryness can harm the lungs easily. It attacks the body through the nose and the mouth, and thus can directly act upon the lungs, making the lungs the most susceptible to the attack of dryness among the internal organs. Because dryness tends to attack the lungs, smoking is particularly harmful to the lungs, making them drier.

Fire (y-scores of 4 within the healthy range and 8 within the pathological range)

Fire affects the human body continually, and it can also attack it from time to time. When fire merely affects the human body, the organs affected may display a y-score of 4, in which case no symptoms are apparent and the organs affected remain in good health. On the other hand, when fire attacks the human body, the organs under attack may display a y-score of 8; in such cases, certain symptoms are observed and the organs under attack have become sick. Although all the internal organs are susceptible to fire, one is particularly vulnerable: the liver. When fire affects the liver, the y-score of the liver is 4; when fire attacks the liver, the y-score of the liver is 8.

Fire is a yang pathogen, because its nature is to flare upward and it spreads quickly. As fire burns upward, it often causes skin eruptions on the face and around the eyes, red and swollen eyes, and canker sores on the tongue and in the mouth, all of which occur in the upper region. Because fire spreads quickly, when it causes disease the symptoms develop and diminish very rapidly. Such symptoms include high fever, severe headache, coma, vomiting of blood, and discharge of blood from the mouth.

Internal Factors Shaping the Internal Organs

All the internal organs are also affected by internal factors, which include sluggish conditions of energy and blood, the accumulation of phlegm, and energy, blood, yin, and yang deficiencies.

Sluggishness (y-scores of -3 within the healthy range and -7 within the pathological range)

Blood Coagulation (y-scores of -3 within the healthy range and -7 within the pathological range)

When mild blood coagulation occurs, the organs affected may display a y-score of -3, in which case no symptoms are apparent and the organs affected remain in good health. But when more severe blood coagulation takes place, the organs involved may display a y-score of -7; in this case, some symptoms are observed and the organs involved have become sick. The organ most frequently under the influence of blood coagulation is the heart. When blood coagulation involves the heart, in mild cases the y-score of the heart is -3 and in severe cases -7.

Blood should circulate within the meridians. It should be free from obstructions, the attack of cold or hot pathogens, stagnation, energy deficiency, damp phlegm, water retention or stoppage, and the influence of external forces. When the above factors are present, blood coagulation will occur.

The major symptoms of blood coagulation are local swelling, pain, needles of pain, pain in fixed regions, swelling inside the body, a blackish face and blackish eyes, bluish-purple lips and tongue, and blood clots that appear purplish-black or that recur frequently. When blood coagulation attacks the heart, this will cause incoherent speech and delirium, as if the sufferer has a mental disorder.

Energy Congestion (y-scores of -3 within the healthy range and -7 within the pathological range)

With mild energy congestion, the organs affected may display a y-score of -3; in this case, no symptoms are apparent and the organs affected continue to be healthy. On the other hand, when energy congestion is more severe, the organs involved may display a y-score of -7; now some symptoms are observed and the organs involved have become sick. Of the internal organs, the liver is most frequently under the influence of energy congestion. When energy congestion involves the liver, in mild cases the y-score of the liver is -3 and in severe cases -7.

Energy congestion refers to the obstruction of energy flow in a particular organ, and it can be due to emotional discomfort, external injuries, and other causes. Energy should travel throughout the body without difficulty, but various factors, including emotional stress, irregular eating, the attack of external energies, and external injuries, can exert a negative impact on energy circulation. This can cause energy sluggishness to occur in the chest or in the stomach and intestine. In the latter case, there can be swelling of the stomach and the abdomen with pain. Wandering pain is characteristic, and generally the swelling becomes more serious than the pain. In addition, there can be intestinal rumbling, pain that gets better on belching, and painful swelling of breasts in women.

Accumulation of Phlegm (y-scores of -1 within the healthy range and -5 within the pathological range)

When light phlegm occurs in the human body, the organs affected may display a y-score of -1, in which case no symptoms are seen and the organs affected remain in good health. However, when copious phlegm occurs in the human body, the organs under attack may display a y-score of -5; at this point, certain symptoms are observed and the organs involved are now sick. Among the organs, the lungs are most often under the influence of phlegm. When light phlegm affects the lungs, the y-score of the lungs is -1; when copious phlegm attacks the lungs, the y-score of the lungs is -5.

Phlegm is an accumulation and gathering of water in a local region. It is due to disorders in the energy transformation of the lungs, the spleen, and the kidneys, impairing the normal distribution

and excretion of body fluids, which results in an abnormal accumulation of water.

The production of phlegm can be traced back not only to the
inability of the lungs to expand and clean up but also to the inca-
pacity of the spleen to transport, affecting the distribution of body
fluids and resulting in the gathering of water to become phlegm.
Common symptoms caused by phlegm are a cough, panting, shortness of breath, and chest congestion. In Chinese medicine, it is said
that "the spleen produces phlegm and the lungs store it away."

Deficiency (y-scores fluctuating with energy, blood, yang, and yin)

Energy Deficiency (y-scores of -2 within the healthy range and -6 within the pathological range)

When there is a mild energy deficiency, the organs affected may display a y-score of -2, with no apparent symptoms and the organs
affected remaining in good health. But when a more severe energy
deficiency occurs, the organs involved may display a y-score of -6, in
which case some symptoms are observed and the organs involved
are now sick. Of all the internal organs, the spleen is the one most
often influenced by energy deficiency. When energy deficiency
involves the spleen, in mild cases the y-score of the spleen is -2 and
in severe cases -6.

Energy deficiency refers to a short supply of vital energy in the
body, possibly due to a functional decline in the internal organs and a
low resistance of the organism against the attack of disease. Chronic
illness, aging, genetics, malnutrition, and excessive fatigue are all
contributing factors. Energy deficiency involves symptoms of the
whole body, but especially fatigue and weakness. Because the internal organs have their respective traits, energy deficiency can display
different symptoms in relation to the various organs. For example,
shortness of breath and a low voice are symptoms of Lungs Energy
Deficiency; poor appetite, indigestion, and prolapse of the organs are
symptoms of spleen and stomach deficiencies; and enuresis and seminal sliding are symptoms of Kidneys Energy Deficiency.

Blood Deficiency (y-scores of 1 within the healthy range and 5 within the pathological range)

When there is a mild blood deficiency, the organs affected may display a y-score of 1, in which case no symptoms are apparent and the organs affected continue to be healthy. On the other hand, when a more severe blood deficiency occurs, the organs involved may display a y-score of 5; in this case, certain symptoms are observed and the organs involved are now sick. The organ most frequently under the influence of a blood deficiency is the heart. When a blood deficiency involves the heart, in mild cases the y-score of the heart is 1 and in severe cases 5.

Blood deficiency refers to a shortage of blood that gives rise to symptoms involving the whole body. It is chiefly due to fatigue, internal injuries, excessive thought, a weak spleen and stomach, and a slow production of energy and blood in the body. The major symptoms of a blood deficiency are dizziness, palpitations, a poor or yellowish complexion, pale lips and tongue, a fine pulse, insomnia, blurred vision, twitching of tendons, dry skin, and withered hair on the head.

Yang Deficiency (y-scores of -4 within the healthy range and -8 within the pathological range)

When there is a mild yang deficiency, the organs affected may display a y-score of -4; in this case, no symptoms are detected and the organs affected remain in good health. But when a more severe yang deficiency occurs, the organs involved may display a y-score of -8, and now certain symptoms are observed and the organs involved have become sick. The kidneys are the organ most often under the influence of a yang deficiency. When a yang deficiency involves the kidneys, in mild cases the y-score of the kidneys is -4 and in severe cases -8.

Yang deficiency refers to insufficient yang energy in the body that gives rise to various kinds of cold symptoms, primarily due to innate deficiency, chronic illness, or the attack of external pathogenic cold that causes harm to yang energy. In addition to the kidneys, yang deficiency primarily affects the heart and the spleen.

Yin Deficiency (y-scores of 3 within the healthy range and 7 within the pathological range)

Yin deficiency refers to a shortage of pure essence and blood or a shortage of body fluids, making yin energy incapable of controlling yang. When a mild yin deficiency occurs, the organs affected may display a y-score of 3, in which case no symptoms are seen and the organs affected stay healthy. On the other hand, when a more severe yin deficiency takes place, the organs involved may display a y-score of 7; in this case, some symptoms are observed and the organs involved have become sick. The organ most often influenced by a yin deficiency is the stomach. When a yin deficiency involves the stomach, in mild cases the y-score of the stomach is 3 and in severe cases 7.

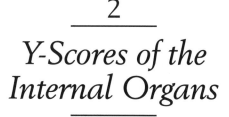

2

Y-Scores of the Internal Organs

This chapter includes a list of all the syndromes discussed in this book accompanied by their respective y-scores. But before you look it over, it will be helpful to have an understanding of the four key concepts: common symptoms, Western diseases, clinical signs, and syndromes.

COMMON SYMPTOMS

A common symptom is an abnormal change in the body. Abdominal pain, headache, diarrhea, hiccups, dizziness, constipation, stomachache, blood in urine, diminished urination, nosebleed, and shortage of milk in nursing mothers can all be considered common symptoms. Other examples of common symptoms are chest pain, cough, indigestion, itch, ringing in the ears and deafness, thirst, and vomiting. Some symptoms require medical treatment.

WESTERN DISEASES

Hypertension, hepatitis, enteritis, and herpes zoster are examples of Western diseases, because they have been diagnosed as such through established clinical and laboratory procedures. Western diseases are the diagnosed diseases in Western medicine.

CLINICAL SIGNS

A clinical sign need not be a common symptom, and it is not a Western disease. A clinical sign refers to a manifestation that points to a particular syndrome in traditional Chinese medicine. A clinical sign may not be a symptom, because it may only point to a possible syndrome. Some clinical signs often used in Chinese medicine are turbid urine, dry stool, pale complexion, aversion to the cold, being prone to anger, and jumpiness, none of which require medical treatment. Clinical signs and symptoms form the very foundation for diagnosis in Chinese medicine, because they indicate, for each patient, what syndrome is involved and needs to be treated. Therefore, when Chinese doctors make a diagnosis, clinical signs and symptoms are looked at in great detail. For example, not only will doctors ask their patients about their urination in general, but they will also be interested in all the particulars regarding their urination.

SYNDROMES

A syndrome refers to a fundamental condition of the body that needs to be treated, and it is indicated by a group of clinical signs and symptoms. For a patient with diarrhea, for example, although diarrhea is the chief complaint to be dealt with, the treatment should be aimed at correcting the syndrome responsible for the diarrhea. However, there are quite a few different syndromes that are responsible for diarrhea, so how does a Chinese doctor know which syndrome to treat? The doctor will have to go through the patient's clinical signs and symptoms to determine which syndrome is involved and then treat that particular syndrome accordingly.

Doctors of Chinese medicine treat syndromes—not diseases, symptoms, or clinical signs—because syndromes alone can determine the y-scores of the internal organs. Each syndrome has a particular y-score that tells us what organ is sick and to what extent. Take blood in urine as an example. This symptom can be due to the following syndromes, each with a particular y-score: Kidneys Yang Deficiency (Kidneys -8), Heart Fire Flaming (Heart 8), or Excessive Heat in the Small Intestine (S. intestine 7). Assuming that three patients with blood in their urine have a different syndrome responsible for this symptom, and because the three syndromes involve three different organs with three different y-scores, it follows that each patient should follow a specially tailored treatment program.

Now here is the list of syndromes accompanied by their respective y-scores:

SYNDROMES

Syndromes and Their Organ Y-Scores	Pathological Range of Y-Scores to Be Applied When You Are Ill	Healthy Range of Y-Scores to Be Applied When You Are Healthy
5.1 Lungs Energy Deficiency	Lungs -6	Lungs -2
5.2 Lungs Yin Deficiency	Lungs 7	Lungs 3
5.3 Lungs under the Attack of Wind and Cold	Lungs -7	Lungs -3
5.4 Deficient and Cold Lungs	Lungs -8	Lungs -4
5.5 Phlegm Dampness Obstructing the Lungs	Lungs -5	Lungs -1
5.6 Wind and Heat Attacking the Lungs	Lungs 7	Lungs 3
5.7 Hot Lungs (Lungs Fire)	Lungs 8	Lungs 4
5.8 Dry Lungs	Lungs 5	Lungs 1
6.1 Large Intestine Damp Heat	L. intestine 6	L. intestine 2
6.2 Large Intestine Fluid Exhaustion	L. intestine 5	L. intestine 1
6.3 Large Intestine Deficiency and Slippery Diarrhea	L. intestine 6	L. intestine 2
7.1 Spleen Energy Deficiency	Spleen -6	Spleen -2
7.2 Spleen Yang Deficiency	Spleen -8	Spleen -4
7.3 Middle Energy Cave-in	Spleen -6	Spleen -2
7.4 Spleen Unable to Govern Blood	Spleen -8	Spleen -4
7.5 Cold Dampness Troubling the Spleen	Spleen -7	Spleen -3
7.6 Damp Heat Steaming the Spleen	Spleen 6	Spleen 2
8.1 Stomach Yin Deficiency	Stomach 7	Stomach 3
8.2 Food Stagnation in Stomach	Stomach -7	Stomach -3

Syndromes and Their Organ Y-Scores	Pathological Range of Y-Scores to Be Applied When You Are Ill	Healthy Range of Y-Scores to Be Applied When You Are Healthy
8.3 Cold Stomach	Stomach -8	Stomach -4
8.4 Hot Stomach	Stomach 7	Stomach 3
9.1 Liver Energy Congestion	Liver -7	Liver -3
9.2 Liver Fire Flaming Upward	Liver 8	Liver 4
9.3 Liver Blood Deficiency	Liver 5	Liver 1
9.4 Liver Yin Deficiency	Liver 7	Liver 3
9.5 Liver Yang Upsurging	Liver 7	Liver 3
9.6 Internal Liver Wind Blowing	Liver 6	Liver 2
9.7 Cold Obstructing the Liver Meridian	Liver -8	Liver -4
9.8 Damp Heat Attacking the Liver and Gallbladder	Liver 6, Gallbladder 6	Liver 2, Gallbladder 2
10.1 Gallbladder Excessive Heat	Gallbladder 7	Gallbladder 3
10.2 Gallbladder Energy Deficiency	Gallbladder -6	Gallbladder -2
11.1 Kidneys Yang Deficiency	Kidneys -8	Kidneys -4
11.2 Kidneys Yin Deficiency	Kidneys 7	Kidneys 3
11.3 Insufficient Kidneys Essence	Kidneys 7	Kidneys 3
11.4 Loosening of Kidneys Energy	Kidneys -6	Kidneys -2
11.5 Kidneys Unable to Absorb Inspiration	Kidneys -7	Kidneys -3
12.1 Bladder Damp Heat	Bladder 5	Bladder 1
12.2 Bladder Cold and Deficiency	Bladder -8	Bladder -4
13.1 Heart Energy Deficiency	Heart -6	Heart -2
13.2 Heart Yang Deficiency	Heart -8	Heart -4
13.3 Heart Yin Deficiency	Heart 7	Heart 3

Syndromes and Their Organ Y-Scores	Pathological Range of Y-Scores to Be Applied When You Are Ill	Healthy Range of Y-Scores to Be Applied When You Are Healthy
13.4 Heart Blood Deficiency	Heart 5	Heart 1
13.5 Heart Fire Flaming	Heart 8	Heart 4
13.6 Phlegm Fire Disturbing the Heart	Heart 8	Heart 4
14.1 Excessive Heat in the Small Intestine	S. intestine 7	S. intestine 3
14.2 Small Intestine Energy Congestion	S. intestine -7	S. intestine -3
15.1 No Communication between the Kidneys and Heart	Kidneys 7, Heart 8	Kidneys 3, Heart 4
15.2 Simultaneous Deficiency of the Heart and Spleen	Heart 5, Spleen 6	Heart 1, Spleen 2
15.3 Yang Deficiency of the Heart and Kidneys	Heart - 8, Kidneys -8	Heart - 4, Kidneys -4
15.4 Energy Deficiency of the Spleen and Lungs	Spleen -6, Lungs -6	Spleen -2, Lungs -2
15.5 Yang Deficiency of the Spleen and Kidneys	Spleen -8, Kidneys -8	Spleen -4, Kidneys -4
15.6 Yin Deficiency of the Lungs and Kidneys	Lungs, 7 Kidneys 7	Lungs 3, Kidneys 3
15.7 Yin Deficiency of the Liver and Kidneys	Liver 7, Kidneys 7	Liver 3, Kidneys 3
15.8 Disharmony between the Liver and Spleen	Liver -7, Spleen -6	Liver -3, Spleen -2
15.9 Disharmony between the Liver and Stomach	Liver -7, Stomach -6	Liver -3, Stomach -2
15.10 Liver Fire Offending the Lungs	Liver 8, Lungs 7	Liver 4, Lungs 3

You can determine the y-scores of your internal organs by going through the four steps of diagnosis, discussed later, to come up with a particular syndrome or syndromes applicable to you. The ancient Chinese did not have sophisticated facilities and instruments such as laboratories and X-ray examinations, but they did develop a theory about the condition of the internal organs by which the y-scores of the internal organs involved are determined.

According to the chart below, the y-scores of your internal organs can be as low as +1 or -1 and as high as +8 or -8. When the y-scores of your internal organs reach +4 or -4, you may not show any symptoms, which means that the y-scores of your internal organs are within the healthy range and you are not sick. But when the y-scores of your internal organs reach beyond -5 or +5, you are sick and you may have some symptoms that need to be treated.

If you examine the contents of the syndromes listed above, you will notice that the syndromes are associated with the following concepts: fire, heat, yin deficiency, wind, dryness, blood deficiency, cold, yang deficiency, sluggishness, energy deficiency, dampness, and phlegm. Each syndrome is assigned two y-scores, with the lesser ones' being within the healthy range and the greater ones' pointing to a sickness.

The scores between -4 and +4 are considered within the healthy

RANGE OF Y-SCORES

+8 +7 +6 +5	+4 +3 +2 +1 0 -1 -2 -3 -4	-5 -6 -7 -8
Pathological range of y-scores	Healthy range of y-scores	Pathological range of y-scores
Yang		Yin
$\Rightarrow$	Food cures are designed to bring y-scores toward the middle and stay within this healthy range.	$\Leftarrow$
$\Leftarrow$	Y-scores within the healthy range may gradually move toward the pathological range, unless they are regulated by eating the right foods.	$\Rightarrow$

range of y-scores, at least technically. But even though the y-scores within this range do not cause any symptoms, they may gradually move toward the pathological range to give rise to symptoms. As an example, someone's y-score may be Liver 4 initially, but gradually it may move toward Liver 8, at which point the person will begin to display symptoms like headaches and hypertension.

In the two charts immediately following, each concept is assigned a y-score ranging from -1 to +8. When a concept is connected to a particular organ, the y-score of the concept becomes that of the organ in question. For example, the concept "yin deficiency" is assigned a y-score of +3, so the y-score of Kidneys Yin Deficiency would be Kidneys 3.

Y-Scores of the Internal Organs (Yang Scores)

Fire	Heat/Yin Deficiency	Wind	Dry/Blood Deficiency
+4/+8	+3/+7	+2/+6	+1/+5

Y-Scores of the Internal Organs (Yin Scores)

Cold/Yang Deficiency	Sluggishness or Congestion	Energy Deficiency	Damp/Phlegm
-4/-8	-3/-7	-2/-6	-1/-5

EXAMPLES SHOWING HOW Y-SCORES OF SYNDROMES ARE ESTABLISHED

Syndromes	Y-Scores Indicating Sickness	Y-Scores within the Healthy Range
9.1 Liver Energy Congestion Energy Congestion = -7 or -3 (Liver and -7) = Liver -7 (Liver and -3) = Liver -3	Liver -7	Liver -3
9.2 Liver Fire Flaming Upward Fire = 8 or 4 (Liver and 8) = Liver 8 (Liver and 4) = Liver 4	Liver 8	Liver 4
9.3 Liver Blood Deficiency Blood Deficiency = 5 or 1 (Liver and 5) = Liver 5 (Liver and 1) = Liver 1	Liver 5	Liver 1
9.4 Liver Yin Deficiency Yin Deficiency = 7 or 3 (Liver and 7) = Liver 7 (Liver and 3) = Liver 3	Liver 7	Liver 3

3

Identifying Your Own Signs and Symptoms

Follow the four steps below to figure out the y-scores of your internal organs:

Step 1: Identify the signs and symptoms applicable to you, using Chart One on page 34.

Step 2: Record the number indicated within the parentheses at the end of each sign or symptom, and then add them up to arrive at the sum, by using Chart Two on page 52. Perform this step only when you are in good health (you are not ill), but want to determine the y-scores of your internal organs. If you are sick and want to know the y-scores of your internal organs, skip this step and go directly to Step 3.

Step 3: Use Chart Three on page 58 to go through this step the same way as you would Step 2, except that you are ill.

Step 4: If you have been diagnosed in Western medicine as having a particular disease, carry out this step by using Chart Four on page 62, to find out the syndrome responsible for your disease as well as the y-score of your internal organs.

All of these steps will be discussed in greater detail later. Once you have identified the y-scores of your internal organs, you will need to go to Part III to select the right foods to promote the health of your affected organs.

STEP 1

These are the categories of signs and symptoms to be recorded along with their numbers and relevant syndromes: 1. Abdomen, 2.Anus and genitals, 3. Appetite, 4. Back, 5. Belching, 6. Bleeding, 7. Bowel movement, 8. Chest, 9. Children's symptoms, 10. Cold and hot sensations, 11. Cough and phlegm, 12. Ears, 13. Emotions and mental states, 14. Eyes, 15. Face, 16. Habits and preferences, 17. Head and neck, 18. Hiccups, 19. Limbs, 20. Men's symptoms, 21. Mouth and lips, 22. Nose, 23. Pain, 24. Perspiration, 25. Respiration, 26. Skin, 27. Sleep, 28. Teeth, 29. Throat, 30. Tongue, 31. Urination, 32. Voice, 33. Vomiting, 34. Whole body, 35. Women (childbirth and pregnancy), 36. Women (vaginal discharge), 37. Women (menstruation), and 38. Women (miscellaneous).

After you have checked certain signs or symptoms, it is important to know how to record the numbers and add them up to arrive at the sum in Step 2 or Step 3. A few examples follow to show you how the recording and the calculating are done.

First Example

Suppose you have checked "discharge of blood from the anus (4), 15.5" as applicable to you, here (4) is the number you should record in the second column and in the same row as 15.5, which represents Yang Deficiency of the Spleen and Kidneys. Here is how this would look:

Syndromes	Numbers	Sum	Y-Scores
15.5 Yang Deficiency of the Spleen and Kidneys	4	4	Spleen -4, Kidneys -4

Second Example

Suppose "prolapse of the anus" is applicable to you. Because there are two listings for "prolapse of the anus," you need to include them both: "prolapse of the anus (1), 6.1" and "prolapse of the anus (4), 6.3, 7.3." The numbers are recorded in the second column in different rows this way:

Syndromes	Numbers	Sum	Y-scores
6.1 Large Intestine Damp Heat	1	1	L. intestine 2
6.3 Large Intestine Deficiency and Slippery Diarrhea	4	4	L. intestine 2
7.3 Middle Energy Cave-in	4	4	Spleen -2

Third Example

Assuming that you have checked the following items as applicable to yourself, you will need to record their numbers and add them up to arrive at the sum, as shown in the chart below. Again, remember that when "poor appetite," for example, is applicable to you, it's important to check all the listings and record them all, because the four numbers within the parentheses have different implications: (1) indicates a minor sign or symptom of a particular syndrome, (2) indicates a median sign or symptom of a particular syndrome, (3) indicates a major sign or symptom of a particular syndrome, and (4) indicates a symptom to be treated under a particular syndrome. These are the items let's say you have selected, followed by the proper way they should be recorded in the chart:

Poor appetite (1), 5.5, 6.1, 9.8, 11.1, 15.2, 15.5
Poor appetite (2), 7.4, 15.5, 15.8
Poor appetite (3), 7.1, 7.2, 7.5
Cold limbs (1), 6.3, 11.2, 13.5, 15.5
Cold limbs (2), 8.3, 9.7, 11.5, 15.3
Cold limbs (3), 5.4, 7.2, 13.2

Syndromes	Numbers	Sum	Y-Scores
5.4 Deficient and Cold Lungs	3	3	Lungs -4
5.5 Phlegm Dampness Obstructing the Lungs	1	1	Lungs -1
6.1 Large Intestine Damp Heat	1	1	L. intestine 2
6.3 Large Intestine Deficiency and Slippery Diarrhea	1	1	L. intestine 2
7.1 Spleen Energy Deficiency	3	3	Spleen -2
7.2 Spleen Yang Deficiency	3, 3	6	Spleen -4
7.3 Middle Energy Cave-in			Spleen -2
7.4 Spleen Unable to Govern Blood	2	2	Spleen -4
7.5 Cold Dampness Troubling the Spleen	3	3	Spleen -3

Syndromes	Numbers	Sum	Y-Scores
8.3 Cold Stomach	2	2	Stomach -4
9.7 Cold Obstructing the Liver Meridian	2	2	Liver -4
9.8 Damp Heat Attacking the Liver and Gallbladder	1	1	Liver 2, Gallbladder 2
11.1 Kidneys Yang Deficiency	1	1	Kidneys -4
11.5 Kidneys Unable to Absorb Inspiration	2	2	Kidneys -3
12.2 Bladder Cold and Deficiency	1	1	Bladder -4
13.2 Heart Yang Deficiency	3	3	Heart -4
13.5 Heart Fire Flaming	1	1	Heart 4
15.2 Simultaneous Deficiency of the Heart and Spleen	1	1	Heart 1, Spleen 2
15.3 Yang Deficiency of the Heart and Kidneys	2	2	Heart 4, Kidneys -4
15.5 Yang Deficiency of the Spleen and Kidneys	1, 2, 1	4	Spleen -4, Kidneys -4
15.8 Disharmony between the Liver and Spleen	2	2	Liver -3, Spleen -2

CHART ONE: SIGNS AND SYMPTOMS

1. Abdomen:

Abdominal comfort following bowel movement or flatulence (2), 14.2

Abdominal distension (4), 6.2

Abdominal obstructions and lumps, as in swelling of the liver and spleen (2), 9.1

Abdominal rumbling (2), 15.9

Abdominal swelling (2), 6.1, 8.3, 9.8, 15.4, 15.5, 15.8

Abdominal swelling (3), 7.1, 7.6, 14.2, 15.2

Abdominal swelling after a meal (2), 8.1

Abdominal swelling and fullness (1), 11.1

Abdominal swelling around the navel that gets relieved by giving off gas (1), 14.1

Congested sensation in the stomach (2), 15.8

Congested sensation in the stomach and abdomen (3), 7.6

Discomfort in the stomach and abdomen (3), 7.5

Falling sensation below the umbilicus (3), 7.3

Falling sensation in the abdomen that is intensified after a meal (3), 7.3

Intestinal rumbling (2), 15.8

Intestinal rumbling (3), 14.2

Lumpy object in the lower abdomen that can be felt by touch (3), 6.2

Swelling and fullness in the stomach and abdomen (2), 7.4, 8.2

2. Anus and genitals:

Discharge of blood from the anus (4), 15.5

Eczema in the scrotum (3), 9.8

Falling of testicle on one side, causing walking difficulty (1), 14.2

Flatulence (2), 15.8

Itch in the female genitals (4), 9.8

Itch in the genitals (3), 9.8

Loud flatulence (1), 6.2

Prolapse of the anus (1), 6.1

Prolapse of the anus (4), 6.3, 7.3

Prolapse of the anus after diarrhea (2), 6.3

Scrotal hernia affecting the lower abdomen (3), 9.7

3. Appetite:

Decreased appetite (2), 15.2

Dislike of greasy foods (3), 7.6

Eating a lot but remaining hungry (3), 8.4

Eating a lot but remaining thin (1), 8.4

Eating in the morning and vomiting in the evening (2), 8.3

Fondness for hot drink (1), 8.3

Hungry with good appetite (1), 8.4

Hungry with no appetite (1), 15.8

Hungry with no appetite (3), 8.1

Indigestion (1), 8.1, 15.4

Indigestion (4), 8.2

Loss of appetite (2), 15.4

Morbid hunger (1), 15.6

No appetite (3), 7.6

Poor appetite (1), 5.5, 6.1, 9.8, 11.1, 15.2, 15.5

Poor appetite (2), 7.4, 15.5, 15.8

Poor appetite (3), 7.1, 7.2, 7.5

Swallowing difficulty (4), 8.1

4. Back:

Weak loins and knees (3), 11.5

Weak loins and tibia (3), 15.7

Weakness in the lower back (3), 15.1

5. Belching:

Acid regurgitation (4), 9.2

Acid swallowing (2), 15.8

Acid swallowing (3), 8.4

Acid swallowing and belching of bad air (3), 8.2

Belching (1), 8.3

Belching (2), 8.2, 15.8, 15.9

Belching after a meal (3), 7.1

Belching with poor appetite (3), 8.2

6. Bleeding:

Bleeding (4), 7.4, 9.2, 15.2, 15.7

Bleeding from gums (1), 13.5

Bleeding from gums and the space between teeth with pain (2), 8.4

Bleeding from the stomach (1), 9.2

Bleeding in small quantity (3), 7.4

Blood in urine (2), 12.1

Blood in urine (3), 7.4

Blood in urine (4), 11.2, 13.5, 14.1

Coughing up blood (4), 5.6

Discharge of blood from the anus (4), 7.4

Discharge of blood from the mouth (4), 5.8, 15.10

Menstrual bleeding (1), 13.4

Nosebleed (1), 5.7, 8.4

Nosebleed (2), 9.2, 13.5

Nosebleed (4), 5.6, 5.8

Vaginal bleeding (1), 11.4

Vaginal bleeding (4), 7.3, 7.4, 9.4, 11.2

7. Bowel movement:

Acute diarrhea with red and white and foul-smelling stools (3), 6.1

Chronic diarrhea (1), 11.1, 15.8

Chronic diarrhea (4), 6.3, 7.3

Constipation (1), 8.1

Constipation (2), 8.2, 8.4, 13.6

Constipation (4), 6.2

Constipation after childbirth (4), 6.2

Constipation or difficult bowel movement with watery stools (2), 7.6

Constipation with dry stool (2), 5.7

Constipation with stools as dry as sheep dung (3), 6.2

Diarrhea (2), 7.4

Diarrhea (4), 6.1, 7.1, 7.2, 7.5, 7.6, 8.2, 8.3, 11.1, 15.5, 15.8

Diarrhea at dawn (3), 15.5

Diarrhea before dawn (1), 11.1

Diarrhea with foul-smelling and turbid stools (1), 11.1, 15.5

Diarrhea with foul-smelling and turbid stools (2), 15.4

Diarrhea with foul-smelling and turbid stools (3), 6.3

Diarrhea with pus and blood (2), 6.1

Diarrhea with thin, yellowish water (3), 6.1

Difficult defecation and urination (1), 15.7

Discharge of dry stools (1), 13.3

Discharge of dry stools (2), 8.1, 9.2, 13.5

Discharge of foul-smelling and turbid stools (2), 7.4

Discharge of soft stools (2), 7.5

Discharge of soft stools (3), 7.1

Frequent bowel movements with little stool (3), 6.1

Frequent desire to empty the bowels (3), 7.3

Irregular bowel movements (1), 15.9

One bowel movement in several days (3), 6.2

Sliding diarrhea (3), 6.3

Stools containing undigested foods (2), 15.5

Stools with an offensive smell (2), 8.2

Stools with an offensive smell (3), 6.1

Watery stools (1), 7.2

Watery stools (2), 7.2, 9.7, 15.8

Watery stools (3), 7.5, 15.2

Watery, thin stools (1), 5.5, 11.1, 15.3

Watery, thin stools (2), 8.2

8. Chest:

Chest discomfort (2), 9.1, 13.6, 15.9

Chest discomfort (3), 13.1

Choking sensation in the chest (3), 13.2

Congested chest (1), 5.3, 5.4

Congested chest (3), 5.5

Congested chest with discomfort in the stomach (1), 10.1

Feeling oppressed in the heart and chest (3), 15.3

Swelling of rib region (2), 15.8

9. Children's symptoms:

Bed-wetting (1), 11.4

Fever and malnutrition (1), 8.2

Fontanel not closed on time (2), 11.3

Incapable of sound sleep (1), 8.4

Malnutrition (1), 7.1

Screaming during sleep (1), 8.4

Slow growth (4), 11.3

Vomiting and diarrhea (1), 8.2

10. Cold and hot sensations:

Aversion to being chilled (1), 11.5

Aversion to being chilled (2), 15.3

Aversion to the cold (3), 11.1, 13.2

Burning sensation in the anus (2), 6.1

Burning sensation in the face (2), 9.5

Chill (2), 9.7

Cold and weak lower limbs (3), 11.1

Cold feet (1), 11.1

Cold limbs (1), 6.3, 11.2, 13.5, 15.5

Cold limbs (2), 8.3, 9.7, 11.5, 15.3

Cold limbs (3), 5.4, 7.2, 13.2

Cold loins and legs (1), 11.1

Cold sensation (1), 11.1

Cold sensation alternating with hot sensation (3), 10.1

Cold sensation in the chest and back (2), 5.4

Coldness on the forehead that does not warm up (1), 7.2

Fondness for cold drink (2), 13.6

Fondness for massage and warmth (1), 8.3

Hot sensations in palms of hands and soles of feet (2), 5.2, 13.3, 15.7

Hot sensation in the body (1), 5.7

Hot sensation in the body (2), 6.1

Hot sensation in the body (3), 9.5, 11.2

Hot sensation in the center of palms (1), 13.5

Hot sensation in the center of palms (3), 11.2

Hot sensation in the soles of feet (3), 11.2

Hot sensations as if heat were coming from the bones (3), 15.6

Shivering with cold (3), 5.8

Shivering with cold sensations of limbs (2), 15.5

11. Cough and phlegm:

Acute attack of cough and panting (3), 5.4

Acute onset of cough (3), 5.7

Blood in phlegm (1), 5.2, 5.6, 15.10

Blood in phlegm (2), 11.2, 15.6

Cough (4), 5.1, 5.2, 5.3, 5.6, 5.7, 5.8, 15.10, 15.6

Cough and panting (1), 11.1

Cough with heavy and unclear sound (1), 5.3

Cough with meager phlegm (3), 5.2

Cough with oppressed sound (2), 5.7

Cough with weak sound (3), 5.1

Cough without phlegm or with little phlegm (3), 15.6

Coughing up and spitting up phlegm and saliva (2), 15.4

Coughing up blood (4), 5.2

Coughing up copious, watery sputum (4), 5.5

Coughing up copious, whitish phlegm easily (3), 5.5

Coughing up fresh blood (2), 11.2, 15.10

Coughing up meager phlegm with difficulty (3), 5.8

Coughing up phlegm easily (1), 5.7

Coughing up pus and blood with a fishy smell (2), 5.7

Coughing up thin, white phlegm (3), 5.3

Coughing up yellowish phlegm (3), 15.10

Coughing up yellowish, sticky phlegm (2), 13.6

Coughing up yellowish, sticky phlegm (3), 5.6, 5.7

Coughing with loud sound (3), 5.6

Discharge of copious, thin, white phlegm (4), 5.4

Discharge of copious, white phlegm (3), 15.4

Discharge of meager, sticky phlegm (1), 5.2

Discharge of meager, sticky phlegm (2), 15.10

Discharge of thin, watery phlegm (1), 5.1

Discharge of thin, whitish phlegm (2), 5.3

Discharge of watery phlegm that is difficult to cough up (2), 5.4

Discharge of white, watery phlegm (1), 13.6

Dry cough (1), 8.1

Dry cough (3), 5.2, 5.8

Phlegm (1), 15.3

Phlegm rumbling in the throat (1), 13.6

Phlegm rumbling in the throat (2), 5.5

Phlegm rumbling in the throat (3), 5.5, 13.6

Phlegm rumbling with panting (1), 15.5

12. Ears:

Deafness (1), 15.1

Deafness (2), 14.1

Deafness (3), 10.1

Deafness (4), 9.2, 9.5

Deafness or decreased hearing (2), 11.3

Ringing in the ears (2), 9.4, 11.3, 15.1, 15.7

Ringing in the ears (4), 9.2, 9.5

Ringing in the ears and deafness (2), 11.1, 11.2

Ringing in the ears like the sound of a cicada (1), 9.3

Ringing in the ears or deafness (2), 11.4

13. Emotions and mental states:

Anger (2), 9.3

Cowardice and getting scared easily (3), 10.2

Delirium (2), 13.5

Delirium (3), 13.6

Depressed, quick tempered, and insecure (1), 8.4

Easily in shock (2), 13.1

Emotional disturbances (3), 13.6

Fatigued spirits (1), 15.8

Feeling miserable (1), 13.5, 15.1

Forgetfulness (1), 11.3

Forgetfulness (2), 9.5, 13.1, 13.3

Forgetfulness (3), 13.4

Forgetfulness (4), 15.1, 15.2

Getting scared easily with rapid heartbeat (1), 13.2

Incoherent speech (2), 13.6

Insanity (2), 13.5

Irregular laughter and crying (2), 13.6

Jumpiness (2), 9.1

Jumpiness (3), 9.2, 9.5

Jumpiness and being prone to anger (1), 15.8

Jumpiness and being prone to anger (2), 15.10

Loss of consciousness (3), 13.6

Love of sighing (3), 10.2

Maniac behavior (3), 13.6
Maniac-type mental illness (4), 9.2
Many dreams (1), 9.3
Many dreams (2), 9.5, 13.6, 15.2, 15.7
Many dreams (3), 13.3, 13.4
Mental depression (1), 10.1
Mental depression (2), 15.2
Mental depression (3), 9.6, 13.3, 13.5, 13.6, 14.1
Mental illness (4), 9.1, 13.6
Mentally confused (2), 13.1
Mentally depressed (3), 9.5
Mentally fatigued (2), 13.1
Nervousness (1), 15.1, 15.2
Nervousness (2), 9.3
Nervousness (3), 13.1
Nervousness (4), 13.3, 13.4, 15.3
Not alert mentally (1), 13.5, 13.6
Prone to anger (2), 10.1
Prone to anger (3), 9.2, 9.5
Prone to sadness and crying (2), 13.1
Prone to shock and fear (1), 9.3
Shock (1), 15.3
Sudden illogical talking (1), 7.3

14. Eyes:
Blurred vision (1), 11.2
Blurred vision (2), 9.3
Both eyes flickering or looking sideways or upward (2), 9.4
Both eyes looking upward (3), 9.6
Dizziness and blurred vision (3), 9.4
Dry and obstructive sensation in the eyes (3), 9.3
Dry eyes (1), 15.7
Misty vision (1), 9.5
Misty vision (3), 10.2
Night blindness (1), 15.7
Night blindness (3), 9.4
Night blindness (4), 9.3

Pink eyes (2), 5.6
Pink eyes (3), 9.2
Pink eyes (4), 5.6
Red eyes (2), 15.10
Wry eyes and mouth (3), 9.6

15. Face:
Blackish complexion (1), 12.2
Complexion and eyes the color of a fresh orange (3), 7.6
Dark and yellowish complexion (1), 7.5
Dark complexion (1), 13.2
Edema of face (3), 11.5
Face becoming red when fatigued or working hard (1), 15.1
Greenish complexion (2), 11.5
Idiotic look (1), 11.3
Pale complexion (1), 9.3, 13.1, 13.2, 15.6, 15.7
Pale complexion (2), 5.1, 9.7, 11.4, 13.1, 13.4, 15.5
Puffy face and limbs (3), 15.5
Purely white complexion (1), 7.4
Red and tender zygomatic regions (2), 15.7
Red complexion (1), 9.5
Red complexion (2), 13.5, 13.6, 15.10
Red complexion (3), 9.2, 9.5
Red complexion with depression (2), 11.5
Red zygomatic regions (2), 13.3, 15.6
White complexion (1), 5.4
Withered and white complexion (1), 6.3
Withered and yellowish complexion (1), 7.2, 7.4, 15.2
Withered and yellowish complexion (2), 7.1, 9.3, 13.4, 15.2

Withered and yellowish complexion (3), 9.6

Zygomatic regions' appearing red in the afternoon (1), 5.2

16. Habits and preferences:

Aversion to being chilled (1), 5.4

Aversion to being chilled (3), 5.3, 7.2

Aversion to wind and being chilled (2), 5.1

Desire for warmth and massage (3), 7.2

Dislike of light (1), 10.1

Love of darkness (1), 10.1

Love of darkness and dislike of light (1), 15.1

Slight aversion to being chilled (3), 5.6

17. Head and neck:

Dizziness (1), 7.3, 7.4, 11.4

Dizziness (2), 9.2, 11.1, 13.4, 13.6, 15.10

Dizziness (3), 11.2, 15.7

Dizziness (4), 9.3, 9.4, 9.5, 9.6, 10.1, 11.3, 15.2, 15.7

Dizziness with a desire to lie down (3), 10.2

Hair falling out easily (1), 11.1

Heavy sensation in the head and the body as a whole (3), 7.5

Heavy sensation in the head with light sensation in the leg (2), 9.5

Neck swelling (1), 11.1

Stiff neck (3), 9.6

Sudden fainting (3), 9.6

Vertigo and feeling about to faint (3), 9.6

18. Hiccups:

Hiccups (1), 13.3

Hiccups (2), 8.3

Hiccups (4), 8.1, 15.9

19. Limbs:

Difficulty in flexing and extending (2), 15.7

Dry and withered nails (1), 9.3

Fatigue of the four limbs (1), 15.4

Nails becoming thin or broken (1), 9.3

Numbness of fingers (1), 9.5

Numbness of the four limbs (1), 9.4

Numbness of limbs (2), 15.7

Numbness of limbs (3), 9.6

Spasm or tremor of limbs (3), 9.6

Weak legs (2), 11.4, 15.1

20. Men's symptoms:

Impotence (1), 15.2

Impotence (2), 9.8

Impotence (4), 11.1, 11.3

Inability to control ejaculation (3), 11.4

Infertility (2), 11.1

Premature ejaculation (2), 11.1, 11.2

Premature ejaculation (3), 11.4

Seminal emission (1), 13.5

Seminal emission (2), 11.1, 15.6, 15.7

Seminal emission (4), 11.2, 11.4, 15.1

Seminal emission with erotic dreams (2), 11.2, 15.1

Seminal emission without erotic dreams (1), 11.4

Sexual decline (3), 11.3

Sliding ejaculation (3), 11.4

Strong penis with easy erection (1), 15.7

21. Mouth and lips:

Absence of thirst (1), 7.2

Absence of thirst (2), 5.4, 7.5

Bad breath (1), 6.2

Bad breath (2), 8.4

Bitter taste in the mouth (1), 9.5

Bitter taste in the mouth (2), 5.7, 7.6, 8.4, 15.10

Bitter taste in the mouth (3), 10.1

Blue ring of lips (1), 7.3

Bluish-purple nails and lips (2), 15.3

Copious spitting (1), 8.3

Dry lips (2), 5.8

Dry lips (3), 8.1

Dry mouth (1), 8.4

Dry mouth (2), 5.2, 5.6, 5.7, 5.8, 6.2, 11.5, 13.3

Dry mouth (3), 8.1

Dry mouth at night (1), 15.6

Dry mouth and drinking little (2), 15.6

Dry sensation in the mouth (2), 9.2

Dry sensation in the mouth and throat (2), 9.5

Dry sensation in the mouth with no desire to drink (2), 11.2

Excessive, clear saliva (2), 7.2

Greasy and tasteless sensation in the mouth (3), 7.5

Lips rolled up (1), 7.1

Mouth canker sore (2), 13.5

Mouth closed as if screwed up (1), 9.4

Mouth ulcer (1), 8.4

Pale lips (2), 9.3, 13.4

Plentiful saliva (3), 5.4

Sour and bad breath (1), 8.2

Thirst (1), 11.2

Thirst (2), 6.1, 6.2, 13.5

Thirst (3), 5.7, 9.6

Thirst with a desire for cold drink (3), 8.4

Thirst with a desire to drink (2), 5.6

Thirst with no desire to drink (1), 15.8

Thirst with no desire to drink (2), 7.6, 9.8

Too lazy to talk (2), 15.5

Unable to speak (3), 9.6

Wry mouth and eyes (3), 9.4

22. Nose:

Clear nasal discharge (2), 5.4

Dry sensation in the nose (2), 5.8

Exhaling hot air from the nose (1), 5.7

Flickering of the nostril (1), 5.6

Flickering of the nostril (3), 5.7

Nasal congestion (2), 5.3, 5.6

Nasal congestion and discharge (4), 5.3

Nasal discharge (2), 5.3

23. Pain:

Abdominal pain (2), 6.1

Abdominal pain (4), 6.1, 7.1, 7.2, 9.1, 9.7

Abdominal pain and swelling (3), 6.2

Abdominal pain preceding diarrhea (3), 15.8

Abdominal pain reduced after diarrhea (3), 15.8

Abdominal pain with discharge of watery stool (1), 7.5

Acute pain in lower abdomen below the navel affecting the back and testicles (3), 14.2

Acute stomachache that gets worse with cold and better with warmth (3), 8.3

Burning pain in the chest and hypochondrium (3), 15.10

Burning pain in the ribs (2), 9.2

Burning pain in the stomach (3), 8.4

Burning pain on urination (4), 14.1

Chest pain (1), 5.5, 5.6, 5.7

Chest pain (3), 5.7

Chest pain (4), 5.1, 5.5, 5.8, 13.1, 13.2, 15.3

Chest pain intensified by labor (3), 13.2

Chest pain on coughing (2), 5.8

Cold pain in the lower back and knees (3), 15.5

Gums' swelling with pain (4), 8.4

Headache (4), 5.6, 9.2, 9.4, 9, 5, 9.6

Headache as if being pulled (3), 9.6

Headache in women (2), 9.5

Headache involving the top of head (3), 9.7

Headache on both sides of head and in corners of eyes (3), 9.2

Headache on the side of head (2), 9.5

Headache that drags on and on (3), 9.4

Headache with dizziness (2), 9.5

Headache with pain in the eyebrows (1), 15.7

Hernia pain in the scrotum (3), 14.2

Lumbago (2), 11.4, 15.1

Lumbago (3), 11.1

Lumbago (4), 15.7

Lumbago with weak legs (3), 11.2

Mild pain in the hypochondrium (3), 9.3

Mild stomachache (2), 7.5

Mild stomachache (3), 8.1

Pain affecting the testes or vagina (2), 14.2

Pain and obstruction in the white of the eye (4), 9.4

Pain and swelling in the chest and hypochondrium regions (3), 15.9

Pain and swelling in the ribs (1), 9.5

Pain and swelling of testicle (4), 9.8

Pain around the umbilicus with hardness (2), 6.2

Pain at top of head or temple that is intensified by cold (2)15.9

Pain in the anus with swelling and burning sensation (1), 6.1

Pain in the body (1), 5.6

Pain in the chest and hypochondrium (4), 9.1

Pain in the eyes (2), 9.8

Pain in the heart (1), 13.1

Pain in the heel (2), 11.2

Pain in the hypochondrium (4), 9.4, 9.8, 10.1, 15.7, 15.8

Pain in the inner part of stomach (1), 15.9

Pain in the lower abdomen (3), 9.1

Pain in the lower abdomen (4), 14.2

Pain in the lower abdomen affecting the lumbar spine and testicles (1), 14.1

Pain in the lower abdomen with swelling (3), 9.7

Pain in the penis (4), 14.1

Pain in the ribs (1), 9.5

Pain in the skin with desire for warm massage (1), 6.3

Pain in the throat with dry sensation (1), 5.7

Pain in the throat with redness and swelling (1), 8.4

Pain in the tibia (2), 11.2

Pain on urination (1), 13.5

Pain on urination (3), 12.1

Period pain (4), 9.3, 9.7, 15.7

Periodic stomachache with burning sensation (2), 8.4

Severe headache (3), 9.2

Short and red urine (2), 12.1

Skin ulcer with redness and pain (2), 13.5
Sore loins and weak legs (2), 15.6
Sore throat (1), 5.7
Sore throat (3), 5.7, 14.1
Sore throat (4), 5.6
Stomachache (2), 15.8
Stomachache (4), 7.1, 7.2, 8.1, 8.2, 8.3, 8.4, 9.1, 15.9
Stomachache that gets better after vomiting (2), 8.3
Stomachache with burning pain (3), 8.1
Stretching pain in the scrotum (3), 9.7
Swelling and pain in the breast (3), 9.1
Toothache (2), 11.2
Toothache (4), 8.4

24. Perspiration:
Absence of perspiration (1), 5.3
Excessive perspiration (1), 11.1
Excessive perspiration (2), 11.5, 13.1, 13.2
Excessive perspiration (4), 5.1, 9.4
Night sweats (1), 15.2
Night sweats (2), 11.2, 13.3, 15.1, 15.6, 15.7
Night sweats (4), 5.2
Perspiration on the forehead (1), 11.1

25. Respiration:
Acute panting with high-pitched sound (2), 5.5, 5.7
Breathing difficulty (1), 5.1, 11.5
Chronic shortness of breath (4), 11.5
Light wheezing (1), 5.1
More expiration than inspiration (3), 11.5
Oppressed and rapid breathing (1), 5.7
Palpitations (1), 7.4, 11.1

Palpitations (2), 9.5
Palpitations (3), 13.6, 15.2
Palpitations (4), 13.1, 13.2, 13.3, 13.4, 13.5, 15.3
Palpitations with nervousness (4), 15.1, 15.2
Panting (1), 5.3, 11.1
Panting (3), 5.5, 11.5
Panting and shortness of breath and perspiration at the same time (1), 13.1
Rapid breath (1), 15.10
Rapid expiration (2), 5.5, 5.7
Rough breath (2), 13.6
Shortness of breath (1), 7.4, 15.2
Shortness of breath (3), 5.1, 13.2, 15.4
Shortness of breath on movement (1), 15.6
Shortness of breath that gets worse with labor (3), 13.1
Urgent panting (1), 15.6
Weak breathing (3), 5.1
Wheezing (1), 11.5, 15.6

26. Skin:
Edema (1), 12.2
Edema (4), 5.1, 5.6, 7.6, 11.1, 15.3, 15.5
Edema in the four limbs (4), 7.1
Edema in the lower limbs (4), 7.2
Edema in the whole body (1), 15.5
Edema in the whole body (2), 7.2
Jaundice (4), 7.5
Skin itch (1), 7.6

27. Sleep:
Feeling insecure over sleep (1), 9.5
Feeling insecure over sleep (2), 10.1
Insomnia (1), 5.2, 8.2, 9.8, 15.6
Insomnia (4), 5.2, 9.2, 9.3, 9.4, 10.1, 11.2, 13.1, 13.3, 13.4, 13.5, 13.6, 15.1, 15.2

Insomnia with forgetfulness (2), 15.7

Poor sleep (3), 15.1

Sleepiness (2), 13.2

28. Teeth:

Clinching and grinding the teeth (1), 9.4

Loose teeth (1), 11.1, 11.2

Loose teeth (2), 11.3

29. Throat:

Dry throat (1), 11.2, 15.7

Dry throat (2), 5.8, 6.2, 11.5, 13.3

Dry throat (3), 5.2, 8.1

Itch in the throat (2), 5.3

Itch in the throat (3), 5.2

Sensation of something in the throat (2), 9.1

30. Tongue:

Dry tongue (1), 7.6, 13.3

Dry tongue (2), 5.8, 6.2, 8.1

Pale and fat tongue (1), 7.5

Pale tongue (1), 7.2

Pale tongue (2), 6.3

Pulpy and decayed tongue (1), 13.5

Red color of the tongue (1), 6.1, 7.6

Red tip of the tongue (1), 5.6

Red tip of the tongue (3), 5.8

Stiff tongue (3), 9.6

Swollen sensation at tip of tongue causing a desire to stick it out (1), 13.6

Tooth marks on the tongue (1), 7.1

Ulcer on the tongue (3), 13.5

Ulcer or soreness on the tongue (4), 14.1

White coating on the tongue (1), 5.3, 7.2

31. Urination:

Burning sensation on urination (3), 12.1

Clear and long stream of urine (1), 11.4

Clear and long stream of urine (2), 9.7

Clear and long stream of urine (3), 12.2

Diminished urination (1), 15.6

Diminished urination (2), 7.2, 12.2

Discharge of red urine with urination difficulty (2), 7.6

Dribbling after urination (1), 13.5

Dribbling after urination (2), 7.3, 11.1, 12.2

Escape of urine on coughing (4), 5.1

Frequent urination (1), 15.3

Frequent urination (3), 12.1, 12.2

Frequent urination at night (1), 11.1

Frequent urination at night (2), 11.1

Frequent urination particularly at night (3)11.4

Frequent urination with clear or white urine (1), 15.5

Inability to retain urine (3), 11.4

Incontinence of urination (4), 12.2

Incontinence of urination with dribbling (3), 11.4

Meager urine (3), 9.8, 15.3

Meager urine accompanied by puffiness of skin (2), 15.5

Red urine (2), 13.6

Red urine (3), 14.1

Red, short streams of urine (2), 6.1

Retention of urine (1), 11.2

Short stream of urine (1), 7.5

Sudden interruption during urination (3), 12.1

Suppression of urination (4), 9.8, 11.1, 12.1, 12.2

Turbid urine (1), 12.1

Urination difficulty (2), 14.1

Urination difficulty (3), 9.8
Urination difficulty (4), 12.1
Urination disorders (4), 11.4
Yellowish urine (2), 9.2, 13.5
Yellowish-red urine (1), 9.8

32. Voice:
Hoarseness (3), 5.2
Loss of voice (4), 5.3, 5.8, 15.6
Low and weak voice (2), 11.5
Low voice (3), 5.1

33. Vomiting:
Dry vomiting (1), 8.1
Dry vomiting (2), 8.1
Nausea (2), 15.8
Nausea (3), 7.5
Nausea and vomiting (2), 9.8
Vomiting (1), 6.1
Vomiting (2), 15.8
Vomiting (4), 7.5, 8.2, 8.3, 8.4, 15.9
Vomiting of acid (1), 15.9
Vomiting of acid (3), 7.1
Vomiting of bitter water (2), 10.1
Vomiting of blood (1), 7.1, 8.1, 8.4, 9.1, 15.9
Vomiting of blood (2), 9.2, 13.5
Vomiting of clear saliva (1), 8.3, 9.7
Vomiting of decomposed acid (2), 8.2
Vomiting of pus and blood with a fishy smell (2), 5.7
Vomiting of sour-smelling foods with desire for cold drink (1), 8.2
Vomiting right after eating (1), 8.4

34. Whole body:
Chronic fatigue (4), 5.1, 5.2, 7.1, 9.3, 9.4, 11.1, 11.2, 11.3, 13.1, 13.2, 13.3, 13.4, 15.2, 15.5, 15.6, 15.7
Common cold (4), 5.1, 5.3, 5.6, 5.8

Contractions of tendons and muscles (1), 9.7
Convulsions (2), 9.1
Easily susceptible to common cold (2), 5.1
Fainting (3), 9.6
Fatigue (1), 11.1, 11.2
Fatigue (2), 5.1, 7.1, 7.3, 11.4, 11.5, 13.2
Fever (1), 8.4
Fever (2), 5.3, 6.1, 13.5
Fever (3), 5.6, 5.7, 5.8
Fever at night (1), 11.2
Fever due to an internal injury (4), 9.4
Fever that comes and goes and persists after perspiration (1)7.6
Heavy sensation in the body (1), 5.5, 7.6
High fever (3), 9.6, 13.6
Inability to lie on back (1), 5.4, 5.5
Inability to lie on back (3), 5.5
Jumping of muscles (1), 9.3
Jumping of muscles (2), 15.7
Jumping of muscles (3), 9.6
Light tidal fever (1), 5.7, 8.1, 15.1
Low fever (1), 7.3, 8.1, 13.3
Meager energy (2), 13.1
Mentally fatigued (1), 6.3, 7.4
Muscular twitching and cramps (2), 15.3
Numbness (1), 9.1
Numbness (4), 9.3
Overweight (2), 7.5
Paralysis (1), 15.7
Paralysis (4), 5.8, 15.5
Premature aging (3), 11.3
Skinniness (2), 5.2, 7.1, 11.2, 15.6
Skinny and weak (1), 15.4
Sudden fainting (1), 7.3
Tidal fever (3), 5.2, 15.6

Tidal fever in the afternoon (2), 13.3

Too lazy to talk (2), 7.1, 13.1, 13.2

Twitching (2), 9.4, 13.1

Weak bones (1), 11.3

Weakness (2), 15.2, 15.5

35. Women (pregnancy and childbirth):

Fainting after childbirth (3), 9.4, 13.4

Fetus motion (1), 11.4

Miscarriage (2), 7.3

Miscarriage (4), 11.4

Morning sickness (1), 8.4, 13.5, 15.9

Morning sickness (2), 9.1

Prone to miscarriage (3), 11.4

Shortage of milk secretion after childbirth (1), 9.1

36. Women (vaginal discharge):

Clear and watery vaginal discharge (1), 11.4

Excessive, whitish vaginal discharge (1), 7.5

Plentiful, whitish discharge (2), 7.2

Vaginal discharge (1), 7.1, 15.7

Vaginal discharge (4), 9.8, 11.1, 11.4, 15.8

Whitish vaginal discharge (1), 9.1

37. Woman (menstruation):

Delayed period (4), 9.4

Discharge of blood from the anus before periods (1), 15.3

Excessive menstrual bleeding (3), 7.4

Extended menstruation (1), 15.2

Irregular menstruation (1), 11.2, 13.4, 15.2, 15.7

Irregular menstruation (2), 9.1

Irregular menstruation (4), 9.3, 15.8

Meager menstrual flow (2), 9.3, 15.7

Menstrual disorders (1), 9.3

Menstrual disorders (4), 9.1

Menstrual flow slightly insufficient (1), 9.3

Overdue period (1), 9.4

Premature menstruation (1), 9.1

Premature menstruation (4), 15.7

Suppression of menses (1), 11.2

Suppression of menses (2), 9.3, 9.4, 11.2

Suppression of menses (3), 9.1

Suppression of menses (4), 9.4, 15.7

38. Woman (miscellaneous):

Infertility (2), 11.1, 11.2

Prolapse of the uterus (4), 7.3

Sexual decline (3), 11.3

STEP 2

Specifically for healthy people, Step 2 involves recording the numbers and the sum for each sign or symptom.

First Example: David

A thirty-five-year-old man named David is in good health, but he wants to know the y-scores of his internal organs. He has gone through Step 1 and checked the following items from Chart One as applicable to him:

Eating a lot but remaining thin (1), 8.4
Hungry with good appetite (1), 8.4
Constipation (1), 8.1
Constipation (2), 8.2, 8.4, 13.6
Constipation (4), 6.2
Dry stools (1), 13.3
Dry stools (2), 9.2, 13.5
One bowel movement in several days (3), 6.2
Cold limbs (1), 6.3, 11.2, 13.5
Cold limbs (2), 8.3, 11.5, 15.3
Cold limbs (3), 5.4, 7.2, 13.2
Dry and obstructive sensation in the eyes (3), 9.3
Prone to anger (2), 10.1
Prone to anger (3), 9.2, 9.5
Pale complexion (1), 9.3, 13.1, 13.2, 15.6, 15.7
Pale complexion (2), 5.1, 9.7, 11.4, 13.1, 13.4, 15.5
Slight aversion to being chilled (3), 5.6
Thirst with a desire for cold drink (3), 8.4
Dry mouth (1), 8.4
Dry mouth (2), 5.2, 5.6, 5.7, 5.8, 6.2, 11.5, 13.3
Excessive perspiration (1), 11.1
Excessive perspiration (2), 11.5, 13.1, 13.2
Excessive perspiration (4), 5.1, 9.4
Loose teeth (1), 11.1, 11.2
Loose teeth (2), 11.3
Red tongue (1), 7.6
Yellowish urine (2), 9.2, 13.5
Skinniness (2), 5.2, 7.1, 11.2, 15.6

David then recorded the above signs and symptoms with their numbers and sums in a chart that looks like this:

Syndromes and Their Organ Y-Scores	Numbers Chart One	Sum	Y-Scores of the Internal Organs
5.1 Lungs Energy Deficiency	**2, 4**	**6**	**Lungs -2**
5.2 Lungs Yin Deficiency	2, 2	4	Lungs 3
5.4 Deficient and Cold Lungs	3	3	Lungs -4

Syndromes and Their Organ Y-Scores	Numbers Chart One	Sum	Y-Scores of the Internal Organs
5.6 Wind and Heat Attacking the Lungs	3, 2	5	Lungs 3
5.7 Hot Lungs (Lungs Fire)	2	2	Lungs 4
5.8 Dry Lungs	2	2	Lungs 1
6.2 Large Intestine Fluid Exhaustion	**4, 3, 2**	**9**	**L. intestine 1**
6.3 Large Intestine Deficiency and Slippery Diarrhea	1	1	L. intestine 2
7.1 Spleen Energy Deficiency	2	2	Spleen -2
7.2 Spleen Yang Deficiency	**3**	**3**	**Spleen -4**
7.6 Damp Heat Steaming the Spleen	1	1	Spleen 2
8.1 Stomach Yin Deficiency	1	1	Stomach 3
8.2 Food Stagnation in Stomach	2	2	Stomach -3
8.3 Cold Stomach	2	2	Stomach -4
8.4 Hot Stomach	**1, 1, 2, 3, 1**	**8**	**Stomach 3**
9.2 Liver Fire Flaming Upward	**2, 3, 2**	**7**	**Liver 4**
9.3 Liver Blood Deficiency	3, 1	4	Liver 1
9.4 Liver Yin Deficiency	4	4	Liver 3
9.5 Liver Yang Upsurging	3	3	Liver 3
9.7 Cold Obstructing the Liver Meridian	2	2	Liver -4
10.1 Gallbladder Excessive Heat	**2**	**2**	**Gallbladder 3**
11.1 Kidneys Yang Deficiency	1, 1	2	Kidneys -4
11.2 Kidneys Yin Deficiency	1, 1, 2	4	Kidneys 3
11.3 Insufficient Kidneys Essence	2	2	Kidneys 3
11.4 Loosening of Kidneys Energy	2	2	Kidneys -2
11.5 Kidneys Unable to Absorb Inspiration	**2, 2, 2**	**6**	**Kidneys -3**

Syndromes and Their Organ Y-Scores	Numbers Chart One	Sum	Y-Scores of the Internal Organs
13.1 Heart Energy Deficiency	1, 2, 2	5	Heart -2
13.2 Heart Yang Deficiency	3, 1, 2	6	Heart -4
13.3 Heart Yin Deficiency	1, 2	3	Heart 3
13.4 Heart Blood Deficiency	2	2	Heart 1
13.5 Heart Fire Flaming	**2, 1, 2**	**5**	**Heart 4**
13.6 Phlegm Fire Disturbing the Heart	2	2	Heart 4
15.3 Yang Deficiency of the Heart and Kidneys	2	2	Heart 4, Kidneys -4
15.4 Energy Deficiency of the Spleen and Lungs			Spleen -2, Lungs -2
15.5 Yang Deficiency of the Spleen and Kidneys	2	2	Spleen -4, Kidneys -4
15.6 Yin Deficiency of the Lungs and Kidneys	1, 2	3	Lungs 3, Kidneys 3
15.7 Yin Deficiency of the Liver and Kidneys	1	1	Liver 3, Kidneys 3

We can determine the y-scores of eight internal organs for David as follows (with the greatest sum in the chart for each organ in bold-face): Lungs -2, L. intestine 1, Spleen -4, Stomach 3, Liver 4, Gall-bladder 3, Kidneys -3, and Heart 4. With knowledge of the y-scores of his internal organs, David can proceed to Step 5, to choose the right foods from Chart Five, beginning on page 230. Because the y-score of his liver is 4, he should choose to eat foods with Liver -1 through Liver -8 and avoid foods with Liver 4 or higher, in order to prevent the y-score of his liver from getting higher, as his liver is on the verge of becoming sick.

Although David is in good health, three of his internal organs are somewhat vulnerable to disease: the liver (with a score of 4), the spleen (with a score of -4), and the heart (with a score of 4). Thus, the potential hazards for David lie in the above three organs' possibly becoming sick, characterized respectively by Liver Fire Flaming Upward (8), Spleen Yang Deficiency (-8), and Heart Fire Flaming

(8). We can predict that if one day David does become ill, he will most likely develop symptoms and diseases related to the above three syndromes. Among the healthiest organs in David's body are the small intestine and the bladder, neither of which shows a number in the chart, which means that their y-score is zero.

After David has identified the y-scores of his internal organs, he can go through Step 5, in order to select the right foods from Chart Five to promote the good health of his affected organs.

Second Example: Judy

Although Judy, a thirty-year-old woman, is in good health, she wants to find out the y-scores of her internal organs. Having gone through Step 1, she has checked the following items from Chart One as applicable to her:

> Mentally depressed (3), 9.5
> Prone to sadness and crying (2), 13.1
> Fondness for massage with heat (3), 7.2
> Absence of perspiration (1), 5.3
> Red zygomatic regions (2), 13.3, 15.6
> Frequent urination (1), 15.3
> Frequent urination (3), 12.1, 12.2
> Frequent urination at night (1), 11.1
> Frequent urination at night (2), 11.1
> Low and weak voice (2), 11.5
> Low voice (3), 5.1

She then recorded the numbers and the sums of her signs and symptoms in a chart:

Syndromes	Numbers	Sum	Y-Scores
5.1 Lungs Energy Deficiency	3	3	Lungs -2
5.3 Lungs under the Attack of Wind and Cold	1	1	Lungs -3
7.2 Spleen Yang Deficiency	3	3	Spleen -4
9.5 Liver Yang Upsurging	3	3	Liver 3
11.1 Kidneys Yang Deficiency	1, 2	3	Kidneys -4

Syndromes	Numbers	Sum	Y-Scores
11.5 Kidneys Unable to Absorb Inspiration	2	2	Kidneys -3
12.1 Bladder Damp Heat	3	3	Bladder 1
12.2 Bladder Cold and Deficiency	**3**	**3**	**Bladder -4**
13.1 Heart Energy Deficiency	**2**	**2**	**Heart -2**
13.3 Heart Yin Deficiency	**2**	**2**	**Heart 3**
15.3 Yang Deficiency of the Heart and Kidneys	1	1	Heart 4, Kidneys -4
15.6 Yin Deficiency of the Lungs and Kidneys	2	2	Lungs 3, Kidneys 3

We can determine the y-scores of six internal organs for Judy as follows (with the greatest sum in the chart for each organ in bold-face): Lungs Energy Deficiency (Lungs -2), Spleen Yang Deficiency (Spleen -4), Liver Yang Upsurging (Liver 3), Kidneys Yang Deficiency (Kidneys -4), Bladder Cold and Deficiency (Bladder -4), and Heart Energy Deficiency (Heart -2) or Heart Yin Deficiency (Heart 3).

Three internal organs in Judy's body are most vulnerable to the attack of disease: the spleen (with a y-score of -4), the kidneys (with a y-score of -4), and the bladder (with a y-score of -4). Therefore, Judy runs the risk of the above three organs' some day becoming sick, characterized respectively by Spleen Yang Deficiency (-8), Kidneys Yang Deficiency (8), and Bladder Cold and Deficiency (-8). Should she become ill, she will most likely develop symptoms and diseases related to these three syndromes. Among Judy's healthiest organs are the large intestine, the small intestine, the stomach, and the gallbladder; none of these organs show a number in the chart, which means that their y-score is zero.

Once Judy has identified the y-scores of her internal organs, she can go through Step 5, to select the right foods to promote the health of her affected organs.

4

Recording and Calculating the Y-Scores of Your Internal Organs

Use this chart if you are in good health to figure out the y-scores of your internal organs.

Chart Two: Recording and Calculating for Healthy Individuals

Syndromes and Their Organ Y-Scores	Numbers Chart One	Sum	Y-Scores of the Internal Organs
5.1 Lungs Energy Deficiency			Lungs -2
5.2 Lungs Yin Deficiency			Lungs 3
5.3 Lungs under the Attack of Wind and Cold			Lungs -3
5.4 Deficient and Cold Lungs			Lungs -4
5.5 Phlegm Dampness Obstructing the Lungs			Lungs -1
5.6 Wind and Heat Attacking the Lungs			Lungs 3
5.7 Hot Lungs (Lungs Fire)			Lungs 4
5.8 Dry Lungs			Lungs 1
6.1 Large Intestine Damp Heat			L. intestine 2
6.2 Large Intestine Fluid Exhaustion			L. intestine 1

Syndromes and Their Organ Y-Scores	Numbers Chart One	Sum	Y-Scores of the Internal Organs
6.3 Large Intestine Deficiency and Slippery Diarrhea			L. intestine 2
7.1 Spleen Energy Deficiency			Spleen -2
7.2 Spleen Yang Deficiency			Spleen -4
7.3 Middle Energy Cave-in			Spleen -2
7.4 Spleen Unable to Govern Blood			Spleen -4
7.5 Cold Dampness Troubling the Spleen			Spleen -3
7.6 Damp Heat Steaming the Spleen			Spleen 2
8.1 Stomach Yin Deficiency			Stomach 3
8.2 Food Stagnation in Stomach			Stomach -3
8.3 Cold Stomach			Stomach -4
8.4 Hot Stomach			Stomach 3
9.1 Liver Energy Congestion			Liver -3
9.2 Liver Fire Flaming Upward			Liver 4
9.3 Liver Blood Deficiency			Liver 1
9.4 Liver Yin Deficiency			Liver 3
9.5 Liver Yang Upsurging			Liver 3
9.6 Internal Liver Wind Blowing			Liver 2
9.7 Cold Obstructing the Liver Meridian			Liver -4
9.8 Damp Heat Attacking the Liver and Gallbladder			Liver 2, Gallbladder 2
10.1 Gallbladder Excessive Heat			Gallbladder 3
10.2 Gallbladder Energy Deficiency			Gallbladder -2
11.1 Kidneys Yang Deficiency			Kidneys -4
11.2 Kidneys Yin Deficiency			Kidneys 3

Syndromes and Their Organ Y-Scores	Numbers Chart One	Sum	Y-Scores of the Internal Organs
11.3 Insufficient Kidneys Essence			Kidneys 3
11.4 Loosening of Kidneys Energy			Kidneys -2
11.5 Kidneys Unable to Absorb Inspiration			Kidneys -3
12.1 Bladder Damp Heat			Bladder 1
12.2 Bladder Cold and Deficiency			Bladder -4
13.1 Heart Energy Deficiency			Heart -2
13.2 Heart Yang Deficiency			Heart -4
13.3 Heart Yin Deficiency			Heart 3
13.4 Heart Blood Deficiency			Heart 1
13.5 Heart Fire Flaming			Heart 4
13.6 Phlegm Fire Disturbing the Heart			Heart 4
14.1 Excessive Heat in the Small Intestine			S. intestine 3
14.2 Small Intestine Energy Congestion			S. intestine -3
15.1 No Communication between the Kidneys and Heart			Kidneys 3, Heart 4
15.2 Simultaneous Deficiency of the Heart and Spleen			Heart 1, Spleen 2
15.3 Yang Deficiency of the Heart and Kidneys			Heart - 4, Kidneys -4
15.4 Energy Deficiency of the Spleen and Lung			Spleen -2, Lungs -2
15.5 Yang Deficiency of the Spleen and Kidneys			Spleen -4, Kidneys -4
15.6 Yin Deficiency of the Lungs and Kidneys			Lungs 3, Kidneys 3

Syndromes and Their Organ Y-Scores	Numbers Chart One	Sum	Y-Scores of the Internal Organs
15.7 Yin Deficiency of the Liver and Kidneys			Liver 3, Kidneys 3
15.8 Disharmony between the Liver and Spleen			Liver -3, Spleen -2
15.9 Disharmony between the Liver and Stomach			Liver -3, Stomach -2
15.10 Liver Fire Offending the Lungs			Liver 4, Lungs 3

STEP 3

When you are ill, you need to record the numbers and the sum of the signs and symptoms applicable to you to figure out the y-scores of your internal organs. To illustrate how to do this, let's use two clinical cases as examples:

First Example: Chen

A forty-year-old male patient with the surname of Chen was suffering from a chronic cough and had asthma for a long time. He could not lie down on his back, because this would intensify the symptoms, and he coughed frequently, coughing up a little sticky, yellowish phlegm. A doctor of traditional Chinese medicine diagnosed his condition as Lungs Yin Deficiency.

For Chen, the following four signs or symptoms should be recorded in Step 3:

> Cough (4), 5.1, 5.2, 5.3, 5.6, 5.7, 5.8, 15.6, 15.10
> Coughing up yellowish and sticky phlegm (2), 13.6
> Coughing up yellowish and sticky phlegm (3), 5.6, 5.7
> Cough with meager phlegm (3), 5.2

Then the numbers and the sum should be recorded in a chart to determine the y-score of his internal organs:

Syndromes	Numbers	Sum	Y-Scores
5.1 Lungs Energy Deficiency	4	4	Lungs -6
5.2 Lungs Yin Deficiency	4, 3	7	Lungs 7
5.3 Lungs under the Attack of Wind and Cold	4	4	Lungs -7
5.6 Wind and Heat Attacking the Lungs	4, 3	7	Lungs 7
5.7 Hot Lungs (Lungs Fire)	4, 3	7	Lungs 8
5.8 Dry Lungs	4	4	Lungs 5
13.6 Phlegm Fire Disturbing the Heart	2		Heart 8
15.6 Yin Deficiency of the Lungs and Kidneys	4		Lungs 7, Kidneys 7
15.10 Liver Fire Offending the Lungs	4	4	Liver 8, Lungs 7

It is obvious from the above information that Chen has either Lungs 7 or Lungs 8, because 7 is the greatest sum and is recorded for 5.2 Lungs Yin Deficiency, 5.6 Wind and Heat Attacking the Lungs, and 5.7 Hot Lungs. As the patient has been diagnosed as having asthma, we can proceed to Step 4, to determine what syndrome is responsible for asthma in this case according to Chart Four.

Second Example: Zhuang

A forty-six-year-old male patient with the surname of Zhuang displayed the following signs and symptoms: vertigo with ringing in the ears, flying spots in front of the eyes, a spinning sensation as if in a boat or on a train, stomach discomfort, nausea, palpitations, and poor sleep. He was diagnosed by a doctor of Western medicine as having Ménière's disease. A doctor of traditional Chinese medicine diagnosed his condition as the syndrome Liver Yang Upsurging.

The following ten signs and symptoms should be recorded in Step 3:

Vertigo and feeling about to faint (3), 9.6
Ringing in the ears (2), 9.4, 11.3, 15.1, 15.7

Ringing in the ears (4), 9.2, 9.5
Discomfort in the stomach and abdomen (3), 7.5
Nausea and vomiting (2), 9.8
Palpitations (1), 7.4, 11.1
Palpitations (2), 9.5
Palpitations (3), 13.6, 15.2
Palpitations (4), 13.1, 13.2, 13.3, 13.4, 13.5, 15.3
Poor sleep (3), 15.1

Now the numbers and the sum of the signs and symptoms should be recorded in a chart this way:

Syndromes	Numbers	Sum	Y-Scores
7.4 Spleen Unable to Govern Blood	1	1	Spleen -8
7.5 Cold Dampness Troubling the Spleen	3	3	Spleen -7
9.2 Liver Fire Flaming Upward	4	4	Liver 8
9.4 Liver Yin Deficiency	2	2	Liver 7
9.5 Liver Yang Upsurging	4, 2	6	Liver 7
9.6 Internal Liver Wind Blowing	3	3	Liver 6
9.8 Damp Heat Attacking the Liver and Gallbladder	2	2	Liver 6, Gallbladder 6
11.1 Kidneys Yang Deficiency	1	1	Kidneys -8
11.3 Insufficient Kidneys Essence	2	2	Kidneys 7
13.1 Heart Energy Deficiency	4	4	Heart -6
13.2 Heart Yang Deficiency	4	4	Heart -8
13.3 Heart Yin Deficiency	4	4	Heart 7
13.4 Heart Blood Deficiency	4	4	Heart 5
13.5 Heart Fire Flaming	4	4	Heart 8
13.6 Phlegm Fire Disturbing the Heart	3	3	Heart 8
15.1 No Communication between the Kidneys and Heart	2, 3	5	Kidneys 7, Heart 8

Syndromes	Numbers	Sum	Y-Scores
15.2 Simultaneous Deficiency of the Heart and Spleen	3	3	Heart 5, Spleen 6
15.3 Yang Deficiency of the Heart and Kidneys	4	4	Heart 8, Kidneys -8
15.7 Yin Deficiency of the Liver and Kidneys	2	2	Liver 7, Kidneys 7

It appears from the above chart that the greatest sum is 6, which refers to 9.5 Liver Yang Upsurging, followed by the sum of 5, referring to 5.1 No Communication between the Kidneys and Heart. Because Zhuang has been diagnosed as having Ménière's disease, we can proceed to Step 4, to determine what syndrome is responsible for Ménière's disease in this case according to Chart Four.

CHART THREE: RECORDING AND CALCULATING FOR INDIVIDUALS WHO ARE ILL

Syndromes and Their Organ Y-Scores	Numbers Chart One	Sum	Y-Scores of the Internal Organs
5.1 Lungs Energy Deficiency			Lungs -6
5.2 Lungs Yin Deficiency			Lungs 7
5.3 Lungs under the Attack of Wind and Cold			Lungs -7
5.4 Deficient and Cold Lungs			Lungs -8
5.5 Phlegm Dampness Obstructing the Lungs			Lungs -5
5.6 Wind and Heat Attacking the Lungs			Lungs 7
5.7 Hot Lungs (Lungs Fire)			Lungs 8
5.8 Dry Lungs			Lungs 5
6.1 Large Intestine Damp Heat			L. intestine 6
6.2 Large Intestine Fluid Exhaustion			L. intestine 5

Syndromes and Their Organ Y-Scores	Numbers Chart One	Sum	Y-Scores of the Internal Organs
6.3 Large Intestine Deficiency and Slippery Diarrhea			L. intestine 6
7.1 Spleen Energy Deficiency			Spleen -6
7.2 Spleen Yang Deficiency			Spleen -8
7.3 Middle Energy Cave-in			Spleen -6
7.4 Spleen Unable to Govern Blood			Spleen -8
7.5 Cold Dampness Troubling the Spleen			Spleen -7
7.6 Damp Heat Steaming the Spleen			Spleen 6
8.1 Stomach Yin Deficiency			Stomach 7
8.2 Food Stagnation in Stomach			Stomach -7
8.3 Cold Stomach			Stomach -8
8.4 Hot Stomach			Stomach 7
9.1 Liver Energy Congestion			Liver -7
9.2 Liver Fire Flaming Upward			Liver 8
9.3 Liver Blood Deficiency			Liver 5
9.4 Liver Yin Deficiency			Liver 7
9.5 Liver Yang Upsurging			Liver 7
9.6 Internal Liver Wind Blowing			Liver 6
9.7 Cold Obstructing the Liver Meridian			Liver -8
9.8 Damp Heat Attacking the Liver and Gallbladder			Liver 6, Gallbladder 6
10.1 Gallbladder Excessive Heat			Gallbladder 7
10.2 Gallbladder Energy Deficiency			Gallbladder -6
11.1 Kidneys Yang Deficiency			Kidneys -8
11.2 Kidneys Yin Deficiency			Kidneys 7

Syndromes and Their Organ Y-Scores	Numbers Chart One	Sum	Y-Scores of the Internal Organs
11.3 Insufficient Kidneys Essence			Kidneys 7
11.4 Loosening of Kidneys Energy			Kidneys -6
11.5 Kidneys Unable to Absorb Inspiration			Kidneys -7
12.1 Bladder Damp Heat			Bladder 5
12.2 Bladder Cold and Deficiency			Bladder -8
13.1 Heart Energy Deficiency			Heart -6
13.2 Heart Yang Deficiency			Heart -8
13.3 Heart Yin Deficiency			Heart 7
13.4 Heart Blood Deficiency			Heart 5
13.5 Heart Fire Flaming			Heart 8
13.6 Phlegm Fire Disturbing the Heart			Heart 8
14.1 Excessive Heat in the Small Intestine			S. intestine 7
14.2 Small Intestine Energy Congestion			S. intestine -7
15.1 No Communication between the Kidneys and Heart			Kidneys 7, Heart 8
15.2 Simultaneous Deficiency of the Heart and Spleen			Heart 5, Spleen 6
15.3 Yang Deficiency of the Heart and Kidneys			Heart 8, Kidneys -8
15.4 Energy Deficiency of the Spleen and Lungs			Spleen -6, Lungs -6
15.5 Yang Deficiency of the Spleen and Kidneys			Spleen -8, Kidneys -8
15.6 Yin Deficiency of the Lungs and Kidneys			Lungs 7, Kidneys 7

Syndromes and Their Organ Y-Scores	Numbers Chart One	Sum	Y-Scores of the Internal Organs
15.7 Yin Deficiency of the Liver and Kidneys			Liver 7, Kidneys 7
15.8 Disharmony between the Liver and Spleen			Liver -7, Spleen -6
15.9 Disharmony between the Liver and Stomach			Liver -7, Stomach -6
15.10 Liver Fire Offending the Lungs			Liver 8, Lungs 7

STEP 4

If you have been diagnosed with a disease in Western medicine, in this step you will identify the syndrome responsible for it along with the y-score of your internal organs.

In many cases, the y-score of the internal organs can be determined instantly. For example, if you have been diagnosed as having acute bacillary dysentery, the y-score of your large intestine is 6; if you have been diagnosed as having chronic infectious hepatitis, the y-score of your liver is -7, or if you have been diagnosed as having acute cystitis, the y-score of your bladder is 5.

There are many diseases with more than one possible syndrome responsible for them, and in these cases you will be confronted with a number of choices and will have to select the syndrome most applicable to you. In this situation, you must go through Step 1 and Step 3 to make a more accurate choice.

Let's use the previous case of the forty-year-old man named Chen as an example. Having gone through Step 3, three syndromes are most likely applicable to him: 5.2 Lungs Yin Deficiency, 5.6 Wind and Heat Attacking the Lungs, and 5.7 Hot Lungs.

Chen has been diagnosed as having asthma, and, when we look through Chart Four (which follows), containing a list of Western diseases, we immediately find that a number of syndromes can be responsible for asthma: 5.2 Lungs Yin Deficiency (Lungs 7), 5.5 Phlegm Dampness Obstructing the Lungs (Lungs -5), 5.6 Wind and Heat Attacking the Lungs (Lungs 7), 11.1 Kidneys Yang Deficiency (Kidneys -8), 11.5 Kidneys Unable to Absorb Inspiration (Kidneys -

7), 15.4 Energy Deficiency of the Spleen and Lungs (Spleen -6, Lungs -6), and 15.6 Yin Deficiency of the Lungs and Kidneys (Lungs 7, Kidneys 7). The question is, which of these seven syndromes is applicable in this case? Any syndrome we select must be one of the three syndromes that have been found to be most likely applicable to the patient according to Step 3. Therefore, we can conclude that it is either 5.2 Lungs Yin Deficiency or 5.6 Wind and Heat Attacking the Lungs.

Using the previous case of the forty-six-year-old patient named Zhuang as another example, having gone through Step 3, we have identified 9.5 Liver Yang Upsurging as being most likely applicable to him.

As Zhuang has been diagnosed as having Ménière's disease, when we look through Chart Four we find that two syndromes could be responsible for it: 9.4 Liver Yin Deficiency (Liver 7) or 9.6 Internal Liver Wind Blowing (Liver 6). Obviously, neither of them is Liver Yang Upsurging (Liver 7). But we can see that both of the two possible syndromes involve the liver. It can be concluded that Liver Yin Deficiency is the right syndrome to be chosen for two reasons: First, Liver Yang Upsurging and Liver Yin Deficiency both have Liver 7— that is, the y-score of the liver is "7" in both syndromes; second, when liver yin is deficient, liver yang can easily upsurge, which means that Liver Yin Deficiency and Liver Yang Upsurging are very close to each other.

CHART FOUR: WESTERN DISEASES WITH THEIR POSSIBLE SYNDROMES

Accessory nasal sinusitis: 5.7 Hot Lungs (Lungs Fire) (Lungs 8), 10.1 Gallbladder Excessive Heat (Gallbladder 7)

Acute and chronic amebic intestine: 6.1 Large Intestine Damp Heat (L. intestine 6)

Acute and chronic bacillary dysentery: 6.1 Large Intestine Damp Heat (L. intestine 6)

Acute and chronic enteritis: 6.1 Large Intestine Damp Heat (L. intestine 6)

Acute and chronic gastritis: 8.3 Cold Stomach (Stomach -8), 15.9 Disharmony between the Liver and Stomach (Liver -7, Stomach -6)

Acute and chronic gastroenteritis: 7.2 Spleen Yang Deficiency (Spleen -8)

Acute and chronic hepatitis: 15.9 Disharmony between the Liver and Stomach (Liver -7, Stomach -6)

Acute appendicitis: 6.1 Large Intestine Damp Heat (L. intestine 6)

Acute bronchitis: 5.3 Lungs under the Attack of Wind and Cold (Lungs -7)

Acute cerebrovascular disease: 13.6 Phlegm Fire Disturbing the Heart (Heart 8)

Acute cholecystitis: 7.6 Damp Heat Steaming the Spleen (Spleen 6), 9.8 Damp Heat Attacking the Liver and Gallbladder (Liver 1, Gallbladder 1), 10.1 Gallbladder Excessive Heat (Gallbladder 7), 13.5 Heart Fire Flaming (Heart 8)

Acute cholecystitis and cholecys-tolithiasis: 9.1 Liver Energy Congestion (Liver -7)

Acute conjunctivitis: 5.7 Hot Lungs (Lungs Fire) (Lungs 8), 9.2 Liver Fire Flaming Upward (Liver 8)

Acute cystitis: 12.1 Bladder Damp Heat (Bladder 5)

Acute enteritis: 7.5 Cold Dampness Troubling the Spleen (Spleen -7), 8.2 Food Stagnation in Stomach (Stomach -7)

Acute epidemic icterohepatitis: 7.1 Spleen Energy Deficiency (Spleen -6), 9.1 Liver Energy Congestion (Liver -7)

Acute gastritis: 8.4 Hot Stomach (Stomach 7), 10.1 Gallbladder Excessive Heat (Gallbladder 7)

Acute gastroenteritis: 8.2 Food Stagnation in Stomach (Stomach -7)

Acute glomerulonephritis: 5.6 Wind and Heat Attacking the Lungs (Lungs 7)

Acute hepatitis: 9.8 Damp Heat Attacking the Liver and Gallbladder (Liver 1, Gallbladder 1)

Acute hepatitis with jaundice: 7.6 Damp Heat Steaming the Spleen (Spleen 6)

Acute icterohepatitis: 9.8 Damp Heat Attacking the Liver and Gallbladder (Liver 1, Gallbladder 1)

Acute intestinal obstruction: 8.2 Food Stagnation in Stomach (Stomach -7)

Acute myelitis: 5.8 Dry Lungs (Lungs 5)

Acute pancreatitis: 8.4 Hot Stomach (Stomach 7), 9.1 Liver Energy Congestion (Liver -7), 9.2 Liver Fire Flaming Upward (Liver 8)

Acute tracheitis: 5.6 Wind and Heat Attacking the Lungs (Lungs 7)

Acute urethritis: 12.1 Bladder Damp Heat (Bladder 5)

Acute urinary infection: 13.5 Heart Fire Flaming (Heart 8)

Acute viral jaundice type hepatitis: 7.6 Damp Heat Steaming the Spleen (Spleen 6)

Addison's disease: 11.2 Kidneys Yin Deficiency (Kidneys 7)

Adnexitis: 11.4 Loosening of Kidneys Energy (Kidneys -6)

Algia: 9.4 Liver Yin Deficiency (Liver 7), 9.6 Internal Liver Wind Blowing (Liver 6)

Amenorrhea: 11.1 Kidneys Yang Deficiency (Kidneys -8), 11.2 Kidneys Yin Deficiency (Kidneys 7)

Anal rectal prolapse: 6.3 Large Intestine Deficiency and Slippery Diarrhea (L. intestine -6)

Anaphylactoid purpura: 7.1 Spleen Energy Deficiency (Spleen -6), 7.4 Spleen Unable to Govern Blood (Spleen -8)

Anemia: 7.1 Spleen Energy Deficiency, (Spleen -6), 9.3 Liver Blood Deficiency (Liver 5), 13.1 Heart Energy Deficiency (Heart -6), 13.3 Heart Yin Deficiency (Heart 7), 15.5 Yang Deficiency of the Spleen and Kidneys (Spleen -8, Kidneys -8), 15.7 Yin Deficiency of the Liver and Kidneys (Liver 7, Kidneys 7)

Angina pectoris: 11.1 Kidneys Yang Deficiency (Kidneys -8), 13.2 Heart Yang Deficiency (Heart -8), 15.2 Simultaneous Deficiency of the Heart and Spleen (Heart 5, Spleen -6), 15.7 Yin Deficiency of the Liver and Kidneys (Liver 7, Kidneys 7)

Aphtha: 14.1 Excessive Heat in the Small Intestine (S. intestine 7)

Aplastic anemia: 7.4 Spleen Unable to Govern Blood (Spleen -8), 9.4 Liver Yin Deficiency (Liver 7), 11.2 Kidneys Yin Deficiency (Kidneys 7), 15.2 Simultaneous Deficiency of the Heart and Spleen (Heart 5, Spleen -6), 15.5 Yang Deficiency of the Spleen and Kidneys (Spleen -8, Kidneys -8)

Arrhythmia: 13.1 Heart Energy Deficiency (Heart -6), 13.3 Heart Yin Deficiency (Heart 7), 13.6 Phlegm Fire Disturbing the Heart (Heart 8), 15.1 No Communication between the Kidneys and Heart (Kidneys 7, Heart 8), 15.2 Simultaneous Deficiency of the Heart and Spleen (Heart 5, Spleen -6), 15.3 Yang Deficiency of the Heart and Kidneys (Heart -8, Kidneys -8)

Arteriosclerosis: 11.3 Insufficient Kidneys Essence (Kidneys 7)

Ascites due to cirrhosis: 7.5 Cold Dampness Troubling the Spleen (Spleen -7), 15.5 Yang Deficiency of the Spleen and Kidneys (Spleen -8, Kidneys -8)

Asthma: 5.2 Lungs Yin Deficiency (Lungs 7), 5.5 Phlegm Dampness Obstructing the Lungs (Lungs -5), 5.6 Wind and Heat Attacking the Lungs (Lungs 7), 11.1 Kidneys Yang Deficiency (Kidneys -8), 11.5 Kidneys Unable to Absorb Inspiration (Kidneys -7), 15.4 Energy Deficiency of the Spleen and Lungs (Spleen -6, Lungs -6), 15.6 Yin Deficiency of the Lungs and Kidneys (Lungs 7, Kidneys 7)

Atelectasis: 5.2 Lungs Yin Deficiency (Lungs 7)

Atrophic rhinitis: 5.8 Dry Lungs (Lungs 5)

Auditory vertigo: 15.7 Yin Deficiency of the Liver and Kidneys (Liver 7, Kidneys 7)

Bacterial food poisoning: 6.1 Large Intestine Damp Heat (L. intestine 6)

Bleeding from upper digestive tract: 8.4 Hot Stomach (Stomach 7)

Bleeding in gastric and duodenalbulbar ulcer: 7.4 Spleen Unable to Govern Blood (Spleen -8)

Bronchial asthma: 5.1 Lungs Energy Deficiency (Lungs -6), 5.4 Deficient and Cold Lungs (Lungs -8), 5.5 Phlegm Dampness Obstructing the Lungs (Lungs -5), 5.7 Hot Lungs (Lungs Fire) (Lungs 8), 7.1 Spleen Energy Deficiency (Spleen -6), 11.1 Kidneys Yang

Deficiency (Kidneys -8), 11.5 Kidneys Unable to Absorb Inspiration (Kidneys -7), 15.6 Yin Deficiency of the Lungs and Kidneys (Lungs 7, Kidneys 7)

Bronchiectasis: 5.3 Lungs under the Attack of Wind and Cold (Lungs -7), 5.4 Deficient and Cold Lungs (Lungs -8), 5.8 Dry Lungs (Lungs 5), 15.10 Liver Fire Offending the Lungs (Liver 8, Lungs 7)

Bronchitis: 5.5 Phlegm Dampness Obstructing the Lungs (Lungs -5), 5.8 Dry Lungs (Lungs 5), 15.10 Liver Fire Offending the Lungs (Liver 8, Lungs 7)

Cancer of esophagus: 9.1 Liver Energy Congestion (Liver -7)

Cancer of uterine cervix: 9.1 Liver Energy Congestion (Liver -7), 9.4 Liver Yin Deficiency (Liver 7), 11.2 Kidneys Yin Deficiency (Kidneys 7), 15.5 Yang Deficiency of the Spleen and Kidneys (Spleen -8, Kidneys -8)

Cardiac asthma: 11.5 Kidneys Unable to Absorb Inspiration (Kidneys -7)

Cardiac neurosis: 13.2 Heart Yang Deficiency (Heart -8)

Cardiomyopathy: 13.1 Heart Energy Deficiency (Heart -6)

Cardiopathy: 13.2 Heart Yang Deficiency (Heart -8)

Cerebrovascular accidents: 9.4 Liver Yin Deficiency (Liver 7), 9.6 Internal Liver Wind Blowing (Liver 6), 13.6 Phlegm Fire Disturbing the Heart (Heart 8)

Cervical cancer: 15.5 Yang Deficiency of the Spleen and Kidneys

(Spleen -8, Kidneys -8), 15.7 Yin Deficiency of the Liver and Kidneys (Liver 7, Kidneys 7)

Cervicitis: 9.8 Damp Heat Attacking the Liver and Gallbladder (Liver 1, Gallbladder 1)

Cholecystolithiasis: 9.8 Damp Heat Attacking the Liver and Gallbladder (Liver 1, Gallbladder 1)

Cholera: 7.5 Cold Dampness Troubling the Spleen (Spleen -7)

Choroiditis: 9.2 Liver Fire Flaming Upward (Liver 8), 11.2 Kidneys Yin Deficiency (Kidneys 7), 13.5 Heart Fire Flaming (Heart 8)

Chronic active hepatitis: 9.4 Liver Yin Deficiency (Liver 7)

Chronic asthmatic bronchitis: 11.5 Kidneys Unable to Absorb Inspiration (Kidneys -7)

Chronic bronchitis: 5.1 Lungs Energy Deficiency (Lungs -6), 5.2 Lungs Yin Deficiency (Lungs 7), 5.3 Lungs under the Attack of Wind and Cold (Lungs -7), 5.6 Wind and Heat Attacking the Lungs (Lungs 7), 5.7 Hot Lungs (Lungs Fire) (Lungs 8), 7.1 Spleen Energy Deficiency (Spleen -6), 11.1 Kidneys Yang Deficiency (Kidneys -8), 15.4 Energy Deficiency of the Spleen and Lungs (Spleen -6, Lungs -6), 15.6 Yin Deficiency of the Lungs and Kidneys (Lungs 7, Kidneys 7)

Chronic cholecystitis: 15.9 Disharmony between the Liver and Stomach (Liver -7, Stomach -6)

Chronic conjunctivitis: 5.2 Lungs Yin Deficiency (Lungs 7)

Chronic cor pulmonale: 13.6 Phlegm Fire Disturbing the Heart (Heart 8), 15.5 Yang Deficiency of the Spleen and Kidneys (Spleen -8, Kidneys -8), 15.6 Yin Deficiency of the Lungs and Kidneys (Lungs 7, Kidneys 7)

Chronic diseases associated with the lungs: 5.1 Lungs Energy Deficiency (Lungs -6)

Chronic dysentery: 6.3 Large Intestine Deficiency and Slippery Diarrhea (L. intestine -6), 7.2 Spleen Yang Deficiency (Spleen -8), 15.5 Yang Deficiency of the Spleen and Kidneys (Spleen -8, Kidneys -8)

Chronic enteritis: 6.3 Large Intestine Deficiency and Slippery Diarrhea (L. intestine -6), 7.3 Middle Energy Cave-in (Spleen -6), 11.1 Kidneys Yang Deficiency (Kidneys -8), 15.2 Simultaneous Deficiency of the Heart and Spleen (Heart 5, Spleen -6), 15.5 Yang Deficiency of the Spleen and Kidneys (Spleen -8, Kidneys -8), 15.8 Disharmony between the Liver and Spleen (Liver -7, Spleen -6), 15.9 Disharmony between the Liver and Stomach (Liver -7, Stomach -6)

Chronic gastritis: 8.1 Stomach Yin Deficiency (Stomach 7)

Chronic glometrulonephritis: 11.2 Kidneys Yin Deficiency (Kidneys 7), 15.5 Yang Deficiency of the Spleen and Kidneys (Spleen -8, Kidneys -8)

Chronic hepatitis: 9.3 Liver Blood Deficiency (Liver 5), 15.7 Yin Deficiency of the Liver and Kidneys (Liver 7, Kidneys 7), 15.8 Disharmony between the Liver and Spleen (Liver -7, Spleen -6)

Chronic infectious hepatitis: 9.1 Liver Energy Congestion (Liver -7)

Chronic leukemia: 13.4 Heart Blood Deficiency (Heart 5)

Chronic nephritis: 7.1 Spleen Energy Deficiency (Spleen -6), 7.2 Spleen Yang Deficiency (Spleen -8), 11.1 Kidneys Yang Deficiency (Kidneys -8), 11.2 Kidneys Yin Deficiency (Kidneys 7), 15.2 Simultaneous Deficiency of the Heart and Spleen (Heart 5, Spleen -6), 15.3 Yang Deficiency of the Heart and Kidneys (Heart -8, Kidneys -8), 15.5 Yang Deficiency of the Spleen and Kidneys (Spleen -8, Kidneys -8), 15.6 Yin Deficiency of the Lungs and Kidneys (Lungs 7, Kidneys 7), 15.7 Yin Deficiency of the Liver and Kidneys (Liver 7, Kidneys 7)

Chronic nonspecific ulcerative colitis: 6.1 Large Intestine Damp Heat (L. intestine 6), 15.5 Yang Deficiency of the Spleen and Kidneys (Spleen -8, Kidneys -8)

Chronic obstructive emphysema: 5.1 Lungs Energy Deficiency (Lungs -6)

Chronic orchitis: 9.7 Cold Obstructing the Liver Meridian (Liver -8)

Chronic pancreatitis: 10.1 Gallbladder Excessive Heat (Gallbladder 7)

Chronic prostatitis: 11.1 Kidneys Yang Deficiency (Kidneys -8)

Chronic pyelonephritis: 11.2 Kidneys Yin Deficiency (Kidneys 7)

Chronic red nose: 5.7 Hot Lungs (Lungs Fire) (Lungs 8), 8.4 Hot Stomach (Stomach 7)

Chronic renal failure: 11.1 Kidneys Yang Deficiency (Kidneys -8)

Chronic tracheitis: 6.3 Large Intestine Deficiency and Slippery Diarrhea (L. intestine -6)

Chyluria: 12.1 Bladder Damp Heat (Bladder 5)

Cirrhosis: 7.1 Spleen Energy Deficiency (Spleen -6), 9.1 Liver Energy Congestion (Liver -7), 15.7 Yin Deficiency of the Liver and Kidneys (Liver 7, Kidneys 7), 15.8 Disharmony between the Liver and Spleen (Liver -7, Spleen -6)

Cirrhotic ascites: 7.1 Spleen Energy Deficiency (Spleen -6)

Circulatory failure: 13.2 Heart Yang Deficiency (Heart -8)

Climacteric melancholia: 9.1 Liver Energy Congestion (Liver -7), 15.2 Simultaneous Deficiency of the Heart and Spleen (Heart 5, Spleen -6)

Congestive cardiac failure: 15.2 Simultaneous Deficiency of the Heart and Spleen (Heart 5, Spleen -6)

Consumptive diseases: 15.7 Yin Deficiency of the Liver and Kidneys (Liver 7, Kidneys 7)

Cor pulmonale: 5.1 Lungs Energy Deficiency (Lungs -6), 5.3 Lungs under the Attack of Wind and Cold (Lungs -7), 15.3 Yang Deficiency of the Heart and Kidneys (Heart -8, Kidneys -8)

Corneal opacity: 9.2 Liver Fire Flaming Upward (Liver 8), 15.2 Simultaneous Deficiency of the Heart and Spleen (Heart 5, Spleen -6), 15.7 Yin Deficiency of the Liver and Kidneys (Liver 7, Kidneys 7)

Coronary heart disease: 13.2 Heart Yang Deficiency (Heart -8), 15.3 Yang Deficiency of the Heart and Kidneys (Heart -8, Kidneys -8)

Diabetes insipidus: 5.8 Dry Lungs (Lungs 5), 11.2 Kidneys Yin Deficiency (Kidneys 7), 11.4 Loosening of Kidneys Energy (Kidneys -6), 15.6 Yin Deficiency of the Lungs and Kidneys (Lungs 7, Kidneys 7)

Diabetes mellitus: 5.7 Hot Lungs (Lungs Fire) (Lungs 8), 8.1 Stomach Yin Deficiency (Stomach 7), 8.4 Hot Stomach (Stomach 7), 11.1 Kidneys Yang Deficiency (Kidneys -8), 11.2 Kidneys Yin Deficiency (Kidneys 7), 15.6 Yin Deficiency of the Lungs and Kidneys (Lungs 7, Kidneys 7)

Diphtheria: 5.2 Lungs Yin Deficiency (Lungs 7), 5.7 Hot Lungs (Lungs Fire) (Lungs 8), 8.4 Hot Stomach (Stomach 7), 13.2 Heart Yang Deficiency (Heart -8), 13.3 Heart Yin Deficiency (Heart 7)

Diphtheritis: 5.7 Hot Lungs (Lungs Fire), (Lungs 8)

Disorder of testes and epididymis: 9.7 Cold Obstructing the Liver Meridian (Liver -8)

Dysentery: 6.1 Large Intestine Damp Heat (L. intestine 6), 15.5 Yang Deficiency of the Spleen and Kidneys (Spleen -8, Kidneys -8)

Dysfunctional uterine bleeding: 15.2 Simultaneous Deficiency of the Heart and Spleen (Heart 5, Spleen -6)

Dysphagia: 8.1 Stomach Yin Deficiency (Stomach 7)

Eclampsia: 9.4 Liver Yin Deficiency (Liver 7), 9.5 Liver Yang Upsurging (Liver 7), 9.6 Internal Liver Wind Blowing (Liver 6)

Eczema: 7.6 Damp Heat Steaming the Spleen (Spleen 6)

Edema of pregnancy: 7.1 Spleen Energy Deficiency (Spleen -6)

Emphysema: 5.3 Lungs under the Attack of Wind and Cold (Lungs -7), 11.5 Kidneys Unable to Absorb Inspiration (Kidneys -7), 15.6 Yin Deficiency of the Lungs and Kidneys (Lungs 7, Kidneys 7)

Encephalitis B: 9.4 Liver Yin Deficiency (Liver 7)

Endocrine disturbances: 11.1 Kidneys Yang Deficiency (Kidneys -8)

Enterocele: 14.2 Small Intestine Energy Congestion (S. intestine -7)

Enteroncus (tumor of the intestine): 6.2 Large Intestine Fluid Exhaustion (L. intestine 5)

Enterospasm: 14.2 Small Intestine Energy Congestion (S. intestine -7)

Enuresis: 9.2 Liver Fire Flaming Upward (Liver 8), 11.4 Loosening of Kidneys Energy (Kidneys -6), 12.2 Bladder Cold and Deficiency (Bladder -8)

Enuresis in children: 7.1 Spleen Energy Deficiency (Spleen -6)

Epidemic encephalitis: 9.4 Liver Yin Deficiency (Liver 7)

Epilepsy: 9.1 Liver Energy Congestion (Liver -7), 9.2 Liver Fire Flaming Upward (Liver 8), 13.1 Heart Energy Deficiency (Heart -6), 13.6 Phlegm Fire Disturbing the Heart (Heart 8), 15.7 Yin Deficiency of the Liver and Kidneys (Liver 7, Kidneys 7)

Erythema multiforme: 7.1 Spleen Energy Deficiency (Spleen -6), 15.9 Disharmony between the Liver and Stomach (Liver -7, Stomach -6)

Fissure of anus: 6.2 Large Intestine Fluid Exhaustion (L. intestine 5)

Flaccid paralysis: 5.7 Hot Lungs (Lungs Fire) (Lungs 8), 15.7 Yin Deficiency of the Liver and Kidneys (Liver 7, Kidneys 7)

Flu: 5.3 Lungs under the Attack of Wind and Cold (Lungs -7), 5.6 Wind and Heat Attacking the Lungs (Lungs 7), 5.8 Dry Lungs (Lungs 5)

Functional low fever: 13.3 Heart Yin Deficiency (Heart 7)

Functional metrorrhagia: 7.1 Spleen Energy Deficiency (Spleen -6), 7.4 Spleen Unable to Govern Blood (Spleen -8)

Gallbladder disease: 9.4 Liver Yin Deficiency (Liver 7)

Gastroduodenal ulcer: 8.3 Cold Stomach (Stomach -8)

Gastric and duodenal bulbar ulcer: 15.9 Disharmony between the Liver and Stomach (Liver -7, Stomach -6)

Gastric neurosis: 8.1 Stomach Yin Deficiency (Stomach 7), 8.3 Cold Stomach (Stomach -8)

Gastric ulcer: 7.2 Spleen Yang Deficiency (Spleen -8)

Gastroduodenal ulcer: 8.4 Hot Stomach (Stomach 7)

Gastrointestinal neurosis: 15.9 Disharmony between the Liver and Stomach (Liver -7, Stomach -6)

Gastrointestinal spasm: 14.2 Small Intestine Energy Congestion (S. intestine -7)

Gastroptosis: 7.2 Spleen Yang Deficiency (Spleen -8), 7.3 Middle Energy Cave-in (Spleen -6)

General infection: 9.2 Liver Fire Flaming Upward (Liver 8), 13.5 Heart Fire Flaming (Heart 8)

General lupus erythematosus: 11.2 Kidneys Yin Deficiency (Kidneys 7)

Glossitis: 13.5 Heart Fire Flaming (Heart 8)

Haematuria: 9.2 Liver Fire Flaming Upward (Liver 8), 12.1 Bladder Damp Heat (Bladder 5), 13.5 Heart Fire Flaming (Heart 8)

Haemoptysis: 5.7 Hot Lungs (Lungs Fire) (Lungs 8), 11.2 Kidneys Yin Deficiency (Kidneys 7)

Heart disease: 13.2 Heart Yang Deficiency (Heart -8), 13.3 Heart Yin Deficiency (Heart 7), 13.4 Heart Blood Deficiency (Heart 5)

Hemiplegia: 9.4 Liver Yin Deficiency (Liver 7)

Hemorrhage: 13.4 Heart Blood Deficiency (Heart 5)

Hemorrhage of retina: 9.2 Liver Fire Flaming Upward (Liver 8)

Hemorrhage of upper digestive tract: 13.5 Heart Fire Flaming (Heart 8)

Hemorrhoids: 6.1 Large Intestine Damp Heat (L. intestine 6)

Hepatic cirrhosis: 7.2 Spleen Yang Deficiency (Spleen -8), 11.1 Kidneys Yang Deficiency (Kidneys -8), 11.2 Kidneys Yin Deficiency (Kidneys 7), 15.5 Yang Deficiency of the Spleen and Kidneys (Spleen -8, Kidneys -8)

Hepatic conjunctivitis: 5.2 Lungs Yin Deficiency (Lungs 7)

Hepatitis: 7.1 Spleen Energy Deficiency (Spleen -6)

Hernia: 7.3 Middle Energy Cave-in (Spleen -6), 14.2 Small Intestine Energy Congestion (S. intestine -7)

Herpes zoster: 9.8 Damp Heat Attacking the Liver and Gallbladder (Liver 1, Gallbladder 1)

Herpetic stomatitis: 8.4 Hot Stomach (Stomach 7)

Herpes zoster: 9.1 Liver Energy Congestion (Liver -7)

Hyperaldosteronism: 11.1 Kidneys Yang Deficiency (Kidneys -8), 15.3 Yang Deficiency of the Heart and Kidneys (Heart -8, Kidneys -8)

Hypertension: 7.1 Spleen Energy Deficiency (Spleen -6), 9.2 Liver Fire Flaming Upward (Liver 8), 9.3 Liver Blood Deficiency (Liver 5), 9.4 Liver Yin Deficiency (Liver 7), 9.5 Liver Yang Upsurging (Liver 7), 11.2 Kidneys Yin Deficiency (Kidneys 7), 15.7 Yin Deficiency of the Liver and Kidneys (Liver 7, Kidneys 7)

Hypoadrenocorticism: 11.1 Kidneys Yang Deficiency (Kidneys -8)

Hyperthyroidism: 9.1 Liver Energy Congestion (Liver -7), 9.2 Liver Fire Flaming Upward (Liver 8), 9.4 Liver Yin Deficiency (Liver 7), 9.5 Liver Yang Upsurging (Liver 7), 9.6 Internal Liver Wind Blowing (Liver 6), 11.2 Kidneys Yin Deficiency (Kidneys 7), 13.3 Heart Yin Deficiency (Heart 7), 13.4 Heart Blood Deficiency (Heart 5), 15.1 No Communication between the Kidneys and Heart (Kidneys 7, Heart 8)

Hypothyroidism: 11.1 Kidneys Yang Deficiency (Kidneys -8), 15.3 Yang Deficiency of the Heart and Kidneys (Heart -8, Kidneys -8)

Hysteria: 9.2 Liver Fire Flaming Upward (Liver 8), 15.2 Simultaneous Deficiency of the Heart and Spleen (Heart 5, Spleen -6)

Hysteroptosis: 7.3 Middle Energy Cave-in (Spleen -6)

Incarcerated hernia at early stage: 14.2 Small Intestine Energy Congestion (S. intestine -7)

Infectious hepatitis: 9.4 Liver Yin Deficiency (Liver 7)

Infertility: 11.3 Insufficient Kidneys Essence (Kidneys 7)

Inflammation of auricular cartilage: 9.2 Liver Fire Flaming Upward (Liver 8)

Innate malnutrition in children: 11.3 Insufficient Kidneys Essence (Kidneys 7)

Insanity: 13.6 Phlegm Fire Disturbing the Heart (Heart 8)

Insomnia: 15.1 No Communication between the Kidneys and Heart (Kidneys 7, Heart 8), 15.2

Simultaneous Deficiency of the Heart and Spleen (Heart 5, Spleen -6)

Intercostal neuritis: 9.2 Liver Fire Flaming Upward (Liver 8)

Intestinal typhoid fever: 9.5 Liver Yang Upsurging (Liver 7)

Iridocyclitis: 9.2 Liver Fire Flaming Upward (Liver 8), 15.7 Yin Deficiency of the Liver and Kidneys (Liver 7, Kidneys 7)

Jaundice: 9.8 Damp Heat Attacking the Liver and Gallbladder (Liver 1, Gallbladder 1), 10.1 Gallbladder Excessive Heat (Gallbladder 7)

Keratitis: 9.2 Liver Fire Flaming Upward (Liver 8)

Laryngitis: 5.2 Lungs Yin Deficiency (Lungs 7)

Liver cancer: 7.1 Spleen Energy Deficiency (Spleen -6)

Lung cancer: 5.2 Lungs Yin Deficiency (Lungs 7), 15.6 Yin Deficiency of the Lungs and Kidneys (Lungs 7, Kidneys 7)

Lymph gland tuberculosis of neck: 9.1 Liver Energy Congestion (Liver -7)

Mastitis: 8.4 Hot Stomach (Stomach 7), 9.1 Liver Energy Congestion (Liver -7)

Mastofibroma: 9.1 Liver Energy Congestion (Liver -7)

Measles: 5.7 Hot Lungs (Lungs Fire) (Lungs 8)

Ménière's disease: 9.4 Liver Yin Deficiency (Liver 7), 9.6 Internal Liver Wind Blowing (Liver 6)

Menopause: 9.1 Liver Energy Congestion (Liver -7), 9.4 Liver Yin Deficiency (Liver 7), 9.5 Liver

Yang Upsurging (Liver 7), 11.1 Kidneys Yang Deficiency (Kidneys -8), 11.2 Kidneys Yin Deficiency (Kidneys 7), 15.1 No Communication between the Kidneys and Heart (Kidneys 7, Heart 8), 15.5 Yang Deficiency of the Spleen and Kidneys (Spleen -8, Kidneys -8), 15.7 Yin Deficiency of the Liver and Kidneys (Liver 7, Kidneys 7)

Menoxenia: 7.1 Spleen Energy Deficiency (Spleen -6), 15.7 Yin Deficiency of the Liver and Kidneys (Liver 7, Kidneys 7)

Mental illness: 13.4 Heart Blood Deficiency (Heart 5)

Muguet: 8.1 Stomach Yin Deficiency (Stomach 7), 13.5 Heart Fire Flaming (Heart 8)

Multiple neuritis: 5.8 Dry Lungs (Lungs 5)

Muscular atrophy: 5.2 Lungs Yin Deficiency (Lungs 7), 5.7 Hot Lungs (Lungs Fire) (Lungs 8)

Myocarditis: 13.2 Heart Yang Deficiency (Heart -8), 13.3 Heart Yin Deficiency (Heart 7), 15.3 Yang Deficiency of the Heart and Kidneys (Heart -8, Kidneys -8)

Myopia: 13.1 Heart Energy Deficiency (Heart -6)

Nasal sinusitis: 5.3 Lungs under the Attack of Wind and Cold (Lungs -7), 5.7 Hot Lungs (Lungs Fire) (Lungs 8)

Nasopharyngeal cancer: 15.6 Yin Deficiency of the Lungs and Kidneys (Lungs 7, Kidneys 7)

Nephritis: 7.1 Spleen Energy Deficiency (Spleen -6)

Nephroptosis: 7.3 Middle Energy Cave-in (Spleen -6)

Nephrotic syndrome: 11.1 Kidneys Yang Deficiency (Kidneys -8), 15.3 Yang Deficiency of the Heart and Kidneys (Heart -8, Kidneys -8)

Nervous vomiting: 15.9 Disharmony between the Liver and Stomach (Liver -7, Stomach -6)

Neurasthenia: 9.3 Liver Blood Deficiency (Liver 5), 10.2 Gallbladder Energy Deficiency (Gallbladder -6), 11.1 Kidneys Yang Deficiency (Kidneys -8), 11.2 Kidneys Yin Deficiency (Kidneys 7), 11.4 Loosening of Kidneys Energy (Kidneys -6), 13.1 Heart Energy Deficiency (Heart -6), 15.2 Simultaneous Deficiency of the Heart and Spleen (Heart 5, Spleen -6)

Neurosis: 9.1 Liver Energy Congestion (Liver -7), 9.2 Liver Fire Flaming Upward (Liver 8), 11.1 Kidneys Yang Deficiency (Kidneys -8), 13.1 Heart Energy Deficiency (Heart -6), 13.2 Heart Yang Deficiency (Heart -8), 13.3 Heart Yin Deficiency (Heart 7), 13.4 Heart Blood Deficiency (Heart 5), 13.5 Heart Fire Flaming (Heart 8), 13.6 Phlegm Fire Disturbing the Heart (Heart 8), 15.1 No Communication between the Kidneys and Heart (Kidneys 7, Heart 8), 15.2 Simultaneous Deficiency of the Heart and Spleen (Heart 5, Spleen -6), 15.7 Yin Deficiency of the Liver and Kidneys (Liver 7, Kidneys 7)

Neurosis in children: 9.6 Internal Liver Wind Blowing (Liver 6), 9.4 Liver Yin Deficiency (Liver 7)

Nocturia: 11.4 Loosening of Kidneys Energy (Kidneys -6)

Nonjaundice type viral hepatitis: 9.1 Liver Energy Congestion (Liver -7)

Optic nerve disease: 15.7 Yin Deficiency of the Liver and Kidneys (Liver 7, Kidneys 7)

Optic neuritis: 9.4 Liver Yin Deficiency (Liver 7), 9.6 Internal Liver Wind Blowing (Liver 6)

Otitis media: 7.1 Spleen Energy Deficiency (Spleen -6), 10.1 Gallbladder Excessive Heat (Gallbladder 7)

Otogenic vertigo: 9.4 Liver Yin Deficiency (Liver 7), 9.5 Liver Yang Upsurging (Liver 7), 9.6 Internal Liver Wind Blowing (Liver 6), 11.1 Kidneys Yang Deficiency (Kidneys -8), 11.2 Kidneys Yin Deficiency (Kidneys 7)

Papillary fibroma of lactiferous tubule: 9.2 Liver Fire Flaming Upward (Liver 8)

Paroxysmal tachycardia: 13.3 Heart Yin Deficiency (Heart 7)

Pelade: 9.1 Liver Energy Congestion (Liver -7)

Peptic ulcer: 7.2 Spleen Yang Deficiency (Spleen -8), 8.1 Stomach Yin Deficiency (Stomach 7)

Perianal rectal abscess: 6.2 Large Intestine Fluid Exhaustion (L. intestine 5)

Periodonitis: 8.4 Hot Stomach (Stomach 7)

Pertussis (whooping cough): 5.2 Lungs Yin Deficiency (Lungs 7), 15.4 Energy Deficiency of the Spleen and Lungs (Spleen -6, Lungs -6), 5.5 Phlegm Dampness Obstructing the Lungs (Lungs -5)

Pharyngitis: 5.2 Lungs Yin Deficiency (Lungs 7)

Phrenospasm: 8.1 Stomach Yin Deficiency (Stomach 7), 8.3 Cold Stomach (Stomach -8), 8.4 Hot Stomach (Stomach 7), 9.2 Liver Fire Flaming Upward (Liver 8)

Pneumonectasis: 5.5 Phlegm Dampness Obstructing the Lungs (Lungs -5)

Pneumonia: 5.3 Lungs under the Attack of Wind and Cold (Lungs -7), 5.5 Phlegm Dampness Obstructing the Lungs (Lungs -5), 5.6 Wind and Heat Attacking the Lungs (Lungs 7), 5.7 Hot Lungs (Lungs Fire) (Lungs 8), 5.8 Dry Lungs (Lungs 5), 15.10 Liver Fire Offending the Lungs (Liver 8, Lungs 7)

Polyneuritis: 5.1 Lungs Energy Deficiency (Lungs -6), 5.7 Hot Lungs (Lungs Fire) (Lungs 8)

Preeclampsia: 9.4 Liver Yin Deficiency (Liver 7), 9.5 Liver Yang Upsurging (Liver 7), 9.6 Internal Liver Wind Blowing (Liver 6)

Primary glaucoma: 7.1 Spleen Energy Deficiency (Spleen -6), 9.2 Liver Fire Flaming Upward (Liver 8), 9.2 Liver Fire Flaming Upward (Liver 8), 9.5 Liver Yang Upsurging (Liver 7), 11.2 Kidneys Yin Deficiency (Kidneys 7), 15.8 Disharmony between the Liver and Spleen (Liver -7, Spleen -6)

Prolapse of gastric mucosa: 8.3 Cold Stomach (Stomach -8)

Prostatic hyperplasia: 12.2 Bladder Cold and Deficiency (Bladder -8)

Prostatitis: 7.3 Middle Energy Cave-in (Spleen -6), 11.2 Kidneys Yin Deficiency (Kidneys 7), 11.4 Loosening of Kidneys Energy (Kidneys -6), 12.1 Bladder Damp Heat (Bladder 5), 15.1 No Communication between the Kidneys and Heart (Kidneys 7, Heart 8), 15.5 Yang Deficiency of the Spleen and Kidneys (Spleen -8, Kidneys -8)

Ptosis: 7.1 Spleen Energy Deficiency (Spleen -6), 7.3 Middle Energy Cave-in (Spleen -6)

Pudendal eczema: 9.8 Damp Heat Attacking the Liver and Gallbladder (Liver 1, Gallbladder 1)

Pulmonary abscess: 5.6 Wind and Heat Attacking the Lungs (Lungs 7), 5.7 Hot Lungs (Lungs Fire) (Lungs 8)

Pulmonary abscess at later stage: 5.2 Lungs Yin Deficiency (Lungs 7)

Pulmonary emphysema: 15.4 Energy Deficiency of the Spleen and Lungs (Spleen -6, Lungs -6)

Pulmonary fibrosis: 5.2 Lungs Yin Deficiency (Lungs 7)

Pulmonary tuberculosis: 5.1 Lungs Energy Deficiency (Lungs -6), 5.2 Lungs Yin Deficiency (Lungs 7), 15.10 Liver Fire Offending the Lungs (Liver 8, Lungs 7), 15.4 Energy Deficiency of the Spleen and Lungs (Spleen -6, Lungs -6), 15.5 Yang Deficiency of the Spleen and Kidneys (Spleen -8, Kidneys -8), 15.6 Yin Deficiency of the Lungs and

Kidneys (Lungs 7, Kidneys 7), 15.7 Yin Deficiency of the Liver and Kidneys (Liver 7, Kidneys 7)

Purpura hemorrhagica: 7.4 Spleen Unable to Govern Blood (Spleen -8)

Purulent otitis media: 9.8 Damp Heat Attacking the Liver and Gallbladder (Liver 1, Gallbladder 1)

Pustule: 7.6 Damp Heat Steaming the Spleen (Spleen 6)

Pyelonephritis: 12.1 Bladder Damp Heat (Bladder 5)

Pyloric spasm and obstruction: 15.9 Disharmony between the Liver and Stomach (Liver -7, Stomach -6)

Recurrent canker sores: 8.2 Food Stagnation in Stomach (Stomach -7), 13.5 Heart Fire Flaming (Heart 8), 15.1 No Communication between the Kidneys and Heart (Kidneys 7, Heart 8)

Recurrent common cold: 5.1 Lungs Energy Deficiency (Lungs -6)

Retinopathy: 9.1 Liver Energy Congestion (Liver -7), 15.7 Yin Deficiency of the Liver and Kidneys (Liver 7, Kidneys 7)

Rheumatic cardiopathy: 15.3 Yang Deficiency of the Heart and Kidneys (Heart -8, Kidneys -8)

Rheumatoid cardiopathy: 11.1 Kidneys Yang Deficiency (Kidneys -8), 13.2 Heart Yang Deficiency (Heart -8), 13.3 Heart Yin Deficiency (Heart 7), 15.2 Simultaneous Deficiency of the Heart and Spleen (Heart 5, Spleen -6)

Rhinitis: 5.7 Hot Lungs (Lungs Fire), (Lungs 8), 10.1 Gallbladder Excessive Heat (Gallbladder 7)

Rickets: 11.3 Insufficient Kidneys Essence (Kidneys 7)

Schistosomial liver disease: 15.8 Disharmony between the Liver and Spleen (Liver -7, Spleen -6)

Schistosomiasis: 15.8 Disharmony between the Liver and Spleen (Liver -7, Spleen -6)

Schizophrenia: 13.5 Heart Fire Flaming (Heart 8), 13.6 Phlegm Fire Disturbing the Heart (Heart 8)

Scleritis: 5.7 Hot Lungs (Lungs Fire) (Lungs 8)

Senile cataract: 9.5 Liver Yang Upsurging (Liver 7), 15.7 Yin Deficiency of the Liver and Kidneys (Liver 7, Kidneys 7)

Senile dementia: 11.3 Insufficient Kidneys Essence (Kidneys 7)

Senile prostatic hyperplasia: 11.4 Loosening of Kidneys Energy (Kidneys -6)

Sexual neurasthenia: 11.1 Kidneys Yang Deficiency (Kidneys -8)

Simple goiter: 9.1 Liver Energy Congestion (Liver -7), 9.2 Liver Fire Flaming Upward (Liver 8), 9.4 Liver Yin Deficiency (Liver 7), 9.6 Internal Liver Wind Blowing (Liver 6)

Stomach cancer: 15.9 Disharmony between the Liver and Stomach (Liver -7, Stomach -6)

Stomatitis: 8.4 Hot Stomach (Stomach 7)

Stroke: 13.6 Phlegm Fire Disturbing the Heart (Heart 8)

Sty: 8.4 Hot Stomach (Stomach 7)

Summer fever in children: 5.7 Hot Lungs (Lungs 8), 8.4 Hot Stomach (Stomach 7)

Suppurative keratitis: 10.1 Gallbladder Excessive Heat (Gallbladder 7)

Tenesmus: 6.1 Large Intestine Damp Heat (L. intestine 6)

Thrombocythenia: 7.1 Spleen Energy Deficiency (Spleen -6)

Thrombocytopenia purpura: 7.1 Spleen Energy Deficiency (Spleen -6), 7.4 Spleen Unable to Govern Blood (Spleen -8), 15.2 Simultaneous Deficiency of the Heart and Spleen (Heart 5, Spleen -6)

Tinea versicolor: 7.4 Spleen Unable to Govern Blood (Spleen -8)

Tonsillitis: 5.2 Lungs Yin Deficiency (Lungs 7), 5.7 Hot Lungs (Lungs Fire) (Lungs 8), 8.4 Hot Stomach (Stomach 7), 11.2 Kidneys Yin Deficiency (Kidneys 7)

Trachoma: 5.7 Hot Lungs (Lungs Fire) (Lungs 8), 9.4 Liver Yin Deficiency (Liver 7), 9.6 Internal Liver Wind Blowing (Liver 6)

Trigeminal neuralgia: 9.5 Liver Yang Upsurging (Liver 7)

Tuberculosis: 11.2 Kidneys Yin Deficiency (Kidneys 7)

Tumors: 15.7 Yin Deficiency of the Liver and Kidneys (Liver 7, Kidneys 7)

Tympanites: 8.2 Food Stagnation in Stomach (Stomach -7), 15.5 Yang Deficiency of the Spleen and Kidneys (Spleen -8, Kidneys -8), 15.7 Yin Deficiency of the Liver and Kidneys (Liver 7, Kidneys 7)

Ulcer: 9.1 Liver Energy Congestion (Liver -7)

Ulcerative blepharitis: 8.4 Hot Stomach (Stomach 7)

Ulcerative colitis: 6.3 Large Intestine Deficiency and Slippery Diarrhea (L. intestine -6)

Upper respiratory tract infection: 5.3 Lungs under the Attack of Wind and Cold (Lungs -7)

Uremia: 15.5 Yang Deficiency of the Spleen and Kidneys (Spleen -8, Kidneys -8), 15.7 Yin Deficiency of the Liver and Kidneys (Liver 7, Kidneys 7)

Urethritis: 12.1 Bladder Damp Heat (Bladder 5)

Urinary calculus: 12.1 Bladder Damp Heat (Bladder 5)

Urinary infection: 12.1 Bladder Damp Heat (Bladder 5)

Urodialysis: 12.1 Bladder Damp Heat (Bladder 5)

Vaginitis: 9.8 Damp Heat Attacking the Liver and Gallbladder (Liver 1, Gallbladder 1)

Vernal conjunctivitis: 5.7 Hot Lungs (Lungs Fire) (Lungs 8)

Vertigo: 9.4 Liver Yin Deficiency (Liver 7), 9.5 Liver Yang Upsurging (Liver 7), 9.6 Internal Liver Wind Blowing (Liver 6)

Viral hepatitis: 7.5 Cold Dampness Troubling the Spleen (Spleen -7), 15.7 Yin Deficiency of the Liver and Kidneys (Liver 7, Kidneys 7), 15.8 Disharmony between the Liver and Spleen (Liver -7, Spleen -6), 15.9 Disharmony between the Liver and Stomach (Liver -7, Stomach -6)

Viral myocarditis: 15.3 Yang Deficiency of the Heart and Kidneys (Heart -8, Kidneys -8)

Zona: 9.2 Liver Fire Flaming Upward (Liver 8)

Part II

THE SYNDROMES

5

Choosing Foods and Herbs to Boost the Lungs and Cure Applicable Symptoms and Diseases

What follow are the different categories used to describe each syndrome.

Definition of the Syndrome. Here, a definition is given to shed light on the meaning and the possible causes of this particular syndrome.

Clinical Signs and Symptoms. In this section, signs and symptoms are listed under three headings: major signs, indicating that the signs listed are among the most important ones for the particular syndrome; median signs, showing that the signs listed are secondary ones for the syndrome; and minor signs, showing that the signs listed are supporting ones for the syndrome.

Applicable Western Diseases. Western diseases that may be due to this particular syndrome are listed here.

Treatment Symptoms. The symptoms that are frequently dealt with by treating the syndrome are listed in this category. In other words, in many cases the symptoms listed here can be dealt with by treating the syndrome.

Clinical Cases. Clinical cases that may be due to the syndrome are presented in this section.

Treatment Principles. The treatment principles by which the syndrome is to be treated are presented here.

Foods Chosen Based on Y-Scores. In this section, foods are chosen on the basis of their y-scores. As an example, a person with Liver 8 will be better off eating any foods with y-scores between Liver 2 and Liver -8, in order for the liver to be balanced.

Generally Beneficial Foods and Other Foods to Be Chosen or Avoided. Here, the foods normally considered beneficial for the syndrome are listed along with other foods to be chosen or avoided. The concept of Chinese food cures can be understood according to different perspectives, and so the foods listed in this section are regarded as supplemental to the foods to be chosen according to their y-scores. Therefore, with the foods listed here on hand as well, you are not only able to select foods based on their y-scores but also on their actions. This way, you get the best of both worlds.

Beneficial Herbs to Be Applied One Herb at a Time. Chinese herbs that are generally considered beneficial for the particular syndrome are listed in this section, along with their pharmaceutical name and recommended dosage. You should select one herb at a time from this category.

Decoct the herb in water using a pot made of something other than iron or bronze, in order to prevent chemical changes from occurring; the Chinese generally use an earthenware pot, which is available in stores where Chinese herbs are sold. Place the herb in the pot, adding just enough cold water to cover the herb, plus an additional cup so that the water level will be a little higher than the herb. Let the herb soak in the water for about twenty minutes. Bring the water to a boil, and then reduce to low heat. The total decoction time depends upon the herb that is being decocted. When ready, the herb should be removed from the heat and strained, to obtain an herbal soup for drinking.

This process should be repeated two or three times daily using the same herb; discard the decocted herb and use a new one every day. In any cases of doubt, the herbalist who sold you the herb should be able to offer you guidance and advice.

Beneficial Herbal Formulas to Be Applied One Formula at a Time. Chinese herbal formulas that are generally considered beneficial for the particular syndrome are listed here. A formula is composed of different herbs, and each one plays a specific role in the formula.

There are four types of herbs in a typical formula: king herbs, which are intended to treat the primary symptoms; minister herbs, which support the king herbs; assistant herbs, which play two different roles, assisting the king and minister herbs and also restraining them from exceeding their limits, making sure that the formula can achieve its therapeutic results satisfactorily; and envoy herbs, which also play two different roles, directing the effects of the other herbs in the formula to reach the affected region as well as harmonizing all the herbs in the formula so that they will not be in conflict.

When you purchase the formulas, which are usually in a patent form, read the instructions on the label, as each manufacturer has specific instructions according to their manufacturing methods.

5.1 Lungs Energy Deficiency

When you are in good health, your y-score is Lungs -2; when you are ill, your y-score is Lungs -6.

Definition of the Syndrome. Because the lungs take charge of respiration, Lungs Energy Deficiency will give rise to symptoms mainly associated with respiration, such as a weak cough and weak panting. In addition, Lungs Energy Deficiency can reduce the body's power of defense against foreign invasion, making it easy to catch a cold. A celebrated Chinese physician from the past said: "Lungs Energy Deficiency means that there is a shortage in the vital energy of the lungs, so the patient may complain about windy weather when in fact there is little wind in the air, or he may complain about cold weather when the weather is not cold at all. Internally, he may display a low voice, shortness of breath, a love of lying down as if sick, a poor appetite, a weak cough, and low spirits."

The lungs are short of energy either because they are not getting sufficient nourishment from foods, they are constantly under the attack of hostile atmospheric energies, or they were weak at birth.

Clinical Signs and Symptoms. Major signs: Shortness of breath, weak breathing, cough with weak sound, low voice. Median signs: Breathing difficulty, being easily susceptible to the common cold, excessive perspiration, fatigue, aversion to wind and cold, pale complexion. Minor signs: Light wheezing, discharge of thin and watery phlegm.

Applicable Western Diseases. Bronchial asthma, chronic bronchitis, chronic diseases associated with the lungs, chronic obstructive emphysema, cor pulmonale, polyneuritis, pulmonary tuberculosis, recurrent common cold.

Treatment Symptoms. Common cold, cough, edema, chest pain, escape of urine on coughing, excessive perspiration, chronic fatigue.

Clinical Cases. (1) A fifty-three-year-old male patient with the last name of Zhang was experiencing a gradual weakening in body strength and was also losing weight. In addition, he had a recurrent cold and sore throat, an occasional cough, chest pain when the cough worsened, and a decreased appetite, and he felt fatigued generally and tended to be depressed in the afternoon. Zhang was diagnosed by a doctor of Western medicine as having upper-right tuberculoma, right tuberculous pleurisy, and laryngitis (as an aftereffect from earlier tuberculosis). On examination by a doctor of traditional Chinese medicine, he appeared skinny, with a poor complexion and in low spirits, and complained of a cough, shortness of breath, a poor appetite, and occasional night sweats; the Chinese doctor diagnosed his condition as Lungs Energy Deficiency. (2) A forty-four-year-old female patient with the last name of Ge suffered from vertigo, and she was diagnosed in Western medicine as having Ménière's disease. Ge basically recovered from the illness after treatment, although she still had profuse perspiration, an aversion to wind, and a cough, and she frequently came down with a cold. A Chinese doctor diagnosed her condition as Lungs Energy Deficiency, primarily because being easily susceptible to the common cold and having excessive perspiration are important signs of this syndrome.

Treatment Principles.   To tone the lungs, benefit energy, and solidify the superficial region.

Foods Chosen Based on Y-Scores.   Chicken egg white (Lungs -2), fishy vegetable (Lungs 0), leaf or brown mustard (Lungs 6), millet (Lungs 2), pork lung (Lungs 2), pumpkin (Lungs 0), rosemary (Lungs 6), royal jelly (Lungs 2), spearmint (Lungs 5), strawberry (Lungs -2), taro leaf (Lungs 2), tobacco (Lungs 6), white fungus (Lungs 2), winter melon (Lungs -1).

Generally Beneficial Foods and Other Foods to Be Chosen or Avoided.   The foods to be chosen must be capable of increasing the energy of the lungs. Such foods are normally called "energy tonics for the lungs" and include broomcorn (L. intestine 2, Spleen 2, Stomach 2), bird's nest (Kidneys 2, Stomach 2), garlic (Spleen 6, Stomach 6), ginkgo (cooked) (Kidneys -2), ginseng (Spleen 1), goose meat (Spleen 2), grape (Kidneys 0, Spleen 0), Job's tears (Kidneys 0, Spleen 0), licorice (Spleen 2, Stomach 2), murrel (Spleen -2, Stomach -2), pork lung (Lungs 2), rock sugar (Spleen 2), sweet rice (Stomach 4), Western ginseng (Stomach -3), whitefish (Liver 2, Stomach 2), and yam (Kidneys 2, Spleen 2).

Beneficial Herbs to Be Applied One Herb at a Time.   Dang shen

(Radix Codonopsis Pilosulae), 15 g; gan cao (Radix Glycyrrhizae), 11 g; huang qi (Radix Astragali Seu Hedysari), 40 g; shan yao (Rhizoma Dioscoreae), 20 g; wu wei zi (Fructus Schisandrae), 4 g.

Beneficial Herbal Formulas to Be Applied One Formula at a Time. Bu Fei Tang, Bu Zhong Yi Qi Tang, Liu Jun Zi Tang, Yu Ping Feng San.

5.2 Lungs Yin Deficiency (Deficient and Hot Lungs)

When you are in good health, your y-score is Lungs 3; when you are ill, your y-score is Lungs 7.

Definition of the Syndrome. When yin deficiency affects the lungs, this can lead to Lungs Yin Deficiency. Yin deficiency gives rise to deficient fire, which burns and steams the lungs, causing the cough; but little or no phlegm is coughed up, because there is a shortage of body fluids. The lungs are burned and damaged, which accounts for the blood in the phlegm. Yin deficiency causes a dry throat, leading to the hoarseness. Deficient fire consumes yin energy in the body, and this is the reason for the skinniness.

Clinical Signs and Symptoms. Major signs: Dry cough or cough with meager phlegm, tidal fever, dry throat, coughing up blood, itchy throat, hoarseness. Median signs: Dry sensation in the mouth, light tidal fever, skinniness. Minor signs: Discharge of meager sticky phlegm, night sweats, palms of hands and soles of feet are both hot, insomnia, blood in phlegm, zygomatic regions' appearing red in the afternoon.

Applicable Western Diseases. Asthma, atelectasis, chronic bronchitis, chronic conjunctivitis, diphtheria, hepatic conjunctivitis, laryngitis, lung cancer, muscular atrophy, pertussis (whooping cough), pharyngitis, pulmonary abscess at later stage, pulmonary fibrosis, pulmonary tuberculosis, tonsillitis.

Treatment Symptoms. Cough, coughing up blood, chronic fatigue, night sweats, insomnia.

Clinical Cases. (1) A forty-year-old male patient by the name of Chen suffered a chronic cough and had asthma for a long time. He found that lying down on his back would intensify the symptoms, and he coughed frequently, coughing up only a little sticky, yellowish phlegm. A doctor of traditional Chinese medicine diagnosed his condition as Lungs Yin Deficiency. (2) One day a thirty-two-year-old male patient named Meng came down with a common cold with an itchy throat, and he coughed up a little phlegm with some blood in it. His other symptoms included an aversion to wind, a fever, pain in the chest, a poor appetite, and a red tongue. A Chinese doctor diagnosed his condition as Lungs Yin Deficiency with slight heat in the lungs. (3) A forty-year-old male patient named Jia spoke in a low, hoarse voice. The more he talked, the worse it became, with a dry throat, vomiting of bubbles, and a congested chest, all of which dragged on for eight months. A Chinese doctor diagnosed his condition as Lungs Yin Deficiency, primarily because hoarseness and a dry throat are major signs of this syndrome.

Treatment Principles. To water the yin and lubricate the lungs.

Foods Chosen Based on Y-Scores. Chicken egg white (Lungs -2), fishy vegetable (Lungs 0), laver (Lungs -5), millet (Lungs 2), pork lung (Lungs 2), pumpkin (Lungs 0), strawberry (Lungs -2), taro leaf (Lungs 2), white fungus (Lungs 2), winter melon (Lungs -1).

Generally Beneficial Foods and Other Foods to Be Chosen or Avoided. 1. Foods that are considered generally good for this syndrome are abalone, air bladder of shark, apple, asparagus, cuttlefish, duck egg, oyster, pork, royal jelly, and sweet rice. 2. Choose from these yin tonics: abalone, air bladder of shark, apple, apricot pit (sweet powder), asparagus (lucid), bean drink, bird's nest, bitter gourd (balsam pear), black-eyed pea, brown sugar, cantaloupe (muskmelon), cheeses, chicken egg, chicken eggshell (inner membrane), clam (freshwater or saltwater), coconut milk, crab, cuttlefish, date, duck, duck egg, fig, frog (river or pond), fungus (white), goose meat, grape, green turtle, honey, kidney bean, kumquat, lard, lemon, litchi nut, loquat, lotus rhizome, maltose, mandarin orange, mango, milk (cow's), mussel, oyster, pea, pear, pineapple, pomegranate (sweet fruit), pork, rabbit, red bayberry, rice (polished), royal jelly, sea cucumber, shrimp, star fruit (carambola), string bean, sugarcane, tofu (bean curd), tomato, turtle egg, walnut, watermelon, white sugar, whitebait, and yam. 3. Foods to be avoided in cases of fire deficiency are garlic, Japanese cassia bark, litchi nut, prickly ash, star anise, and walnut. 4. Foods and drinks to be avoided in cases of deficiency heat are alcohol, cayenne pepper, Chinese chive, eel, and fresh ginger.

Beneficial Herbs to Be Applied One Herb at a Time. Bai he (Bulbus Lilii), 11 g; bai mu er (Tremella), 10 g; bei sha shen (Radix Glehniae), 11 g; E jiao (Colla Corii Asini [Gelatina Nigra]), 11 g;

mai men dong (Radix Ophiopogonis), 11 g; shu di huang (Radix Rehmanniae), cooked, 18 g; tian dong (Radix Asparagi), 14 g; wu wei zi (Fructus Schisandrae), 4 g; yu zhu (Rhizoma Polygonati Odorati), 11 g.

Beneficial Herbal Formulas to Be Applied One Formula at a Time. Bai He Gu Jin Tang, Ma Xing Shi Gan Tang, Qing Zao Jiu Fei Tang, Sha Shen Mai Dong Tang.

5.3 Lungs under the Attack of Wind and Cold

When you are in good health, your y-score is Lungs -3; when you are ill, your y-score is Lungs -7.

Definition of the Syndrome. This syndrome is due to the attack of external wind and cold that restricts the energy of the lungs and prevents the lungs from expanding. Wind and cold have penetrated through the skin, restricting the lungs, which accounts for the cough. The nose is the outlet of the lungs, and the throat is the door to the lungs. The lungs are unable to expand and push downward, causing the nasal congestion and discharge as well as the itch in the throat. The pathogen attacks the defense energy, and this is the reason for the aversion to the cold. A struggle has occurred between the pathogen and the body's energy, which is why there is the slight fever. The attack of wind and cold is the cause of the superficial and tight pulse.

Clinical Signs and Symptoms. Major signs: Cough, aversion to the cold, coughing up thin, white phlegm. Median signs: Fever, nasal congestion, nasal discharge, itch in the throat, thin and whitish phlegm. Minor signs: Cough with heavy and unclear sounds, panting, absence of perspiration, congested chest, whitish coating on the tongue.

Applicable Western Diseases and Conditions. Acute bronchitis, bronchiectasis (bronchodilatation), chronic bronchitis, cor pulmonale, emphysema of the lungs, flu, nasal congestion, nasal sinusitis, pneumonia, upper respiratory tract infection.

Treatment Symptoms. Common cold, cough, loss of voice, itch in the throat, nasal congestion with nasal discharge.

Clinical Cases. (1) Under an attack of trachitis, a forty-three-year-old male patient named Huang was coughing up whitish phlegm. He had come down with a cold two days earlier, with nasal congestion and discharge, fever without perspiration, headache, coughing, shortness of breath, pain all over the body, and a thin, whitish coating on the tongue. A doctor of traditional Chinese medicine diagnosed his condition as Lungs under the Attack of Wind and Cold, primarily because a common cold at an early stage before profuse perspiration occurs is generally due to this syndrome. (2) A male student, age seventeen, Gao had a cold that lasted for more than ten days. He experienced alternating chills and fever, headaches, nasal congestion, and coughing up sticky phlegm. A Chinese doctor diagnosed his condition as Lungs under the Attack of Wind and Cold, mainly because a common cold at an early stage is generally due to this syndrome. (3) Li, a thirty-five-year-old female patient, had suffered from asthma for ten years, and it had attacked her mostly in winter. Recently, she had a cold that triggered the old symptoms: a fear of the cold and an aversion to being chilled, a fever, coughing up whitish bubbles of phlegm, a lack of thirst, a poor appetite, a pale tongue with a whitish and slippery coating, and coughing and panting that made it difficult for her to lie on her back. A Chinese doctor diagnosed her condition as Lungs under the Attack of Wind and Cold, especially because its symptoms are triggered by the common cold with many signs of this syndrome.

Treatment Principles. To disperse wind and cold, expand the lungs, and relieve the cough.

Foods Chosen Based on Y-Scores. Chicken egg white (Lungs -2), fishy vegetable (Lungs 0), leaf or brown mustard (Lungs 6), millet (Lungs 2), pork lung (Lungs 2), pumpkin (Lungs 0), rosemary (Lungs 6), royal jelly (Lungs 2), spearmint (Lungs 5), strawberry (Lungs -2), taro leaf (Lungs 2), tobacco (Lungs 6), white fungus (Lungs 2), winter melon (Lungs -1).

Generally Beneficial Foods and Other Foods to Be Chosen or Avoided. 1. Foods that are normally good for this syndrome are almond, asparagus, cayenne pepper, common button mushroom, fennel, fresh ginger, leaf or brown mustard, mustard seed, peppermint and peppermint oil, prickly ash leaf, rock sugar, spearmint, star anise, sweet basil, tangerine, and walnut. 2. Choose from these foods that can disperse wind: buckwheat, caper, carp (grass), cassia bark (Japanese), celery, chive (Chinese leek), chrysanthemum, coconut meat, green-onion leaf, jellyfish skin, lotus flower, peppermint and peppermint oil, rosin, soybean (black), spearmint, spinach seed, strawberry plant, and sunflower (top of peduncle).

Beneficial Herbs to Be Applied One Herb at a Time. Gan cao (Radix Glycyrrhizae), 11 g; gui zhi (Ramulus Cinnamomi), 10 g; jie geng (Radix Platycodi), 5 g; ma huang (Herba Ephedrae), 10 g; xing ren (Semen Armeniacae Amarae), 11 g; zi su ye (Folium Perillae), 10 g.

Beneficial Herbal Formulas to Be Applied One Formula at a Time. Hua Gai San, Jing Fang Bai Du San, Xing Su San, Zhi Sou San.

5.4 Deficient and Cold Lungs (Lungs Yang Deficiency)

When you are in good health, your y-score is Lungs -4; when you are ill, your y-score is Lungs -8.

Definition of the Syndrome. When the lungs are deficient and also under the attack of external cold energy, Deficient and Cold Lungs will occur as a consequence. The cold takes a heavy toll on yang energy, resulting in a shortage of yang energy in the lungs, which is why this syndrome is also called Lungs Yang Deficiency.

Clinical Signs and Symptoms. Major signs: Acute attack of coughing and panting, cold limbs, discharge of thin and white phlegm, plentiful saliva. Median signs: Absence of thirst, clear nasal discharge, cold sensations in the chest and back, discharge of watery phlegm that is difficult to cough up. Minor signs: Aversion to being chilled, inability to lie on back, white complexion, congested chest.

Applicable Western Diseases. Bronchial asthma, bronchiectasis (bronchodilatation).

Treatment Symptoms. Discharge of copious, thin, whitish phlegm.

Clinical Cases. A seventy-year-old male patient named Huang had previously displayed the following symptoms: fear of being chilled, dizziness, coughing up phlegm, and vomiting of bubbles. A month later, he reported a severe cough, coughing up sticky phlegm, shortness of breath on labor, palpitations, poor sleep, slight puffiness in the face and the feet, soft stools, a clear stream of urine, and a whitish coating on the tongue. A doctor of traditional Chinese medicine diagnosed his condition as Deficient and Cold Lungs mainly because of his fear of being chilled and other symptoms of this syndrome.

Treatment Principles. To warm the lungs and disperse cold, to relieve the cough and shortness of breath.

Foods Chosen Based on Y-Scores. Chicken egg white (Lungs -2), fishy vegetable (Lungs 0), leaf or brown mustard (Lungs 6), millet (Lungs 2), pork lung (Lungs 2), pumpkin (Lungs 0), rosemary (Lungs 6), royal jelly (Lungs 2), spearmint (Lungs 5), strawberry (Lungs -2), taro leaf (Lungs 2), white fungus (Lungs 2), winter melon (Lungs -1).

Beneficial Foods and Foods to Be Chosen or Avoided. 1. Choose from these tonic foods for the lungs: air bladder of shark, cheeses, garlic, ginkgo (cooked), ginseng (Western), Job's tears, milk (cow's), pork lung, pork pancreas, rice (glutinous or sweet), walnut, whitebait, and yam. 2. Choose from the following warm foods: blood clam, caper, caraway seed, cassia bark and fruit (Japanese), chicken, chili-pepper leaf, chili rhizome, chive (Chinese), chive root and bulb (Chinese), chive seed (Chinese), cinnamon twig, clove, date, dill seed, fennel seed, fenugreek seed (Oriental), fresh ginger, green onion (white head), mustard (white or yellow), mustard seed (white or yellow), nutmeg, pepper (black or white), prickly ash, rice (polished, long-grain), shallot (aromatic green onion), small garlic, sorghum, star anise, sword bean (jack bean), and water chestnut. 3. Avoid these cold foods: adzuki bean, aloe vera, asparagus (lucid), bamboo shoots, banana, bitter endive, bitter gourd (balsam pear), brake (fern), burdock, camphor mint, cattail, crab, endive (Chinese), fig, frog (pond), grapefruit, hair vegetable, honey, leaf beet (spinach beet, Swiss chard), lemon, lily flower, mung bean (including powder and sprouts), orchid leaf, peppermint, potato (Irish), preserved duck egg, pricking amaranth (amaranth, pigweed), purslane, rabbit, rambutan, romaine lettuce, Russian olive (oleaster), safflower fruit, salt, soybean paste, squash, star fruit (carambola), strawberry (Indian or mock), sweet basil, tofu, water spinach, wax gourd (Chinese), and wheat.

Beneficial Herbs to Be Applied One Herb at a Time. Ren shen (Radix Ginseng), 10 g; huang qi (Radix Asragali), 25 g; ban xia (Rhzioma Pinelliae), 10 g; chen pi (Pericarpium Citri Reticulatae), 6 g.

Beneficial Herbal Formulas to Be Applied One Formula at a Time. Bu Fei Tang, Ling Gui Zhu Gan Tang, Xiao Qing Long Tang.

5.5 *Phlegm Dampness Obstructing the Lungs*

When you are in good health, your y-score is Lungs -1; when you are ill, your y-score is Lungs -5.

Definition of the Syndrome. Phlegm dampness refers to phlegm that is copious, whitish, and easily coughed up. Phlegm dampness obstructs the lungs and forces the energy of the lungs to upsurge, which accounts for the coughing up of the copious phlegm. It also obstructs the chest, causing a breakdown in the upward and downward functions of the lungs; this is the reason for the congested chest and the sound of phlegm in the throat.

Clinical Signs and Symptoms. Major signs: Coughing up copious and whitish phlegm easily, panting, congested chest, inability to lie on back, sound of phlegm in the throat. Median signs: Acute panting with high-pitched sound, rapid expiration, phlegm rumbling in the throat. Minor signs: Inability to lie on back, chest pain, congested chest, poor appetite, heavy sensation in the body, thin and watery stools.

Applicable Western Diseases. Asthma, bronchial asthma, bronchitis, pertussis (whooping cough), pneumonectasis (emphysema, pulmonary emphysema), pneumonia.

Treatment Symptoms. Coughing up copious and watery phlegm, chest pain.

Clinical Cases. (1) Feng, a fifty-year-old male patient, had developed a cough a year before, and he is still suffering from it. He is vomiting bubbles of phlegm, the sound of water can be heard from his chest when he coughs, and his tongue shows a thick, greasy coating. A doctor of traditional Chinese medicine diagnosed his condition as Phlegm Dampness Obstructing the Lungs. (2) A forty-year-old male patient named Shu had a cough and was panting and coughing up copious, watery phlegm. He felt congested in the chest, and it was difficult for him to lie down, especially on his back. Shu was diagnosed by a Western physician as having pulmonary emphysema; a Chinese doctor diagnosed his condition as Phlegm Dampness Obstructing the Lungs.

Treatment Principles. To transform the phlegm, make the dampness flow, relieve the cough, sedate the lungs, and expel the phlegm.

Foods Chosen Based on Y-Scores. Chicken egg white (Lungs -2), fishy vegetable (Lungs 0), leaf or brown mustard (Lungs 6), millet (Lungs 2), pork lung (Lungs 2), pumpkin (Lungs 0), rosemary (Lungs 6), royal jelly (Lungs 2), spearmint (Lungs 5), strawberry (Lungs -2), taro leaf (Lungs 2), white fungus (Lungs 2), winter melon (Lungs -1).

Generally Beneficial Foods and Other Foods to Be Chosen or Avoided. 1. Choose from these foods that eliminate damp phlegm: adzuki bean, ambergris, asparagus, bamboo shoots, barley, common carp, crown daisy, cucumber, date, fresh ginger, leaf or brown mustard, mustard seed (white or yellow), mung bean, pear, pepper (black or white), seaweed, shepherd's purse, and star fruit. 2. Avoid these foods: bird's nest, brown sugar, green turtle meat, honey, lard, loquat, maltose, pork, red bayberry, sugarcane, white eel, and white sugar. 3. Avoid mandarin orange in cases of cold phlegm and foods that are likely to trigger chronic asthma or intensify an existing attack, such as eggs, fish, milk, and shrimp.

Beneficial Herbs to Be Applied One Herb at a Time. Bai jie zi (Semen Sinapis Albae), 11 g; ban xia (Rhizoma Pinelliae), 12 g; cang zhu (Rhizoma Atractylodis), 11 g; chen pi (Pericarpium Citri Reticulatae), 11 g; dan nan xing (Arisaema Cum Bile), 8 g; fu ling (Poria), 14 g; lai fu zi (Semen Raphani), 11 g; ting li zi (Semen Lepidii Seu Descurainiae), 11 g; zao jia (Spina Gleditsiae), 10 g.

Beneficial Herbal Formulas to Be Applied One Formula at a Time. Er Chen Tang, Qing Fei Yin, Ting Li Da Zao Xie Fei Tang, Yue Bi Jia Zhu Tang.

5.6 *Wind and Heat Attacking the Lungs*

When you are in good health, your y-score is Lungs 3; when you are ill, your y-score is Lungs 7.

Definition of the Syndrome. Wind and heat offending the lungs means that wind and heat are invading the lungs. This is due to the attack of the external pathogens of wind and heat or the attack of the external pathogens of wind and cold gradually transforming into wind and heat. When the lungs are under the attack of wind and heat, they lose their cooling and cleaning effects, which accounts for the cough. Wind and heat team up to burn the fluids of the lungs, and this causes the yellowish, sticky phlegm. Wind and heat consume the body's fluids, which is why there is the yellowish nasal discharge. The lungs correspond to the tip of the tongue, so this accounts for the red tip.

Clinical Signs and Symptoms. Major signs: Coughing up yellowish and sticky phlegm, fever, slight aversion to being chilled, coughing with a loud sound. Median signs: Thirst with a desire to drink, pink eyes, dry mouth, nasal congestion. Minor signs: Flickering of the nostril, chest pain, pain in the body, sore throat, blood in phlegm, red tip of the tongue.

Applicable Western Diseases. Asthma, acute glomerulonehritis, acute tracheitis (trachitis), chronic bronchitis, common cold, flu, pneumonia, pulmonary abscess.

Treatment Symptoms.   Common cold, cough, coughing up blood, nosebleed, edema, sore throat, pink eyes, headache.

Clinical Cases. (1) A former soldier, Zhang, age fifty-four, suddenly experienced pain throughout his entire body overnight, with a fever, an aversion to wind and cold, and a cough. The next day, his temperature reached 40 degrees C (104 degrees F), and he was diagnosed in a Western hospital as having an upper respiratory infection. After being treated in the hospital, Zhang found that his temperature had dropped quickly to normal. But the fever started again the following evening, and he experienced a slight aversion to wind and cold, a headache, coughing up whitish phlegm, a sore and dry throat, nasal discharge, a congested chest, a poor appetite, and pain in the four extremities. Upon examination by a doctor of traditional Chinese medicine, Zhang was diagnosed as having Wind and Heat Attacking the Lungs. (2) Tending to be physically weak, Xu, a twenty-four-year-old woman, frequently came down with a cold and a cough. At a Western hospital, she was suspected of having a lung disease, and medicine was prescribed for her. She was also advised to get plenty of rest and have some chicken soup. Right after this, Xu began to experience an aversion to the cold, a fever, pain all over her body, a terrible headache, ringing in both ears, an incessant cough, nasal congestion and discharge, a dry and itchy throat, a dry cough, and hoarseness. At this point, she was diagnosed by a Chinese doctor as having Wind and Heat Attacking the Lungs. (3) A five-year-old girl named Sheng displayed a fever, a cough, panting, coughing up yellowish and sticky phlegm, a sore throat with redness, hoarseness, and a red tongue. A Chinese doctor diagnosed her condition as Wind and Heat Attacking the Lungs, primarily because a cough is a sign of a lung condition and yellowish phlegm indicates heat.

Treatment Principles. To disperse wind and heat, expand the lungs, and relax the superficial region.

Foods Chosen Based on Y-Scores. Chicken egg white (Lungs -2), fishy vegetable (Lungs 0), millet (Lungs 2), pork lung (Lungs 2), pumpkin (Lungs 0), royal jelly (Lungs 2), strawberry (Lungs -2), taro leaf (Lungs 2), white fungus (Lungs 2), winter melon (Lungs -1).

Generally Beneficial Foods and Other Foods to Be Chosen or Avoided. 1. Foods that are generally good for this syndrome are apple, apple cucumber, coriander, lemon, parsley, sweet potato, sweet rice, tofu, tomato, and white sugar. 2. Avoid irritants such as alcohol, coffee, tea, tobacco, and wine. Not only can they irritate the stomach, but they can also produce damp heat, and fire is harmful to both yin and energy. 3. Avoid these hot and spicy foods and drinks: alcohol, chili pepper (cayenne pepper), chive (Chinese), cinnamon bark (cassia), cinnamon twig, clove, coffee, garlic, ginger (fresh or dried), green onion (leaf and white head), mustard seed, nutmeg, onion, pepper (black or white), tea, and wine. Such foods force yin energy to excrete through perspiration, which is harmful to both yin and energy. 4. Choose from among these yin tonics: abalone, air bladder of shark, apple, apricot pit (sweet powder), asparagus (lucid), bean drink, bird's nest, bitter gourd (balsam pear), black-eyed pea, brown sugar, cantaloupe (muskmelon), cheeses, chicken egg, chicken eggshell (inner membrane), clam (saltwater or freshwater), coconut milk, crab, cuttlefish, date, duck, duck egg, fig, frog (river or pond), fungus (white), goose meat, grape, green turtle, honey, kidney bean, kumquat, lard, lemon, litchi nut, loquat (Japanese medlai), lotus rhizome, maltose, mandarin orange, mango, milk (cow's), mussel, oyster, pea, pear, pearl (powder), pineapple, pomegranate (sweet fruit), pork, rabbit, red bayberry, rice (polished), royal jelly, sea cucumber, shrimp, star fruit (carambola), string bean, sugarcane, tofu, tomato, turtle egg, walnut, watermelon, white sugar, whitebait, and yam. 5. Choose from the following foods and drinks that reduce heat in the lungs: agar, asparagus, asparagus (lucid), bean drink, boiled soybean drink (top layer), broad-leaved epiphythum, burdock, duck egg, epiphyllum, ginseng leaf, longevity fruit (momordica fruit), loquat leaf, olive, preserved duck egg, and Western watercress.

Beneficial Herbs to Be Applied One Herb at a Time. Gan cao (Radix Glycyrrhizae), 11 g; huang qin (Radix Scutellariae), 15 g; ma huang (Herba Ephedrae), 10 g; sang bai pi (Cortex Mori Radicis), 11 g; shi gao (Gypsum Fibrosum), 70 g; ting li zi (Semen Lepidii Seu Descurainiae), 11 g; xing ren (Semen Armeniacae Amarae), 11 g; yu xing cao (Herba Houttuyniae), 18 g; zhi mu (Rhizoma Anemarrhenae), 15 g.

Beneficial Herbal Formulas to Be Applied One Formula at a Time. Qing Re Jie Du Tang, Sang Ju Yin, Xiao Feng San, Yin Qiao San.

5.7 Hot Lungs (Lungs Fire)

When you are in good health, your y-score is Lungs 4; when you are ill, your y-score is Lungs 8.

Definition of the Syndrome. With this syndrome, there is too much heat in the lungs, or fire in the lungs in more severe cases, either due to an excessive and prolonged consumption of hot foods or to external energies of heat that are attacking the lungs.

Clinical Signs and Symptoms. Major signs: Acute onset of cough, fever, thirst, chest pain, sore throat, discharge of yellowish and sticky phlegm, flickering of the nostril. Median signs: Acute panting with high-pitched sound, rapid expiration, bitter taste in the mouth, constipation with discharge of dry stool, cough with oppressed sound, coughing up pus and blood with a fishy smell, dry sensation in the mouth. Minor signs: Hot sensation in the body, light tidal fever, nosebleed, red and swollen throat, oppressed and rapid breathing, pain in the chest, pain in the throat, pain in the throat with a dry sensation, exhaling hot air from the nose, presence of phlegm that can't be coughed up easily, mental depression.

Applicable Western Diseases and Conditions. Accessory nasal sinusitis, acute conjunctivitis, bronchial asthma, chronic bronchitis, chronic red nose, diabetes mellitus, diphtheria, diphtheritis, flaccid paralysis, haemoptysis, measles, muscular atrophy, nasal sinusitis, pneumonia, polyneuritis, pulmonary abscess, rhinitis, scleritis, summer fever in children, tonsillitis, trachoma, vernal conjunctivitis.

Treatment Symptoms. Cough, coughing up pus and blood, discharge of sticky and yellowish phlegm.

Clinical Cases. A twenty-one-year-old male patient named Xiang displayed the following symptoms: coughing up sticky phlegm with difficulty, a burning sensation throughout the whole body, profuse perspiration, chest pain on the right side triggered by coughing, yellowish phlegm with an offensive smell, a thin and yellowish coating on the tongue, and a rapid pulse. A doctor of traditional Chinese medicine diagnosed his condition as Hot Lungs mainly because of the presence of several hot symptoms, including hot sensations, and many symptoms of the lungs, such as a cough and phlegm.

Treatment Principles. To clear the heat in the lungs, transform the phlegm, relieve the cough, and calm down asthma.

Foods Chosen Based on Y-Scores. Chicken egg white (Lungs -2), fishy vegetable (Lungs 0), laver (Lungs -5), pumpkin (Lungs 0), strawberry (Lungs -2), taro leaf (Lungs 2), winter melon (Lungs -1).

Generally Beneficial Foods and Other Foods to Be Chosen or Avoided. 1. Foods that are considered generally good for this syndrome are apple, apple cucumber, apricot, date (red or black), eggplant, fungus (white), ham, jackfruit, lemon, maltose, mandarin orange, mulberry, mung bean, olive, peach, pear, sweet potato, tomato, and white sugar. 2. Choose from the following cool foods and drinks: amaranth, bamboo shoots, barley, beer, bitter bamboo shoots, bottle gourd, cantaloupe (muskmelon), crab, cucumber, eggplant (aubergine), flour, freshwater clam, gluten, jellyfish, Job's tears, kidney bean, kiwifruit (Chinese gooseberry), laver, lotus plumule, lotus sprouts, mare's milk, matrimony-vine leaf, millet, mulberry leaf, mung bean, peach leaf, pear, peppermint, peppermint oil, persimmon (including powder on its surface), pork brain, rice (polished), sea grass, seaweed, small white cabbage, star fruit (carambola), sugarcane, towel gourd (seed and sponge), watercress (water celery), watermelon (including white portion), wax-gourd pulp (Chinese), wheat, wheat (floating), and wheat bran. 3. Avoid these hot and spicy foods and drinks: alcohol, chili pepper (cayenne pepper), chive (Chinese), cinnamon bark (cassia), cinnamon twig, clove, coffee, garlic, ginger (fresh or dried), green onion (leaf and white head), mustard seed, nutmeg, onion, pepper (black or white), tea, and wine. They force yin energy to excrete through perspiration, which is harmful to both yin and energy.

Beneficial Herbs to Be Applied One Herb at a Time. Qing hao (Herba Aremisiae Chinghao), 6 g; bie Jia (Carapax Trionycis), 20 g; di gu pi (Cortex Lycii Radicis), 15 g; qin jiao (Radix Gentianae Macrophyllae), 10 g.

Beneficial Herbal Formulas to Be Applied One Formula at a Time. Wei Jing Tang, Xie Bai San, Xie Fei Tang.

5.8 Dry Lungs

When you are in good health, your y-score is Lungs 1; when you are ill, your y-score is Lungs 5.

Definition of the Syndrome. With this syndrome, the lungs have become overly dry, which can be due to a prolonged consumption of dry foods or to a frequent external attack of dry weather on the lungs. Both can cause harm to lungs yin, with an exhaustion of fluids in the lungs as a result.

The dry pathogen's attack on the lungs causes the dry cough and the meager phlegm that is difficult to cough up. The energy of the lungs is in communication with the skin and the hair, and now that the lungs are under the attack of dryness, there is the aversion to the cold that occurs along with the fever. When dryness transforms into fire, the chest pain and the discharge of blood from the mouth will occur.

Clinical Signs and Symptoms. Major signs: Dry cough without phlegm or with meager phlegm not easily coughed up, red tip of the tongue, fever, shivering with cold. Median signs: Dry sensation in the nose, dry throat, cough causing chest pain, dry tongue, dry mouth, dry lips. Minor signs: Coughing up blood, loss of voice, morbid hunger, thirst, nosebleed, pain in the throat, tickle in the throat, nosebleed, fever, aversion to being chilled.

Applicable Western Diseases. Acute myelitis, atrophic rhinitis, bronchiectasis, bronchitis, common cold and flu, diabetes insipidus, multiple neuritis, pneumonia.

Treatment Symptoms. Cough, loss of voice, paralysis, discharge of blood from the mouth, nosebleed, common cold, chest pain.

Clinical Cases. (1) Zheng, a forty-year-old female patient, had developed a cough two years before and with it displayed insecurity over sleep, red cheeks, and low spirits. The cough got worse in the fall, when she was diagnosed by a Chinese doctor as having Dry Lungs, primarily because it was dry in the fall when the symptoms occurred and the symptoms worsened with the dry climate. (2) A female patient named Yu, age thirty-five, complained of a headache, a fever, a dry cough or coughing up a little sticky phlegm, panting, a dry and sore throat, a dry nose and dry lips, a congested chest and chest pain, and thirst. A Chinese doctor diagnosed her condition as Dry Lungs, mainly because she displayed many dry symptoms. (3) On a warm, dry, and pleasant day in autumn, a thirty-five-year-old male patient named Wang displayed the following symptoms: a headache, hot sensations in the body, a dry cough, coughing up a little sticky phlegm, shortness of breath with panting, a sore and dry throat, dry nose and lips, pain in the ribs region, and thirst. A Chinese doctor diagnosed his condition as Dry Lungs, especially because the symptoms were occurring in the dry autumn and were supported by other symptoms that are important signs of this syndrome.

Treatment Principles.   To lubricate the lungs and relieve the cough, to clear the lungs and nourish and lubricate dryness.

Foods Chosen Based on Y-Scores.   Chicken egg white (Lungs -2), fishy vegetable (Lungs 0), laver (Lungs -5), millet (Lungs 2), pork lung (Lungs 2), pumpkin (Lungs 0), rosemary (Lungs 6), royal jelly (Lungs 2), strawberry (Lungs -2), taro leaf (Lungs 2), white fungus (Lungs 2), winter melon (Lungs -1).

Generally Beneficial Foods and Other Foods to Be Chosen or Avoided.   1. Foods that are normally good for this syndrome are almond, apple, apricot, asparagus, fungus (white), licorice, loquat, peanut, pear peel, rock sugar, and tangerine. 2. Choose from among these lubricating foods and drinks: asparagus, asparagus (lucid), bean drink, bird's nest, cattail, chicken egg, donggui (lavage), fungus (white), hemp, honey, lard, licorice, maltose, milk (cow's, mare's, or human), pear, persimmon powder on its surface, pork, pork pancreas, sea cucumber, sesame oil, sesame seed (white), soybean (yellow), spinach, sugarcane, taro, tofu, and torreya nut. 3. Avoid these hot and spicy foods and drinks: alcohol, chili pepper (cayenne pepper), chive (Chinese), cinnamon bark (cassia), cinnamon twig, clove, coffee, garlic, ginger (fresh or dried), green onion (leaf and white head), mustard seed, nutmeg, onion, pepper (black or white), tea, and wine. They force yin energy to excrete through perspiration, and this is harmful to both yin and energy.

Beneficial Herbs to Be Applied One Herb at a Time.   Bei sha shen (Radix Glehniae), 11 g; dong gua ren (Semen Benincasae), 14 g; E jiao (Colla Corii Asini [Gelatina Nigra]), 11 g; gua lou ren (Semen Trichosanthis), 15 g; mai men dong (Radix Ophiopogonis), 11 g; pi pa ye (Folium Eriobotryae), 11 g; sang ye (Folium Mori), 10 g; sheng di (Radix Rehmanniae), fresh, 35 g; xing ren (Semen Armeniacae Amarae), 11 g; zhi mu (Rhizoma Anemarrhenae), 15 g; zi wan (Radix Asteris), 11 g.

Beneficial Herbal Formulas to Be Applied One Formula at a Time.   Qing Zao Jiu Fei Tang, Sang Xing Tang, Sha Shen Mai Dong Tang, Wu Wei Zi Tang, Xing Su San.

6

Choosing Foods and Herbs to Boost the Large Intestine and Cure Applicable Symptoms and Diseases

6.1 Large Intestine Damp Heat

When you are in good health, your y-score is L. intestine 2; when you are ill, your y-score is L. intestine 6.

Definition of the Syndrome. When damp heat affects the large intestine, Large Intestine Damp Heat can ensue. This syndrome can arise from the attack of seasonal damp heat energy or from the consumption of decomposed or toxic foods. In severe cases, there can be fainting and coma. When damp heat attacks the large intestine, dampness and heat stick together, which accounts for the abdominal pain and tenesmus (distressing but ineffectual urge to urinate or defecate). Damp heat can harm the intestinal tract, producing pus combined with blood, which accounts for the diarrhea with the discharge of red and white and sticky, or thin and yellowish, water. Damp heat flows downward, causing the burning sensation in the anus and the short, red streams of urine.

Clinical Signs and Symptoms. Major signs: Frequent bowel movements with little stool discharged, discharge of stools with an offensive smell, acute diarrhea with discharge of red and white and sticky, or thin and yellowish, water. Median signs: Abdominal pain, abdominal swelling, diarrhea with discharge of pus and blood, burning sensation in the anus, fever, thirst, hot sensation in the body, discharge of short and reddish streams of urine. Minor signs: Prolapse of the anus, pain in the anus with swelling and burning sensation, vomiting, poor appetite, red color of the tongue.

Applicable Western Diseases. Acute and chronic amebic intestine, acute and chronic bacillary dysentery, acute and chronic enteritis, acute appendicitis, bacterial food poisoning, chronic nonspecific ulcerative colitis, dysentery, hemorrhoids, tenesmus.

Treatment Symptoms. Abdominal pain, diarrhea, hemorrhoids.

Clinical Cases. (1) A thirty-year-old male patient named He suffered from diarrhea for three consecutive days, which gradually changed to dysentery, with a discharge of reddish and whitish stools, an evacuation of more than twenty bowel movements a night with abdominal pain, and a frequent desire to empty the bowels but having difficulty in doing so. A Chinese doctor diagnosed his condition as Large Intestine Damp Heat, primarily because two contradictory factors were present: the desire to empty the bowels while having difficulty doing so; this was due to a mixture of dampness and heat in the intestine. (2) Wu, a thirty-one-year-old male patient, was under the attack of dysentery at the beginning of summer, and it lasted for more than a month, with at least ten bowel movements each day, a frequent desire to empty the bowels but having trouble doing so, and the discharge of sticky and bloody stools. A Chinese doctor diagnosed his condition as Large Intestine Damp Heat.

Treatment Principles. To clear heat and benefit dampness, to regulate energy and blood.

Foods Chosen Based on Y-Scores. Amaranth (L. intestine 0), apricot (L. intestine 0), areca nut (L. intestine -2), bean curd (L. intestine 0), black fungus (L. intestine 2), broomcorn (L. intestine 2), buckwheat (L. intestine 0), cabbage (Chinese) (L. intestine 2), Chinese wax gourd (winter melon) (L. intestine 0), coconut meat (L. intestine 2), common button mushroom (L. intestine 0), corn cob (L. intestine 2), cucumber (L. intestine 0), fig (L. intestine 2), honey (L. intestine 2), kohlrabi (L. intestine 1), lettuce (leaf and stalk) (L. intestine -2), lettuce seed (L. intestine -2), ling (L. intestine 0), marjoram (L. intestine 2), millet (L. intestine 2), palm seed (L. intestine -4), peach (L. intestine 2), persimmon (L. intestine -2), salt (L. intestine -7), scallion bulb (L. intestine 2), sesame oil (L. intestine: 0), small white cabbage (L. intestine 2), sorghum (L. intestine 4), soybean (yellow) (L. intestine 2), sweet potato (L. intestine -2), taro flower (L. intestine 0), taro leaf (L. intestine 2), tea melon (L. intestine -2), trifoliate orange (L. intestine -2), water spinach (L. intestine -2), winter melon (L. intestine -1).

Generally Beneficial Foods and Other Foods to Be Chosen or Avoided. 1. Foods that are generally beneficial for this syndrome are abalone, adzuki bean, celery, chicken egg white, day lily, eggplant, hyacinth bean, jellyfish, Job's tears, mackerel, mung bean, and sweet basil. 2. Choose from the following foods that are good for damp heat: adzuki bean sprouts, black soybean sprouts (dried), buckwheat, cantaloupe (muskmelon), carp (common), celery root, Chinese cabbage, coconut shell, corn silk, cucumber vine (stem), day lily, eggplant (aubergine), eggplant calyx, fig leaf, frog (river or pond), green turtle, hawthorn fruit, olive, pricking amaranth (amaranth, pigweed), soybean (yellow), soybean oil, squash (flower and root), star fruit (carambola), sunflower (top of peduncle), turnip seed, water-rice root, wax gourd (Chinese), and wheat seedling. 3. Avoid items that are likely to trigger a chronic damp heat syndrome or intensify an existing one, such as alcohol, maltose, pork, and sweet rice. 4. Choose from these grease-free, bland, and nonirritating foods and drinks: apple, banana, beef, brown sugar, cabbages, carrot, celery, chicken, chicken egg, Chinese cabbage, corn, cottage cheese, cow's milk, fish, fruit, honey, horse beans (broad beans), lean meats, lemon, lettuce, liver, lotus juice (fresh), millet, mung bean, mung bean sprouts, noodle, peach, pea, pear, polished rice, pork, orange, radish, rice, seaweed, skim milk, soybean sprouts, string bean, sweet potato, soybean, sword bean, taro, tofu, tomato, vegetables, watermelon, wheat, white fungus, white sugar, and yam. 5. Avoid greasy and fatty foods, such as animal fats, butter, chicken egg yolk, creams, fatty meats, fish-liver oils, fried foods, and lard. These foods can generate heat and produce phlegm, and they are bad for indigestion, a poor appetite, jaundice, dysentery, and diarrhea.

Beneficial Herbs to Be Applied One Herb at a Time. Sheng di (Radix Rehmanniae), 30 g; huai jiao (Pericarpium Zanthoxyli), 10 g; huang qin (Radix Scutellaria), 15 g; huang lian (Rhizoma Coptidis), 10 g.

Beneficial Herbal Formulas to Be Applied One Formula at a Time. Bai Tou Weng Tang, Ge Gen Qin Lian Tang, Shao Yao Tang.

6.2 Large Intestine Fluid Exhaustion (Dry Large Intestine)

When you are in good health, your y-score is L. intestine 1; when you are ill, your y-score is L. intestine 5.

Definition of the Syndrome. Large Intestine Fluid Exhaustion is also called Dry Large Intestine. The dryness can be due to the attack of external pathogenic heat, old age, or a blood deficiency after childbirth. This syndrome is characterized by dry stools and difficult bowel movements.

Clinical Signs and Symptoms. Major signs: Constipation with stools as dry as sheep dung, one bowel movement in several days, abdominal pain and swelling, lumpy object in the lower abdomen that can be felt by touch. Median signs: Attacks of pain around the umbilicus with sensations of hardness on massage. Minor signs: Loud passing of gas, bad breath, dry mouth, dry throat, thirst, dry tongue.

Applicable Western Diseases. Enteroncus (tumor of the intestine), fissure of the anus, habitual constipation, perianal rectal abscess.

Treatment Symptoms. Constipation, constipation after childbirth, abdominal distension.

Clinical Cases. (1) A female patient named Chang, age eighty-two, suffered from constipation with frequent urination at night. A Chinese doctor diagnosed her condition as Large Intestine Fluid Exhaustion, mainly because most cases of constipation in the elderly are due to this syndrome. (2) Liu, a seventy-two-year-old male patient, had constipation for more than five years, with a discharge of dry stools like balls, discomfort in the lower abdomen, poor sleep, easily waking up in shock, and no coating on the tongue. A Chinese doctor diagnosed his condition as Large Intestine Fluid Exhaustion primarily because of the constipation's occurring in old age and the dry stools. (3) A female patient named Lee, at the age of thirty-four, had suffered from pulmonary tuberculosis on the right lung for more than ten months, but her condition is now stable. Yet she still displays the following signs and symptoms: constipation, abdominal pain that worsens with massage, swelling and pain in the lower abdomen after a bowel movement, insecurity over sleep, and a red tongue. A Chinese doctor diagnosed her condition as Large Intestine Fluid Exhaustion chiefly on account of her constipation and red tongue.

Treatment Principles. To nourish yin and produce fluids, to lubricate the intestine and promote bowel movements.

Foods Chosen Based on Y-Scores. Amaranth (L. intestine 0), apricot (L. intestine 0), areca nut (L. intestine -2), bean curd (L. intestine 0), black fungus (L. intestine 2), broomcorn (L. intestine 2), buckwheat (L. intestine 0), cabbage (Chinese) (L. intestine 2), Chinese wax gourd (winter melon) (L. intestine 0), coconut meat (L. intestine 2), common button mushroom (L. intestine 0), corn cob (L. intestine 2), cucumber (L. intestine 0), fig (L. intestine 2), honey (L. intestine 2), kohlrabi (L. intestine 1), lettuce (leaf and stalk) (L. intestine -2), lettuce seed (L. intestine -2), ling (L. intestine 0), marjoram (L. intestine 2), millet (L. intestine 2), palm seed (L. intestine -4), peach (L. intestine 2), persimmon (L. intestine -2), salt (L. intestine -7), scallion bulb (L. intestine 2), sesame oil (L. intestine 0), small white cabbage (L. intestine 2), sorghum (L. intestine 4), soybean (yellow) (L. intestine 2), sweet potato (L. intestine -2), taro flower (L. intestine 0), taro leaf (L. intestine 2), tea melon (L. intestine -2), trifoliate orange (L. intestine -2), water spinach (L. intestine -2), winter melon (L. intestine -1).

Generally Beneficial Foods and Other Foods to Be Chosen or Avoided. 1. Choose from the following lubricating foods: asparagus, asparagus (lucid), bean drink, bird's nest, cattail, chicken egg, donggui (lavage), fungus (white), hemp, honey, lard, licorice, maltose, milk (cow's, mare's, or human), pear, persimmon powder on its surface, pork, pork pancreas, sea cucumber, sesame oil, sesame seed (white), soybean (yellow), spinach, sugarcane, taro, tofu, and torreya nut. 2. Choose from these foods that can induce bowel movements in cases of constipation: aloe vera, amaranth, amaranth seed, black sesame seed, bog bean (buck bean), bottle gourd (autumn), castor bean, castor bean oil, crown daisy, donggui (lavage), fenugreek seed (Oriental), fig, papaya, sesame oil, sesame seed (white), small white cabbage, soybean oil, sweet potato, tamarind (sour plum), walnut oil, water spinach, and wild rice gall (water-oats gall). 3. Avoid these hot and spicy foods and drinks: alcohol, chili pepper (cayenne pepper), chive (Chinese), cinnamon bark (cassia), cinnamon twig, clove, coffee, garlic, ginger (fresh or dried), green onion (leaf and white head), mustard seed, nutmeg, onion, pepper (black or white), tea, and wine. They force yin energy to excrete through perspiration, which is harmful to both yin and energy.

Beneficial Herbs to Be Applied One Herb at a Time. Tao ren (Semen Persicae), 10 g; huo ma ren (Fructus Cannabis), 15 g; xing ren (Semen Ameniacae Amanum), 10 g; dang gui (Radix Angelicae Sinensis), 15 g; rou cong rong (Herba Cistanchis Caulis Cistanchis), 12 g.

Beneficial Herbal Formulas to Be Applied One Formula at a Time. Ma Zi Ren Wan, Wu Ren Wan, Zeng Yi Tang.

6.3 *Large Intestine Deficiency and Slippery Diarrhea*

When you are in good health, your y-score is L. intestine 2; when you are ill, your y-score is L. intestine 6.

Definition of the Syndrome. With this syndrome, chronic diarrhea can lead to yang deficiency in the large intestine, causing the large intestine to become too loose and to lack adequate control, which in turn can cause prolapse of the anus.

Clinical Signs and Symptoms. Major signs: Sliding diarrhea (continual diarrhea that doesn't stop), diarrhea with discharge of sticky and muddy stool. Median signs: Prolapse of the anus after diarrhea, pale tongue. Minor signs: Mentally fatigued, withered and white complexion, cold limbs, pain in the skin with a desire for warmth and massage.

Applicable Western Diseases. Anal rectal prolapse, chronic dysentery, chronic enteritis, chronic tracheitis (trachitis), ulcerative colitis.

Treatment Symptoms. Chronic diarrhea, prolapse of the anus.

Clinical Cases. (1) A thirty-two-year-old male patient named Yu had suffered from enteritis for five years. The last two weeks, the symptoms worsened, and, at one point, he discharged a lump of something that looked like a big chunk of rotten meat. He also reported a poor appetite, indigestion, pain in the lower abdomen, discharge of red and whitish stools resembling pus, and discharge of eight to nine bowel movements every day with an urgent need to defecate. A Chinese doctor diagnosed Yu's condition as Large Intestine Deficiency and Slippery Diarrhea primarily because of the chronic diarrhea with the frequent bowel movements. (2) Tending to be physically weak, Lin, a fifty-seven-year-old male patient, caught a cold in spring, but he did not want to take medication. The cold turned into diarrhea ten days later, and it dragged on and on until early autumn, when he developed some additional symptoms, such as physical exhaustion, a pale complexion, and a loss of appetite. Lin would get diarrhea after drinking only a little bit of water, and, when he had it, he often yawned and vomited and felt dizzy. A Chinese doctor diagnosed his condition as Large Intestine Deficiency and Slippery Diarrhea, chiefly because the cold had weakened his large intestine causing the diarrhea.

Treatment Principles. To warm and tone the large intestine so that it can exercise an adequate control over its movements, to dry up excessive dampness in the large intestine to stop diarrhea.

Foods Chosen Based on Y-Scores. Amaranth (L. intestine 0), apricot (L. intestine 0), areca nut (L. intestine -2), bean curd (L. intestine 0), black fungus (L. intestine 2), broomcorn (L. intestine 2), buckwheat (L. intestine 0), cabbage (Chinese) (L. intestine 2), Chinese wax gourd (winter melon) (L. intestine 0), coconut meat (L. intestine 2), common button mushroom (L. intestine 0), corn cob (L. intestine 2), cucumber (L. intestine 0), fig (L. intestine 2), honey (L. intestine 2), kohlrabi (L. intestine 1), lettuce (leaf and stalk) (L. intestine -2), lettuce seed (L. intestine -2), ling (L. intestine 0), marjoram (L. intestine 2), millet (L. intestine 2), palm seed (L. intestine -4), peach (L. intestine 2), persimmon (L. intestine -2), salt (L. intestine -7), scallion bulb (L. intestine 2), sesame oil (L. intestine 0), small white cabbage (L. intestine 2), sorghum (L. intestine 4), soybean (yellow) (L. intestine 2), sweet potato (L. intestine -2), taro flower (L. intestine 0), taro leaf (L. intestine 2), tea melon (L. intestine -2), trifoliate orange (L. intestine -2), water spinach (L. intestine -2), winter melon (L. intestine -1).

Generally Beneficial Foods and Other Foods to Be Chosen or Avoided. 1. Choose from the following energy-tonic foods: beef, bird's nest, broomcorn, cherry, chicken, coconut meat, crane meat, date (red or black), eel, ginkgo (cooked), ginseng, goose meat, grape, herring, honey, jackfruit, loach, longan, mackerel, mandarin fish, octopus, pheasant, pigeon (meat and egg), meat, potato (Irish), rabbit, rice (glutinous or sweet), rice (fermented, glutinous), rice (polished), rice (polished, long-grain), rock sugar, shark's fin, sheep or goat meat, shiitake mushroom, snake melon, squash, sturgeon, sweet potato, tofu, turtledove, walnut root, and white string bean. 2. Choose from these foods that can control diarrhea: black-eyed pea, broomcorn, buckwheat sprouts, carrot seed, chestnut flower, common button mushroom, crabapple, cucumber leaf, cucumber root, fig, flour, gorgan fruit, guava (fresh or dried), guava leaf, hyacinth bean (lablab bean), hyacinth-bean leaf, Job's tears, kudzu seed, lotus (fruit and seed), persimmon, persimmon cake, pistachio nut, pomegranate (sour fruit), pomegranate peel, pork skin, prune (including leaf), quail, rabbit liver, rambutan, rice (glutinous, sweet, or polished), rice sprouts, Russian olive (oleaster), sorghum, string bean, sweet potato, vine leaves, and yellow croaker. 3. Avoid these foods that can intensify diarrhea: amaranth, black sesame seed, duck, eel, eggplant, honey, lard, lily (bulb and leaf), purslane, sea cucumber, sesame oil, water spinach, white eel, and wild cabbage.

Beneficial Herbs to Be Applied One Herb at a Time. Mu li (Concha Ostreae), 30 g; wu mei (Fructus Mume), 10 g; shi liu pi (Pericarpium Granati), 15 g; yi zhi ren (Fructus Zigiberis Nigri), 8 g.

Beneficial Herbal Formulas to Be Applied One Formula at a Time. Si Shen Wan, Tao Hua Tang, Yang Zang Tang.

7

Choosing Foods and Herbs to Boost the Spleen and Cure Applicable Symptoms and Diseases

7.1 *Spleen Energy Deficiency*

When you are in good health, your y-score is Spleen -2; when you are ill, your y-score is Spleen -6.

Definition of the Syndrome. When energy deficiency affects the spleen, this can lead to Spleen Energy Deficiency. This syndrome occurs mainly because of irregular eating and excessive thought and fatigue, but can also arise after the attack of acute diseases that consume spleen energy such as acute diarrhea.

The spleen and the stomach are interrelated, so a spleen deficiency will affect the stomach, which accounts for the poor appetite. The spleen cannot mobilize foods efficiently, causing the abdominal swelling that occurs after eating a meal. When the spleen is deficient, it is more susceptible to the attack of dampness, which gives rise to the diarrhea and the edema in the four limbs. In addition, the spleen fails to send the refined substances of water and grains to various parts of the body; this is the reason for the fatigue and the feeling of being too lazy to talk.

Clinical Signs and Symptoms. Major signs: Poor appetite, soft stools, abdominal swelling, belching after a meal, vomiting of acid. Median signs: Withered and yellowish complexion, fatigue, feeling too lazy to talk, skinniness, edema in the four limbs. Minor signs: Abdominal pain, diarrhea, lips rolled up, malnutrition in children, stomachache, vaginal discharge, vomiting of blood, tooth marks on the tongue.

Applicable Western Diseases and Conditions. Acute epidemic icterohepatitis, anaphylactoid purpura, anemia, bronchial asthma, chronic bronchitis, chronic infectious hepatitis, chronic nephritis, cirrhosis, cirrhotic ascites, edema of pregnancy, enuresis in children, erythema multiforme, functional metrorrhagia, hypertension, infectious hepatitis, liver cancer, menoxenia, nephritis, nephrotic edema (nutritional edema), otitis media, primary hepatoma, ptosis, thrombocythenia, thrombocytopenia purpura (thrombopenic purpura), uterine bleeding, vaginal discharge, viral hepatitis (nonjaundice type).

Treatment Symptoms. Diarrhea, stomachache, abdominal pain, edema, chronic fatigue.

Clinical Cases. (1) A thirty-year-old male patient named Wang displayed a decreased appetite for two years, with shortness of breath, fatigue, a pale complexion, and mild abdominal pain that improves with massage. A Chinese doctor diagnosed his condition as Spleen Energy Deficiency. (2) Lee, a thirty-five-year-old male patient, suffered from intermittent diarrhea for more than a month. Over one week, he had four or five bouts of diarrhea every day, losing more than 6 pounds (3 kilograms) in the process; he also complained of fatigue, a poor appetite, abdominal swelling and mild pain, mental depression, insomnia, and dripping of urine. Lee was diagnosed in one Western hospital as having the aftereffects of enteritis and in another as having allergic colitis. A Chinese doctor diagnosed his condition as Spleen Energy Deficiency. (3) A twelve-year-old female patient, Ling was born from a mother with many illnesses. She had poor growth after she was born and, throughout her childhood, tended to be skinny, have shortness of breath, be easily fatigued, be too weak to play, have soft stools, and have a poor appetite. A Chinese doctor diagnosed her condition as Spleen Energy Deficiency, primarily because the spleen is the acquired source of energy and malnutrition in a young child is generally the result of this syndrome.

Treatment Principles. To strengthen the spleen and benefit energy.

Foods Chosen Based on Y-Scores. Apple (Spleen -2), autumn bottle gourd (Spleen 2), banana (Spleen -2), bean curd (Spleen 0), beef (Spleen 2), blood clam (Spleen 4), broad bean (horse bean) (Spleen 2), broomcorn (Spleen 2), brown sugar (Spleen 4), buckwheat (Spleen 0), carp (common) (Spleen 2), carp (gold) (Spleen

2), carp (grass) (Spleen 4), carrot (Spleen 2), cherry (Spleen 4), chestnut (Spleen 4), chicken (Spleen 4), chili pepper (cayenne pepper) (Spleen 8), cinnamon bark (Spleen 7), clove (Spleen 6), clove oil (Spleen 7), coconut meat (Spleen 2), coriander (Chinese parsley) (Spleen 6), crown daisy (Spleen 6), cucumber (Spleen 0), danggui (Spleen 1), date (red or black) (Spleen 4), day lily (Spleen 0), dill seed (Spleen 6), eel (Spleen 4), eggplant (Spleen 0), fig (Spleen 2), garlic (Spleen 6), ginger (dried) (Spleen 8), ginger (fresh) (Spleen 6), ginseng (Spleen 1), goose meat (Spleen 2), gorgan fruit (Spleen 2), grapefruit peel (Spleen 3), grape (Spleen 0), hairtail (Spleen 4), ham (Spleen -1), hawthorn fruit (Spleen 2), herring (Spleen 2), honey (Spleen 2), hyacinth bean (Spleen 2), hyacinth-bean flower (Spleen 2), Japanese cassia bark (Spleen 6), Job's tears (Spleen 0), lard (Spleen 0), licorice (Spleen 2), litchi nut (Spleen 2), loach (Spleen 2), longevity fruit (Spleen 0), longan (Spleen 4), long-kissing sturgeon (Spleen 2), long-tailed anchovy (Spleen 4), loquat (Spleen -2), lotus (fruit, seed, and root) (Spleen 2), lotus-rhizome powder (Spleen -1), mackerel (Spleen 2), malt (Spleen 4), maltose (Spleen 4), mandarin orange (Spleen -2), mandarin-orange peel (dry) (Spleen 2), mango (Spleen -2), milk (mare's) (Spleen 0), millet (Spleen 2), mung bean sprouts (Spleen -2), murrel (snakehead) (Spleen -2), mutton (Spleen 4), nutmeg (Spleen 6), onion (Spleen 6), oxtail (Spleen 1), papaya (Spleen 2), pea (Spleen 2), peanut (Spleen 2), pearl sago (Spleen 4), perch (Spleen 2), pheasant (Spleen 2), pineapple (Spleen 0), pistachio nut (Spleen 7), polished rice (Spleen 2), pork (Spleen -1), potato (Irish) (Spleen 2), prickly ash (Spleen 6), radish leaf (Spleen 0), rape (Spleen 2), red or green pepper (chili pepper or cayenne pepper) (Spleen 2), rock sugar (Spleen 2), royal jelly (Spleen 2), shark's fin: (Spleen -1), shrimp (Spleen 4), silver carp (Spleen 4), sorghum (Spleen 4), sour date (Spleen 0), soybean (black) (Spleen 2), soybean (yellow) (Spleen 2), soybean sprouts (yellow) (Spleen 4), squash (Spleen 4), star anise (Spleen 5), strawberry (Spleen -2), string bean (Spleen 2), sweet basil (Spleen 6), sweet potato (Spleen -2), trifoliate orange (Spleen -2), wheat (Spleen 0), white eel (Spleen 2), white sugar (Spleen 2), whitebait (Spleen 2), wild cabbage (Spleen 2), wild rice gall (Spleen -2), yam (Spleen 2).

Generally Beneficial Foods and Other Foods to Be Chosen or Avoided. 1. Foods that are generally good for this syndrome are apple cucumber, beef, bird's nest, carrot, cherry, chestnut, chicken egg yolk, coconut meat, common button mushroom, date (red or black), Irish potato, mustard seed, rice, rock sugar, sweet potato, tofu, and wheat bran. 2. Choose from the following tonic foods for the spleen and pancreas: apple cucumber, beef, bird's nest, black-eyed pea, broomcorn, caraway seed, carp gall (grass), carrot, cassia bark (Japanese), cherry leaf, chestnut, cinnamon bark (cassia), corn cob, crown daisy, date (red or black), dill seed, frog (pond), garlic, ham, horse bean (broad bean, fava bean), hyacinth bean (lablab bean), hyacinth-bean flower, Job's tears (root), longan, lotus (fruit and seed), mullet (black or striped), pearl sago, perch, pheasant, pineapple, pistachio nut, pork pancreas, rice (glutinous, sweet, or polished), rice sprouts, royal jelly, string bean, white string bean, whitefish, and yam.

Beneficial Herbs to Be Applied One Herb at a Time. Dang shen (Radix Codonopsis Pilosulae), 30 g; bai zhu (Rhizoma Atractylodis Macrocephalae), 10 g; fu ling (Poria), 18 g; gan cao (Radix Gly-cyrrhizae), 10 g; shan yao (Rhizoma Dioscoreae Rhizoma Batatatis), 30 g; huang qi (Radix Astragali), 25 g.

Beneficial Herbal Formulas to Be Applied One Formula at a Time. Bu Zhong Yi Qi Tang, Liu Jun Zi Tang, Si Jun Zi Tang.

7.2 Spleen Yang Deficiency (Deficient and Cold Spleen)

When you are in good health, your y-score is Spleen -4; when you are ill, your y-score is Spleen -8.

Definition of the Syndrome. When yang deficiency affects the spleen, this can lead to Spleen Yang Deficiency. This syndrome mostly arises from a spleen deficiency affecting yang energy, an excessive consumption of cold foods or cold and cool herbs, a decline in the yang energy of the kidneys, or a failure of fire to warm the spleen.

Cold energy accumulates in the spleen, which accounts for the cold abdominal pain, poor appetite, fondness for warmth and massage, aversion to the cold with cold limbs, and diarrhea. Cold damp-ness in the middle region slows down digestion, causing the discharge of watery stools. Water overflows into the skin, and this is the reason for the whitish discharge in women, edema throughout the whole body, and diminished urination.

Clinical Signs and Symptoms. Major signs: Cold abdominal pain, poor appetite, fondness for warmth and massage, aversion to the cold, cold limbs, diarrhea. Median signs: Discharge of watery stools, excessive clear saliva, plentiful whitish discharge in women, edema in the whole body, diminished urination. Minor signs: Withered and yellowish complexion, no thirst, discharge of watery stools, coldness on the forehead that does not warm up, edema in the lower limbs, stomachache, pale tongue, white coating on the tongue.

Applicable Western Diseases. Acute and chronic gastroenteritis, chronic dysentery, chronic nephritis, gastroptosis, gastric ulcer, hepatic cirrhosis, peptic ulcer.

Treatment Symptoms. Diarrhea, stomachache, abdominal pain, edema.

Clinical Cases. (1) A forty-two-year-old female patient by the name of Guo suffered abdominal pain surrounding the umbilicus, followed by diarrhea. This occurred two or three times a day, and the condition dragged on for a couple of months. She was diagnosed at a Western hospital as having chronic colitis and was treated with good results. A Chinese doctor diagnosed her condition as Spleen Yang Deficiency. (2) Zha, a thirty-nine-year-old male patient, displayed edema all over his body that had worsened over the past two weeks. Initially, he had a common cold, and then he exhibited puffiness below the lower eyelids and in the lower extremities, with fatigue, dizziness, an aversion to the cold, and a discharge of thin and watery stools. Zha was diagnosed by a Chinese doctor as having Spleen Yang Deficiency. (3) A thirty-one-year-old male patient named Lin had suffered from a peptic ulcer for more than a year with the following signs and symptoms: a fear of the cold particularly in the stomach region with dull pain, a poor appetite, fatigue, and soft stools. A Chinese doctor diagnosed Lin's condition as Spleen Yang Deficiency, mainly because a peptic ulcer is often a sign of this syndrome and is supported by fear of the cold and soft stools.

Treatment Principles. To warm the middle region and strengthen the spleen.

Foods Chosen Based on Y-Scores. Autumn bottle gourd (Spleen 2), bean curd (Spleen 0), beef (Spleen 2), blood clam (Spleen 4), broad bean (horse bean) (Spleen 2), broomcorn (Spleen 2), brown sugar (Spleen 4), buckwheat (Spleen 0), carp (common) (Spleen 2), carp (gold) (Spleen 2), carp (grass) (Spleen 4), carrot (Spleen 2), cherry (Spleen 4), chestnut (Spleen 4), chicken (Spleen 4), chili pepper (cayenne pepper) (Spleen 8), cinnamon bark (Spleen 7), clove (Spleen 6), clove oil (Spleen 7), coconut meat (Spleen 2), coriander (Chinese parsley) (Spleen 6), crown daisy (Spleen 6), cucumber (Spleen 0), danggui (Spleen 1), date (red or black) (Spleen 4), day lily (Spleen 0), dill seed (Spleen 6), eel (Spleen 4), eggplant (Spleen 0), fig (Spleen 2), garlic (Spleen 6), ginger (dried) (Spleen 8), ginger (fresh) (Spleen 6), ginseng (Spleen 1), goose meat (Spleen 2), gorgan fruit (Spleen 2), grape (Spleen 0), grape-fruit peel (Spleen 3), hairtail (Spleen 4), hawthorn fruit (Spleen 2), herring (Spleen 2), honey (Spleen 2), hyacinth bean (Spleen 2), hyacinth-bean flower (Spleen 2), Japanese cassia bark (Spleen 6), Job's tears (Spleen 0), lard (Spleen 0), licorice (Spleen 2), litchi nut (Spleen 2), loach (Spleen 2), longevity fruit (Spleen 0), longan (Spleen 4), long-kissing sturgeon (Spleen 2), long-tailed anchovy (Spleen 4), loquat (Spleen -2), lotus (fruit, seed, and root) (Spleen 2), mackerel (Spleen 2), malt (Spleen 4), maltose (Spleen 4), man-darin-orange peel (dry) (Spleen 2), milk (mare's) (Spleen 0), millet (Spleen 2), mutton (Spleen 4), nutmeg (Spleen 6), onion (Spleen 6), oxtail (Spleen 1), papaya (Spleen 2), pea (Spleen 2), peanut (Spleen 2), pearl sago (Spleen 4), perch (Spleen 2), pheasant (Spleen 2), pineapple (Spleen 0), pistachio nut (Spleen 7), polished rice (Spleen 2), potato (Irish) (Spleen 2), prickly ash (Spleen 6), radish leaf (Spleen 0), rape (Spleen 2), red or green pepper (chili pepper or cayenne pepper) (Spleen 2), rock sugar (Spleen 2), royal jelly (Spleen 2), shrimp (Spleen 4), silver carp (Spleen 4), sorghum (Spleen 4), sour date (Spleen 0), soybean (black) (Spleen 2), soy-bean (yellow) (Spleen 2), soybean sprouts (yellow) (Spleen 4), squash (Spleen 4), star anise (Spleen 5), string bean (Spleen 2), sweet basil (Spleen 6), wheat (Spleen 0), white eel (Spleen 2), white sugar (Spleen 2), whitebait (Spleen 2), wild cabbage (Spleen 2), yam (Spleen 2).

Generally Beneficial Foods and Other Foods to Be Chosen or Avoided. 1. Foods that are considered usually good for this syn-drome are air bladder of shark, cayenne pepper, chicken, fennel, mustard (white or yellow), mutton, nutmeg, pepper (black or white), prickly ash, and sword bean. 2. Avoid these irritants: alco-hol, coffee, tea, tobacco, and wine. They can irritate the stomach and produce damp heat, and fire is harmful to yin and energy. 3. Choose from the following tonic foods for the spleen and the pan-creas: apple cucumber, beef, bird's nest, black-eyed pea, broomcorn, caraway seed, carp gall (grass), carrot, cassia bark (Japanese), cherry leaf, chestnut, cinnamon bark (cassia), corn cob, crown daisy, date (red or black), dill seed, frog (pond), garlic, ham, horse bean (broad bean, fava bean), hyacinth bean (lablab bean), hyacinth-bean flower, Job's tears (root), longan, lotus (fruit and seed), mullet (black or striped), pearl sago, perch, pheasant, pineapple, pistachio nut, pork pancreas, rice (glutinous, sweet, or polished), rice sprouts, royal jelly, string bean, white string bean, whitefish, and yam. 4. Choose from these yang-tonic foods for the kidneys: air bladder of shark, beef kidney, cassia fruit (Japanese), chestnut, chive seed (Chinese), cinnamon bark (cassia), clove, clove oil, deer kidney, dill seed, fennel (root and seed), fenugreek seed (Oriental), green-onion seed, lobster (sea prawn), mandarin-orange seed, oxtail, pistachio nut, pork testes, prickly ash root, raspberry, sheep or goat kidney, shrimp, sparrow egg, star anise, strawberry, and sword bean (jack bean).

Beneficial Herbs to Be Applied One Herb at a Time. Bai dou kou (Fructus Amomi Cardamomi), 7 g; bai zhu (Rhizoma Atractylodis Macrocephalae), 11 g; dang shen (Radix Codonopsis Pilosulae), 15 g; ding xiang (Flos Caryophylli), 4 g; fu ling (Poria), 14 g; gan cao (Radix Glycyrrhizae), 11 g; gan jiang (Rhizoma Zingiberis), 7 g; rou dou kou (Semen Myristicae), 8 g; wu zhu yu (Fructus Euodiae), 7 g.

Beneficial Herbal Formulas to Be Applied One Formula at a Time. Da Jian Zhong Tang, Fu Zi Li Zhong Tang, Li Zhong Tang, Shi Pi Yin.

7.3 Middle Energy Cave-in (Deficient Spleen with Cave-in of Its Energy)

When you are in good health, your y-score is Spleen -2; when you are ill, your y-score is Spleen -6.

Definition of the Syndrome. This syndrome is characterized by the falling of the internal organs generally due to fatigue, innate deficiency, and chronic illness; the falling symptoms include prolapse of the anus, prolapse of the uterus, and falling of the internal organs.

Clinical Signs and Symptoms. Major signs: Chronic diarrhea, prolapse of the anus, prolapse of the uterus, falling sensation in the abdomen that intensifies after a meal, falling sensation below the umbilicus, frequent desire to empty the bowels. Median signs: Fatigue, low voice, dribbling of urine, vaginal bleeding, miscarriage. Minor signs: Blue ring of lips, dizziness, sudden illogical talking, sudden fainting, low fever.

Applicable Western Diseases and Conditions. Chronic enteritis, gastroptosis (falling of the stomach), hernia, hysteroptosis (prolapse of the uterus), nephroptosis (prolapse of the kidneys), prostatitis, ptosis (drooping of the upper eyelid).

Treatment Symptoms. Chronic diarrhea, vaginal bleeding, prolapse of the uterus, prolapse of the anus, vaginal bleeding.

Clinical Cases. (1) A thirty-six-year-old male patient by the name of Wang suffered from prolapse of the anus for five or six years; the prolapse occurred especially with prolonged standing or walking. A Chinese doctor diagnosed his condition as Middle Energy Cave-in, primarily because Wang did not have sufficient yang energy to support the anus. (2) A fifty-four-year-old female patient named Ho displayed the following signs: a constant sound of water in the stomach, a cold sensation in the stomach region, a poor appetite, a fondness for eating dry dishes like fried rice that bring comfort to her stomach, a stomach disturbance from water intake that causes vomiting once in a while, an absence of thirst, and a bland taste in the mouth. She was diagnosed in Western medicine as having gastroptosis. A Chinese doctor diagnosed her condition as Middle Energy Cave-in, chiefly because gastroptosis is a distinct sign of this syndrome and is supported by other symptoms as well.

Treatment Principles. To tone yang energy so that it can support the internal organs, including the anus.

Foods Chosen Based on Y-Scores. Apple (Spleen -2), autumn bottle gourd (Spleen 2), banana (Spleen -2), bean curd (Spleen 0), beef (Spleen 2), blood clam (Spleen 4), broad bean (horse bean) (Spleen 2), broomcorn (Spleen 2), brown sugar (Spleen 4), buckwheat (Spleen 0), carp (common) (Spleen 2), carp (gold) (Spleen 2), carp (grass) (Spleen 4), carrot (Spleen 2), cherry (Spleen 4), chestnut (Spleen 4), chicken (Spleen 4), chili pepper (cayenne pepper) (Spleen 8), cinnamon bark (Spleen 7), clove (Spleen 6), clove oil (Spleen 7), coconut meat (Spleen 2), coriander (Chinese parsley) (Spleen 6), crown daisy (Spleen 6), cucumber (Spleen 0), danggui (Spleen 1), date (red or black) (Spleen 4), day lily (Spleen 0), dill seed (Spleen 6), eel (Spleen 4), eggplant (Spleen 0), fig (Spleen 2), garlic (Spleen 6), ginger (dried) (Spleen 8), ginger (fresh) (Spleen 6), ginseng (Spleen 1), goose meat (Spleen 2), gorgan fruit (Spleen 2), grapefruit peel (Spleen 3), grape (Spleen 0), hairtail (Spleen 4), ham (Spleen -1), hawthorn fruit (Spleen 2), herring (Spleen 2), honey (Spleen 2), hyacinth bean (Spleen 2), hyacinth-bean flower (Spleen 2), Japanese cassia bark (Spleen 6), Job's tears (Spleen 0), lard (Spleen 0), licorice (Spleen 2), litchi nut (Spleen 2), loach (Spleen 2), longevity fruit (Spleen 0), longan (Spleen 4), long-kissing sturgeon (Spleen 2), long-tailed anchovy (Spleen 4), loquat (Spleen -2), lotus (fruit, seed, and root) (Spleen 2), lotus-rhizome powder (Spleen -1), mackerel (Spleen 2), malt (Spleen 4), maltose (Spleen 4), mandarin orange (Spleen -2), mandarin-orange peel (dry) (Spleen 2), mango (Spleen -2), milk (mare's) (Spleen 0), millet (Spleen 2), mung bean sprouts (Spleen -2), murrel (snakehead) (Spleen -2), mutton (Spleen 4), nutmeg (Spleen 6), onion (Spleen 6), oxtail (Spleen 1), papaya (Spleen 2), pea (Spleen 2), peanut (Spleen 2), pearl sago (Spleen 4), perch (Spleen 2), pheasant (Spleen 2), pineapple (Spleen 0), pistachio nut (Spleen 7), polished rice (Spleen 2), pork (Spleen -1), potato (Irish) (Spleen 2), prickly ash (Spleen 6), radish leaf (Spleen 0), rape (Spleen 2), red or green pepper (chili pepper or cayenne pepper) (Spleen 2), rock sugar (Spleen 2), royal jelly (Spleen 2), shark's fin (Spleen -1), shrimp (Spleen 4), silver carp (Spleen 4), sorghum (Spleen 4), sour date (Spleen 0), soybean (black) (Spleen 2), soybean (yellow) (Spleen 2), soybean sprouts (yellow) (Spleen 4), squash (Spleen 4), star anise (Spleen 5), strawberry (Spleen -2), string bean (Spleen 2), sweet basil (Spleen 6), sweet potato (Spleen -2), trifoliate orange (Spleen -2), wheat (Spleen 0), white eel (Spleen 2), white sugar (Spleen 2), whitebait (Spleen 2), wild cabbage (Spleen 2), wild rice gall (Spleen -2), yam (Spleen 2).

Generally Beneficial Foods and Other Foods to Be Chosen or Avoided. 1. Foods that are normally beneficial for this syndrome are apple cucumber, beef, carp (gold), carrot, chestnut, corn cob, date (red or black), Irish potato, Job's tears, longan nut, mandarin fish, rice, royal jelly, string bean, and yam. 2. Choose from among these digestible foods: areca nut (unripe), asafetida, bog bean (buck bean), buckwheat, cardamom seed, carrot, chicken gizzard, coriander (Chinese parsley), coriander seed, dill seed, distillers' grains, grapefruit (including peel), green-onion white head, hawthorn fruit, jackfruit, kiwifruit (Chinese gooseberry), lime (young trifoliate orange), lobster (sea prawn), longan seed, malt, millet sprouts, orange peel (sweet or sour), papaya, peach, quince, radish, red bay-berry, sorghum, soybean (yellow), sweet basil, tomato, water chest-nut, and whitefish. 3. Choose from these tonic foods for the spleen and pancreas: apple cucumber, beef, bird's nest, black-eyed pea, broomcorn, caraway seed, carp gall (grass), carrot, cassia bark (Japanese), cherry leaf, chestnut, cinnamon bark (cassia), corn cob, crown daisy, date (red or black), dill seed, frog (pond), garlic, ham, horse bean (broad bean, fava bean), hyacinth bean (lablab bean), hyacinth-bean flower, Job's tears (root), longan, lotus (fruit and seed), mullet (black or striped), pearl sago, perch, pheasant, pine-apple, pistachio nut, pork pancreas, rice (glutinous, sweet, or pol-ished), rice sprouts, royal jelly, string bean, white string bean, whitefish, and yam. 4. Choose from these energy-tonic foods: beef, bird's nest, broomcorn, cherry, chicken, coconut meat, crane meat, date (red or black), eel, ginkgo (cooked), ginseng, goose meat, grape, herring, honey, jackfruit, loach, longan, mackerel, mandarin fish, octopus, pheasant, pigeon egg, pigeon meat, potato (Irish), rabbit, rice (fermented, glutinous), rice (glutinous or sweet), rice (polished), rice (polished, long-grain), rock sugar, shark's fin, sheep or goat meat, shiitake mushroom, snake melon, squash, sturgeon, sweet potato, tofu, turtledove, walnut root, and white string bean. 5. Avoid these hot and spicy items: alcohol, chili pepper (cayenne pepper), chive (Chinese), cinnamon bark (cassia), cinnamon twig, clove, coffee, garlic, ginger (fresh or dried), green onion (leaf and white head), mustard seed, nutmeg, onion, pepper (black or white), tea, and wine. They force yin energy to excrete through perspira-tion, which is harmful to both yin and energy. 6. Avoid these irri-tants: alcohol, coffee, tea, tobacco, and wine. They can irritate the stomach and produce damp heat, and fire is harmful to yin and energy.

Beneficial Herbs to Be Applied One Herb at a Time. Bai zhu (Rhizoma Atractylodis Macrocephalae), 11 g; chai hu (Radix Bupleuri), 16 g; chen pi (Pericarpium Citri Reticulatae), 11 g; dang shen (Radix Codonopsis Pilosulae), 15 g; gan cao (Radix Gly-cyrrhizae), 11 g; huang qi (Radix Astragali Seu Hedysari), 40 g; shan yao (Rhizoma Dioscoreae), 20 g; sheng ma (Rhizoma Cimi-cifugae), 10 g.

Beneficial Herbal Formulas to Be Applied One Formula at a Time. Bu Zhong Yi Qi Tang, Huang Qi Jian zhong Tang, Ju Yuan Jian, Sheng Ma Huang Qi Tang.

7.4 Spleen Unable to Govern Blood (Spleen Deficiency and Cold)

When you are in good health, your y-score is Spleen -4; when you are ill, your y-score is Spleen -8.

Definition of the Syndrome. This syndrome is basically due to a deficient spleen that is unable to control the blood, so the blood escapes from the vessels, causing bleeding. Spleen Unable to Govern Blood can be seen in various types of bleeding, such as functional bleeding from the uterus, bleeding from the anus, and hemorrhage diseases like thrombocytopenia purpura and allergic purpura.

In traditional Chinese medicine, a distinction is drawn between bleeding right after a bowel movement, which is called "distant bleeding," and bleeding before a bowel movement, which is called "local bleeding." Distant bleeding refers to bleeding that occurs in the small intestine or the stomach, whereas local bleeding concerns bleeding that takes place in the sigmoidorectum or the anus. The blood from distant bleeding normally looks dark or black, whereas the blood from local bleeding looks fresh and red. Distant bleeding is due to a deficient and cold spleen and stomach; because of this, the spleen cannot control the blood that is excreted after a bowel movement. Local bleeding is normally caused by irregular eating, intoxication, and the consumption of hot and spicy foods, all of which generate heat in the blood so that the blood escapes from the vessels just prior to a bowel movement.

Clinical Signs and Symptoms. Major signs: Bleeding in small quantity, blood in urine, discharge of blood from the anus, excessive menstrual bleeding. Median signs: Poor appetite, stomach and abdomen swelling and fullness, discharge of sticky and muddy stools or diarrhea. Minor signs: Dizziness, mentally fatigued, palpitations, purely white complexion, shortness of breath, withered and yellowish complexion.

Applicable Western Diseases. Anaphylactoid purpura, aplastic anemia, bleeding in gastric and duodenalbulbar ulcer, functional metrorrhagia, purpura hemorrhagica (Werlhof's disease), thrombocytopenia purpura (thrombopenic purpura), tinea versicolor.

Treatment Symptoms. Bleeding, discharge of blood from the anus, vaginal bleeding.

Clinical Cases. (1) A forty-year-old male patient named Xu displayed bleeding from the anus right after a bowel movement, with the blood appearing dark or black; he also showed signs of abdominal swelling and of dizziness triggered by movement. A Chinese doctor diagnosed his condition as Spleen Unable to Govern Blood, mainly because of the bleeding that occurred after the bowel movement and also because abdominal swelling points to this syndrome. (2) At age fifty-one, Lao was still having a menstrual period every month, with heavy bleeding lasting longer than usual, as well as a whitish vaginal discharge. In March of this year, she suddenly experienced heavy bleeding right after her period was over. Other symptoms included low spirits, her four limbs' lacking warmth, soft stools, a whitish coating on the tongue, and puffiness in the face, around the eyes, and at the ankles. A Chinese doctor diagnosed her condition as Spleen Unable to Govern Blood, primarily because menstruation at this age is a distinct sign of this syndrome and is supported by heavy bleeding after the period.

Treatment Principles. To warm and tone spleen energy in order to stop the bleeding.

Foods Chosen Based on Y-Scores. Autumn bottle gourd (Spleen 2), bean curd (Spleen 0), beef (Spleen 2), blood clam (Spleen 4), broad bean (horse bean) (Spleen 2), broomcorn (Spleen 2), brown sugar (Spleen 4), buckwheat (Spleen 0), carp (common) (Spleen 2), carp (gold) (Spleen 2), carp (grass) (Spleen 4), carrot (Spleen 2), cherry (Spleen 4), chestnut (Spleen 4), chicken (Spleen 4), chili pepper (cayenne pepper) (Spleen 8), cinnamon bark (Spleen 7), clove (Spleen 6), clove oil (Spleen 7), coconut meat (Spleen 2), coriander (Chinese parsley) (Spleen 6), crown daisy (Spleen 6), cucumber (Spleen 0), danggui (Spleen 1), date (red or black) (Spleen 4), day lily (Spleen 0), dill seed (Spleen 6), eel (Spleen 4), eggplant (Spleen 0), fig (Spleen 2), garlic (Spleen 6), ginger (dried) (Spleen 8), ginger (fresh) (Spleen 6), ginseng (Spleen 1), goose meat (Spleen 2), gorgan fruit (Spleen 2), grapefruit peel (Spleen 3), grape (Spleen 0), hairtail (Spleen 4), hawthorn fruit (Spleen 2), herring (Spleen 2), honey (Spleen 2), hyacinth bean (Spleen 2), hyacinth-bean flower (Spleen 2), Japanese cassia bark (Spleen 6), Job's tears (Spleen 0), lard (Spleen 0), licorice (Spleen 2), litchi nut (Spleen 2), loach (Spleen 2), longevity fruit (Spleen 0), longan (Spleen 4), long-kissing sturgeon (Spleen 2), long-tailed anchovy (Spleen 4), lotus (fruit, seed, and root) (Spleen 2), mackerel (Spleen 2), malt (Spleen 4), maltose (Spleen 4), mandarin-orange peel (dry) (Spleen 2), milk (mare's) (Spleen 0), millet (Spleen 2), mutton (Spleen 4), nutmeg (Spleen 6), onion (Spleen 6), oxtail (Spleen 1), papaya (Spleen 2), pea (Spleen 2), peanut (Spleen 2), pearl sago (Spleen 4), perch (Spleen 2), pheasant (Spleen 2), pineapple (Spleen 0), pistachio nut (Spleen 7), polished rice (Spleen 2), potato (Irish) (Spleen 2), prickly ash (Spleen 6), radish leaf (Spleen 0), rape (Spleen 2), red or green pepper (chili pepper or cayenne pepper) (Spleen 2), rock sugar (Spleen 2), royal jelly (Spleen 2), shrimp (Spleen 4), silver carp (Spleen 4), sorghum (Spleen 4), sour date (Spleen 0), soybean (black) (Spleen 2), soybean (yellow) (Spleen 2), soybean sprouts (yellow) (Spleen 4), squash (Spleen 4), star anise (Spleen 5), string bean (Spleen 2), sweet basil (Spleen 6), wheat (Spleen 0), white eel (Spleen 2), white sugar (Spleen 2), whitebait (Spleen 2), wild cabbage (Spleen 2), yam (Spleen 2).

Generally Beneficial Foods and Other Foods to Be Chosen or Avoided. 1. Foods that are usually good for this syndrome are apple cucumber, bog bean, carp (gold), carrot, chestnut, chicken, chicken egg yolk, date (red or black), grape, ham, horse bean, hyacinth bean, Irish potato, Job's tears, longan nut, maltose, mandarin fish, mutton, rock sugar, royal jelly, squash, string bean, sweet rice, whitefish, and yam. 2. Choose from among the following tonic foods for the spleen and pancreas: apple cucumber, beef, bird's nest, black-eyed pea, broomcorn, caraway seed, carp gall (grass), carrot, cassia bark (Japanese), cherry leaf, chestnut, cinnamon bark (cassia), corn cob, crown daisy, date (red or black), dill seed, frog (pond), garlic, ham, horse bean (broad bean, fava bean), hyacinth bean (lablab bean), hyacinth-bean flower, Job's tears (root), longan, lotus (fruit and seed), mullet (black or striped), pearl sago, perch, pheasant, pine-apple, pistachio nut, pork pancreas, rice (glutinous, sweet, or polished), rice sprouts, royal jelly, string bean, white string bean, whitefish, and yam. 3. Avoid these hot and spicy items: alcohol, chili pepper (cayenne pepper), chive (Chinese), cinnamon bark (cassia), cinnamon twig, clove, coffee, garlic, ginger (fresh or dried), green onion (leaf and white head), mustard seed, nutmeg, onion, pepper (black or white), tea, and wine. They force yin energy to excrete through perspiration, which is harmful to both yin and energy.

Beneficial Herbs to Be Applied One Herb at a Time. Bai zhu (Rhizoma Atractylodis Macrocephalae), 11 g; da zao (Fructus Ziziphi Jujubae), 18 g; dang gui (Radix Angelicae Sinensis), 11 g; dang shen (Radix Codonopsis Pilosulae), 15 g; fu long gan (Terra

Flava Usta), 35 g; fu shen (Buyury with Pine Root), 15 g; gan cao (Radix Glycyrrhizae), 11 g; huang qi (Radix Astragali Seu Hedysari), 40 g; long yan rou (Arillus Longan), 11 g.

Beneficial Herbal Formulas to Be Applied One Formula at a Time. Gui Pi Tang, Huang Tu Tang, Jiao Ai Tang, Wen Jing She Xue Tang.

7.5 *Cold Dampness Troubling the Spleen (Dampness Troubling Spleen Yang)*

When you are in good health, your y-score is Spleen -3; when you are ill, your y-score is Spleen -7.

Definition of the Syndrome. The spleen is related to the earth, and it loves dryness and dislikes dampness. Cold dampness can invade the spleen when we walk in rain, swim in water, or consume an excessive amount of cold foods, or when dampness is produced inside the body itself.

Cold dampness obstructs the normal function of the spleen in digesting and mobilizing food, which accounts for the discomfort in the stomach and the abdomen as well as the poor appetite. An excessive accumulation of water in the body causes the heavy sensations and the edema in addition to the short streams of urine. The spleen fails to produce sufficient energy and blood to nourish the face, which gives rise to the dark, yellowish complexion.

Clinical Signs and Symptoms. Major signs: Discomfort in the stomach and the abdomen, poor appetite, discharge of watery stools, nausea, sticky and greasy sensation in the mouth, heavy sensation in the head and the body as a whole. Median signs: Absence of thirst, diarrhea, discharge of soft stools, mild stomachache, overweight. Minor signs: Abdominal pain with discharge of watery stools, dark and yellowish complexion, edema in the four limbs, short streams of urine, excessive whitish vaginal discharge, pale and fat tongue.

Applicable Western Diseases. Acute enteritis, ascites due to cirrhosis, cholera, jaundice, viral hepatitis.

Treatment Symptoms. Vomiting, diarrhea, jaundice, edema.

Clinical Cases. (1) A fifty-two-year-old male patient named Chou had four to five bowel movements every day, with a discharge of thin and watery stools. He experienced no abdominal pain, but had a poor appetite. A Chinese doctor diagnosed his condition as

Cold Dampness Troubling the Spleen mainly because of his watery stools and poor appetite. (2) Wong, a twenty-six-year-old male patient, developed a dark and yellowish complexion, including the region around the eyes, and a poor appetite. He was diagnosed in a Western hospital as having viral hepatitis. A Chinese doctor diagnosed his condition as Cold Dampness Troubling the Spleen primarily because of his dark and yellowish skin. (3) Chung, age forty-eight, was a male patient who was in the habit of drinking cold water and lying in a cool and windy place during the hot months of the summer, which apparently prevented him from perspiring. However, this resulted in an accumulation of damp heat inside his body. As time went on, he gradually developed a dark and yellowish cast to his complexion, including the area around the eyes, and to the skin all over his body. He reported feeling neither hot nor thirsty, having soft stools and clear urine, and feeling fatigued and wanting to lie down. A Chinese doctor diagnosed his condition as Cold Dampness Troubling the Spleen mostly because of his yellowish skin, soft stools, and clear urine, all of which are important signs of this syndrome.

Treatment Principles. To warm the middle region and transform dampness.

Foods Chosen Based on Y-Scores. Apple: (Spleen -2), autumn bottle gourd (Spleen 2), banana (Spleen -2), bean curd (Spleen 0), beef (Spleen 2), blood clam (Spleen 4), broad bean (horse bean) (Spleen 2), broomcorn (Spleen 2), brown sugar (Spleen 4), buckwheat (Spleen 0), carp (common) (Spleen 2), carp (gold) (Spleen 2), carp (grass) (Spleen 4), carrot (Spleen 2), cherry (Spleen 4), chestnut (Spleen 4), chicken (Spleen 4), chili pepper (cayenne pepper) (Spleen 8), cinnamon bark (Spleen 7), clove (Spleen 6), clove oil (Spleen 7), coconut meat (Spleen 2), coriander (Chinese parsley) (Spleen 6), crown daisy (Spleen 6), cucumber (Spleen 0), danggui (Spleen 1), date (red or black) (Spleen 4), day lily (Spleen 0), dill seed (Spleen 6), eel (Spleen 4), eggplant (Spleen 0), fig (Spleen 2), garlic (Spleen 6), ginger (dried) (Spleen 8), ginger (fresh) (Spleen 6), ginseng (Spleen 1), goose meat (Spleen 2), gorgan fruit (Spleen 2), grapefruit peel (Spleen 3), grape (Spleen 0), hairtail (Spleen 4), ham (Spleen -1), hawthorn fruit (Spleen 2), herring (Spleen 2), honey (Spleen 2), hyacinth bean (Spleen 2), hyacinth-bean flower (Spleen 2), Japanese cassia bark (Spleen 6), Job's tears (Spleen 0), lard (Spleen 0), licorice (Spleen 2), litchi nut

(Spleen 2), loach (Spleen 2), longevity fruit (Spleen 0), longan (Spleen 4), long-kissing sturgeon (Spleen 2), long-tailed anchovy (Spleen 4), loquat (Spleen -2), lotus (fruit, seed, and root) (Spleen 2), lotus-rhizome powder (Spleen -1), mackerel (Spleen 2), malt (Spleen 4), maltose (Spleen 4), mandarin orange (Spleen -2), mandarin-orange peel (dry) (Spleen 2), mango (Spleen -2), milk (mare's) (Spleen 0), millet (Spleen 2), mung bean sprouts (Spleen -2), murrel (snakehead) (Spleen -2), mutton (Spleen 4), nutmeg (Spleen 6), onion (Spleen 6), oxtail (Spleen 1), papaya (Spleen 2), pea (Spleen 2), peanut (Spleen 2), pearl sago (Spleen 4), perch (Spleen 2), pheasant (Spleen 2), pineapple (Spleen 0), pistachio nut (Spleen 7), polished rice (Spleen 2), pork (Spleen -1), potato (Irish) (Spleen 2), prickly ash (Spleen 6), radish leaf (Spleen 0), rape (Spleen 2), red or green pepper (chili pepper or cayenne pepper) (Spleen 2), rock sugar (Spleen 2), royal jelly (Spleen 2), shark's fin (Spleen -1), shrimp (Spleen 4), silver carp (Spleen 4), sorghum (Spleen 4), sour date (Spleen 0), soybean (black) (Spleen 2), soybean (yellow) (Spleen 2), soybean sprouts (yellow) (Spleen 4), squash (Spleen 4), star anise (Spleen 5), strawberry (Spleen -2), string bean (Spleen 2), sweet basil (Spleen 6), sweet potato (Spleen -2), trifoliate orange (Spleen -2), wheat (Spleen 0), white eel (Spleen 2), white sugar (Spleen 2), whitebait (Spleen 2), wild cabbage (Spleen 2), wild rice gall (Spleen -2), yam (Spleen 2).

Generally Beneficial Foods and Other Foods to Be Chosen or Avoided. 1. Avoid the following cold foods: adzuki bean, aloe vera, asparagus (lucid), bamboo shoots, banana, bitter endive, bitter gourd (balsam pear), brake (fern), burdock, camphor mint, cattail, crab, endive (Chinese), fig, frog (pond), grapefruit, hair vegetable, honey, leaf beet (spinach beet, Swiss chard), lemon, lily flower, mung bean, mung-bean powder, mung bean sprouts, orchid leaf, peppermint, potato (Irish), preserved duck egg, pricking amaranth (amaranth, pigweed), purslane, rabbit, rambutan, romaine lettuce, Russian olive (oleaster), safflower fruit, salt, soybean paste, squash, star fruit (carambola), strawberry (Indian or mock), sweet basil, tofu, water spinach, wax gourd (Chinese), and wheat. 2. Choose from these water-eliminating foods: adzuki bean, bitter bamboo shoots, broad bean (shell), caper, carp (gold), carp gall (grass), celery, corn cob, cuttlebone, duck, fenugreek seed (Oriental), frog (river or pond), ginger peel, ginkgo leaf, grapefruit leaf, horse bean (broad bean, fava bean), hyacinth bean (dried outer skin), hyacinth bean (lablab bean), hyacinth-bean flower, Job's tears, kelp, loach, lotus (flower, leaf, and leaf base), mackerel, mallow seed, marjoram, oregano (wild), peach blossom, plantain, prickly ash, radish root (old and dried), raspberry leaf, rice (polished, long-grain), rosin, sea grass, seaweed, shepherd's purse, soybean (yellow), sweet basil, tangerine peel, taro (flower and stalk), tea oil, tea-seed residue, and watercress (water celery). 3. Choose from these yang-tonic foods for the kidneys: air bladder of shark, beef kidney, cassia fruit (Japanese), chestnut, chive seed (Chinese), cinnamon bark (cassia), clove, clove oil, deer kidney, dill seed, fennel (root and seed), fenugreek seed (Oriental), green-onion seed, lobster (sea prawn), mandarin-orange seed, oxtail, pistachio nut, pork testes, prickly ash root, raspberry, sheep or goat kidney, shrimp, sparrow egg, star anise, strawberry, and sword bean (jack bean).

Beneficial Herbs to Be Applied One Herb at a Time. Ban xia (Rhizoma Pinelliae), 12 g; cang zhu (Rhizoma Atractylodis), 11 g; cao guo (Fructus Tsaoko), 5 g; chen pi (Pericarpium Citri Reticulatae), 11 g; fu ling (Poria), 14 g; gui zhi (Ramulus Cinnamomi), 10 g; hou po (Cortex Magnoliae Officinalis), 11 g; huo xiang (Herba Agastachis), 11 g; pei lan (Herba Eupatorii), 11 g.

Beneficial Herbal Formulas to Be Applied One Formula at a Time. Huo Xiang Zheng Qi San, Ling Gui Zhu Gan Tang, Ping Wei San.

7.6 Damp Heat Steaming the Spleen

When you are in good health, your y-score is Spleen 2; when you are ill, your y-score is Spleen 6.

Definition of the Syndrome. When dampness and heat team up to attack the middle *jiao*, this can cause spleen damp heat. (*Jiao* is a Chinese word meaning "burner," "burning space," or "heater," depending on the translation, but it would be safe to say that middle *jiao* refers to the middle heater that covers the abdominal cavity.) The attack occurs primarily because of an excessive consumption of greasy foods and alcohol, as well as the accumulation of spices in the spleen.

When dampness and heat get mixed together, they become difficult to separate, and the mixture cannot be excreted from the body. Instead, it tends to stay inside the body, steaming the gallbladder with bile boiling and overflowing, which accounts for the itchy skin and the complexion and the eyes' taking on the color of a fresh orange. The symptoms of this syndrome are either symptoms of dampness or those of heat or symptoms of both dampness and heat.

Clinical Signs and Symptoms. Major signs: Abdominal swelling, the complexion and the eyes' becoming the color of a fresh orange, congested sensation in the stomach and the abdomen, no appetite, dislike of greasy foods. Median signs: Bitter taste in the mouth, discharge of red urine with urination difficulty, constipation or difficult bowel movements with discharge of watery stool, thirst with no desire to drink. Minor signs: Fever that comes and goes and persists after perspiration, heavy sensation in the body, itchy skin, red tongue.

Applicable Western Diseases. Acute hepatitis with jaundice, acute cholecystitis, acute viral jaundice type of hepatitis, eczema, pustules.

Treatment Symptoms. Yellowish-orange appearance of face and eyes, diarrhea, edema.

Clinical Cases. (1) Upon a visit to a doctor of traditional Chinese medicine, Sun, a fifty-six-year-old man, reported having a yellowish-orange cast to his face and eyes for a week and a temperature of 38 degrees C (100.4 degrees F) six days before. Although his temperature is now normal, he has the following symptoms: nausea, a poor appetite, yellowish-orange skin all over his body and face, phlegm in his throat, reddish-yellow urine, and dry stools. Sun had been diagnosed previously by a Western physician as having an acute viral jaundice type of hepatitis. The Chinese doctor diagnosed his condition as Damp Heat Steaming the Spleen primarily on account of the yellowish-orange appearance of his face and eyes. (2) Zhao, a female patient who is fifty-two years old, reported having suffered from fatigue six months before, and now displays a yellowish-orange cast to her body and face, a prickling itch all over her body, nausea with a poor appetite, abdominal distention, insomnia, and yellowish urine. At a Western hospital, she was diagnosed as having an acute viral jaundice type of hepatitis. A Chinese doctor diagnosed her condition as Damp Heat Steaming the Spleen mainly because of the yellowish-orange appearance of her face and eyes as well as her yellowish urine, itchy skin, and distended abdomen. (3) A heavy drinker, Ling, age sixty-four, could drink a lot and still not get intoxicated. In June, when the weather was hot and humid, he developed severe jaundice after a bout of drinking, with the following additional symptoms: a high fever that would not subside, a yellowish-orange cast to his face and eyes as well as to his entire body, thirst with a craving to drink, constipation, and retention of urine. The symptoms gradually worsened to the point that he became totally bedridden. A Chinese doctor diagnosed his condition as Damp Heat Steaming the Spleen, chiefly because an excessive consumption of alcohol will give rise to damp heat in the spleen, which is supported by many other symptoms, including a yellowish-orange cast to the skin and retention of urine.

Treatment Principles. To clear up damp heat in the spleen.

Foods Chosen Based on Y-Scores. Autumn bottle gourd (Spleen 2), bean curd (Spleen 0), beef (Spleen 2), blood clam (Spleen 4), broad bean (horse bean) (Spleen 2), broomcorn (Spleen 2), brown sugar (Spleen 4), buckwheat (Spleen 0), carp (common) (Spleen 2), carp (gold) (Spleen 2), carp (grass) (Spleen 4), carrot (Spleen 2), cherry (Spleen 4), chestnut (Spleen 4), chicken (Spleen 4), chili pepper (cayenne pepper) (Spleen 8), cinnamon bark (Spleen 7), clove (Spleen 6), clove oil (Spleen 7), coconut meat (Spleen 2), coriander (Chinese parsley) (Spleen 6), crown daisy (Spleen 6), cucumber (Spleen 0), danggui (Spleen 1), date (red or black) (Spleen 4), day lily (Spleen 0), dill seed (Spleen 6), eel (Spleen 4), eggplant (Spleen 0), fig (Spleen 2), garlic (Spleen 6), ginger (dried) (Spleen 8), ginger (fresh) (Spleen 6), ginseng (Spleen 1), goose meat (Spleen 2), gorgan fruit (Spleen 2), grapefruit peel (Spleen 3), grape (Spleen 0), hairtail (Spleen 4), ham (Spleen -1), hawthorn fruit (Spleen 2), herring (Spleen 2), honey (Spleen 2), hyacinth bean (Spleen 2), hyacinth-bean flower (Spleen 2), Japanese cassia bark (Spleen 6), Job's tears (Spleen 0), lard (Spleen 0), licorice (Spleen 2), litchi nut (Spleen 2), loach (Spleen 2), longevity fruit (Spleen 0), longan (Spleen 4), long-kissing sturgeon (Spleen 2), long-tailed anchovy (Spleen 4), lotus (fruit, seed, and root) (Spleen 2), lotus- rhizome powder (Spleen -1), mackerel (Spleen 2), malt (Spleen 4), maltose (Spleen 4), mandarin-orange peel (dry) (Spleen 2), milk (mare's) (Spleen 0), millet (Spleen 2), mutton (Spleen 4), nutmeg (Spleen 6), onion (Spleen 6), oxtail (Spleen 1), papaya (Spleen 2), pea (Spleen 2), peanut (Spleen 2), pearl sago (Spleen 4), perch (Spleen 2), pheasant (Spleen 2), pineapple (Spleen 0), pistachio nut (Spleen 7), polished rice (Spleen 2), pork (Spleen -1), potato (Irish) (Spleen 2), prickly ash (Spleen 6), radish leaf (Spleen 0), rape (Spleen 2), red or green pepper (chili pepper or cayenne pepper) (Spleen 2), rock sugar (Spleen 2), royal jelly (Spleen 2), shark's fin (Spleen -1), shrimp (Spleen 4), silver carp (Spleen 4), sorghum (Spleen 4), sour date (Spleen 0), soybean (black) (Spleen 2), soybean (yellow) (Spleen 2), soybean sprouts (yellow) (Spleen 4), squash (Spleen 4), star anise (Spleen 5), star fruit (carambola) (Spleen -4), string bean (Spleen 2), sweet basil (Spleen 6), wheat (Spleen 0), white eel (Spleen 2), white sugar (Spleen 2), whitebait (Spleen 2), wild cabbage (Spleen 2), yam (Spleen 2).

Generally Beneficial Foods and Other Foods to Be Chosen or Avoided. 1. Choose from these foods that are good for damp heat: adzuki bean sprouts, buckwheat, cantaloupe (muskmelon), carp (common), celery root, Chinese cabbage, coconut (shell), corn silk, cucumber vine (stem), day lily, eggplant (aubergine), eggplant calyx, fig leaf, frog (river or pond), green turtle, hawthorn fruit, olive, pricking amaranth (amaranth, pigweed), soybean oil, soybean sprouts (dried, black), soybean (yellow), squash (flower and root), star fruit (carambola), sunflower (top of peduncle), turnip seed, water-rice root, wax gourd (Chinese), and wheat seedling. 2. Avoid items that are likely to trigger a chronic damp heat syndrome or intensify an existing one, such as alcohol, maltose, pork, and sweet rice.

Beneficial Herbs to Be Applied One Herb at a Time. Cang zhu (Rhizoma Atractylodis), 11 g; che qian zi (Semen Plantaginis), 11 g; da huang (Radix Et Rhizoma Rhei), 15 g; fu ling (Poria), 14 g; huang bai (Cortex Phellodendri), 15 g; yin chen (Herba Artemisiae Scopariae), 21 g; ze xie (Rhizoma Alismatis), 14 g; zhi zi (Fructus Gardeniae), 16 g; zhu ling (Polyporus Umbellatus [Grifola]), 14 g.

Beneficial Herbal Formulas to Be Applied One Formula at a Time. Si Ling San, Yin Chen Hao Tang.

8

Choosing Foods and Herbs to Boost the Stomach and Cure Applicable Symptoms and Diseases

8.1 Stomach Yin Deficiency (Stomach Deficient Heat)

When you are in good health, your y-score is Stomach 3; when you are ill, your y-score is Stomach 7.

Definition of the Syndrome. Stomach Yin Deficiency means that there is insufficient yin energy in the stomach that can be due to a chronic illness that consumes yin fluids, stomach heat that eats up stomach yin, liver heat that burns up stomach yin, or heart fire that harms stomach yin.

The stomach desires moisture, and it dislikes dryness. Stomach Yin Deficiency produces dryness, which accounts for the dry symptoms, the feeling of hunger with no appetite, and the constipation; this syndrome also generates heat, which is the cause of the burning pain in the stomach.

Clinical Signs and Symptoms. Major signs: Mild stomachache, stomachache with burning pain, dry mouth, dry throat, hungry with no appetite, dry lips, dry sensation in the mouth. Median signs: Abdominal swelling after a meal, discharge of dry stools, dry vomiting, hiccups, dry tongue. Minor signs: Constipation, dry cough, indigestion, light tidal fever or low fever, dry vomiting, vomiting of blood.

Applicable Western Diseases. Chronic gastritis, diabetes mellitus, dysphagia, gastric neurosis, muguet, peptic ulcer, phrenospasm.

Treatment Symptoms. Stomachache, hiccups, swallowing difficulty.

125

Clinical Cases. (1) A fifty-year-old female patient named Sing was diagnosed as having atrophic gastritis and displayed the following symptoms: mild stomachache all day long that gets better on consuming sweet and sour foods but recurs easily, dry mouth, dry stools, and red color of the tongue. A Chinese doctor diagnosed her condition as Stomach Yin Deficiency primarily due to her mild stomachache and number of dry symptoms. (2) Having suffered from a stomachache for three years, Lee, a twenty-nine-year-old male patient, had been hospitalized twice and was diagnosed as having a peptic ulcer. When he came in for an examination at a Chinese medicine clinic, his symptoms included a burning pain in the stomach, feeling hungry with no desire to eat, belching, a dry mouth, and constipation. At the clinic, his condition was diagnosed as Stomach Yin Deficiency, chiefly because he was hungry but had no interest in eating, he had a burning pain in his stomach, and he had dry symptoms. (3) Zhang, a thirty-eight-year-old female patient, suffered a penicillin-allergy shock and displayed the following symptoms after emergency treatment: nervousness and tension beyond control, a loss of appetite, a dry mouth, fatigue, dry stools, and the tongue as shiny as a mirror. These symptoms lasted more than a month. She was subsequently diagnosed by a doctor of Western medicine as having vegetative nerve functional disturbance. After that, a Chinese doctor diagnosed her condition as Stomach Yin Deficiency mainly because of her dry symptoms and loss of appetite.

Treatment Principles. To nourish stomach yin, clear stomach heat, and benefit the stomach.

Foods Chosen Based on Y-Scores. Areca nut (Stomach -2), asparagus (Stomach 1), bamboo shoots (Stomach -2), banana (Stomach -2), barley (Stomach -3), bean curd (Stomach 0), beef (Spleen 2, Stomach 2), bird's nest (Stomach 2), bitter gourd (balsam pear) (Stomach -8), black-bean seed (processed) (Stomach -8), black fungus (Stomach 2), broad bean (Spleen 2, Stomach 2), brome seed (Stomach 0), broomcorn (faxtail millet) (Stomach 2), buckwheat (Stomach 0), celery (Stomach -1), Chinese cabbage (Stomach 2), Chinese toon leaf (Stomach -4), coconut (Stomach 2), common button mushroom (Stomach 0), corn (Stomach 2), cow's milk (Stomach 2), crab (Stomach -7), cucumber (Stomach 0), eggplant (Stomach 0), gold carp (Stomach 2), hami melon (Stomach -2), hawthorn fruit (Stomach 2), hyacinth bean (Stomach 2), kiwifruit (Stomach -4), lard (Stomach 0), lettuce (Stomach -2), ling (Stomach 0), mackerel (Stomach 2), mandarin fish (Stomach 2), mandarin orange (Stomach -2), mango (Stomach -2), mung bean (Stomach 0), mung bean sprouts (Stomach -2), murrel (snakehead) (Stomach -2), muskmelon (cantaloupe) (Stomach -2), olive (Stomach 0), papaya (Stomach 2), pea (Stomach 2), peach (Stomach 2), pear (Stomach -2), pineapple (Stomach 0), polished rice (Stomach 2), pomegranate (sour fruit) (Stomach 2), pork (Stomach -1), potato (Irish) (Stomach 2), radish (Stomach 1), red bayberry (Stomach 2), seaweed (marine alga) (Stomach -8), shiitake mushroom (Stomach 2), soy sauce (Spleen -7, Stomach -7), star fruit (carambola) (Stomach -4), sugarcane (Stomach -2), sweet potato (Stomach -2), tangerine (Stomach -2), tea (Heart -6, Stomach -6), tea melon (Stomach -2), tomato (Stomach -4), towel gourd (Stomach 0), vinegar (Stomach -1), water chestnut (Stomach -2), white cabbage (small) (Stomach 2), white fungus (Stomach 2), whitebait (Stomach 2), wild cabbage (Stomach 2), yam bean (Stomach 0), yellow croaker (Stomach -1).

Generally Beneficial Foods and Other Foods to Be Chosen or Avoided. 1. Foods that are often beneficial for this syndrome are abalone, alfalfa, asparagus, bird's nest, cheeses, chicken egg, cuttlefish, duck, duck egg, ginseng leaf, kidney bean, oyster, pork, royal jelly, and white fungus. 2. Choose from the following yin tonics: abalone, air bladder of shark, apple, apricot pit (sweet powder), asparagus (lucid), bean drink, bird's nest, bitter gourd (balsam pear), black-eyed pea, brown sugar, cantaloupe (muskmelon), cheeses, chicken egg, chicken eggshell (inner membrane), clam (saltwater or freshwater), coconut milk, crab, cuttlefish, date, duck, duck egg, fig, frog (river or pond), goose meat, grape, green turtle, honey, kidney bean, kumquat, lard, lemon, litchi nut, loquat (Japanese), lotus rhizome, maltose, mandarin orange, mango, milk (cow's), mussel, oyster, pea, pear, pearl (powder), pineapple, pomegranate (sweet fruit), pork, rabbit, red bayberry, rice (polished), royal jelly, sea cucumber, shrimp, star fruit (carambola), string bean, sugarcane, tofu, tomato, turtle egg, walnut, watermelon, white fungus, white sugar, whitebait, and yam. 3. Avoid these hot and spicy foods and drinks: alcohol, chili pepper (cayenne pepper), chive (Chinese), cinnamon bark (cassia), cinnamon twig, clove, coffee, garlic, ginger (fresh or dried), green onion (leaf and white head), mustard seed, nutmeg, onion, pepper (black or white), tea, and wine. They force yin energy to excrete through perspiration, which is harmful to both yin and energy.

Beneficial Herbs to Be Applied One Herb at a Time. Bai shao yao (Radix Paeoniae Alba), 11 g; gan cao (Radix Glycyrrhizae), 11 g; mai men dong (Radix Ophiopogonis), 11 g; shi hu (Herba Dendrobii), 14 g; yu zhu (Rhizoma Polygonati Odorati), 11 g.

Beneficial Herbal Formulas to Be Applied One Formula at a Time. Gan Lu Yin, Mai Men Dong Tang, Sha Shen Mai Dong Tang.

8.2 Food Stagnation in the Stomach (Stomach Energy Congestion)

When you are in good health, your y-score is Stomach -3; when you are ill, your y-score is Stomach -7.

Definition of the Syndrome. The stomach is the sea of water and grains, and it is in charge of digesting food. Irregular or excessive eating or chronic stomach deficiency can cause stomach indigestion. Energy congestion of the stomach due to indigestion accounts for the stomachache associated with this syndrome. Stomach energy should go down, but it goes up instead, because of the obstruction of food, causing the vomiting and belching. Decomposed foods move downward undigested, which leads to the offensive-smelling diarrhea.

Clinical Signs and Symptoms. Major signs: Swallowing acid and belching bad air, belching with poor appetite, stomachache. Median signs: Swelling of stomach and abdomen, vomiting of decomposed acid, belching, discharge of watery and thin stools or constipation, discharge of stools with an offensive smell. Minor signs: Fever and malnutrition in children, insomnia, sour and bad breath, vomiting and diarrhea in children, vomiting of sour-smelling foods with a desire for cold drink.

Applicable Western Diseases. Acute enteritis, acute gastroenteritis, acute intestinal obstruction, recurrent canker sores, tympanities.

Treatment Symptoms. Diarrhea, vomiting, indigestion, stomachache.

Clinical Cases. (1) A forty-five-year-old male patient named Ou said that he experienced abdominal distension and discomfort the previous night due to an excessive consumption of food and alcohol, and that the symptoms gradually intensified into the night until they became almost unbearable. He also said that the symptoms seemed to worsen on massage, with the belching of rotten-smelling foods. A Chinese doctor diagnosed his condition as Food Stagnation in the Stomach, primarily because the symptoms developed after eating and belching points to this syndrome as well. (2) As a result of overeating, a fifty-seven-year-old female patient named Lin experienced a swollen stomach, swallowing of acid with belching of bad air, a poor appetite, and loose stools for more than a month. She was diagnosed in a Western hospital as having acute gastroenteritis, but a Chinese doctor diagnosed her condition as Food Stagnation in the Stomach.

Treatment Principles. To promote digestion.

Foods Chosen Based on Y-Scores. Asparagus (Stomach 1), bean curd (Stomach 0), beef (Stomach 2), bird's nest (Stomach 2), bitter gourd (balsam pear) (Stomach -8), black and white pepper (Stomach 8), black fungus (Stomach 2), blood clam (Stomach 4), broad bean (Stomach 2), brome seed (Stomach 0), broomcorn (faxtail millet) (Stomach 2), brown sugar (Stomach 4), buckwheat (Stomach 0), catfish (Stomach 4), chestnut (Stomach 4), chicken (Stomach 4), Chinese cabbage (Stomach 2), coconut (Stomach 2), common button mushroom (Stomach 0), corn (Stomach 2), cow's milk (Stomach 2), crown daisy (Stomach 8), cucumber (Stomach 0), eggplant (Stomach 0), fresh ginger (Stomach 6), freshwater shrimp (Stomach 4), garlic (Stomach 6), ginkgo (Stomach 6), gold carp (Stomach 2), grass carp (Stomach 4), green-onion white head (Stomach 6), hawthorn fruit (Stomach 2), hyacinth bean (Stomach 2), lard (Stomach 0), leaf or brown mustard (Stomach 6), ling (Stomach 0), mackerel (Stomach 2), maltose (Stomach 4), mandarin fish (Stomach 2), mung bean (Stomach 0), mutton (Stomach 4), olive (Stomach 0), onion (Stomach 6), papaya (Stomach 2), pea (Spleen 2, Stomach 2), peach (Stomach 2), pineapple (Stomach 0), polished rice (Stomach 2), pomegranate (sour fruit) (Stomach 2), pork (Stomach -1), potato (Irish) (Stomach 2), radish (Stomach 1), red bayberry (Stomach 2), red date (Stomach 4), goat's milk (Stomach 4), shiitake mushroom (Stomach 2), silver carp (Stomach 4), small white cabbage (Stomach 2), small-eyed carp (Stomach 4), sorghum (Stomach 4), squash (Stomach 4), sweet rice (and glutinous rice) (Stomach 4), sword bean (Stomach 4), taro (Stomach 3), towel gourd (Stomach 0), white fungus (Stomach 2), whitebait (Stomach 2), wild cabbage (Stomach 2), wine (Liver 3, Stomach 3), yam bean (Stomach 0).

Generally Beneficial Foods and Other Foods to Be Chosen or Avoided. 1. Foods that are generally good for this syndrome are asafetida, buckwheat, cardamom seed, castor bean, cayenne pepper, coriander, grapefruit, jackfruit, jellyfish, malt, peach, radish, sweet basil, tea, tomato, and water chestnut. 2. Avoid foods that can cause indigestion, such as fried pea, goose, mango, raw chestnut, red date, sweet rice, taro, and yellow soybean.

Beneficial Herbs to Be Applied One Herb at a Time. Shan zha (Fructus Crataegi), 25 g; zhi shi (Fructus Aurantii Immaturus), 10 g; chen pi (Pericarpium Citri Reticulatae), 6 g; bai zhu (Rhizoma Atractylodis Macrocephalae), 10 g; shen qu (Mass Medicata Fermentata), 12 g.

Beneficial Herbal Formulas to Be Applied One Formula at a Time. Jian Pi Wan, Zhi Shi Dao Zhi Wan, Zhi Zhu Wan.

8.3 *Cold Stomach*

When you are in good health, your y-score is Stomach -4; when you are ill, your y-score is Stomach -8.

Definition of the Syndrome. Cold Stomach means that the stomach has come under the attack of a cold pathogen due to an excessive consumption of cold foods or an exposure to external coldness.

The stomach's coming under the attack of coldness accounts for the acute, cold stomachache that worsens with coldness and gets better with warmth. Vomiting can remove cold energy from the stomach, which is why the stomachache gets better after vomiting. Cold energy reduces the strength of stomach yang, causing the cold limbs.

Clinical Signs and Symptoms. Major signs: Cold stomachache that is acute in force and gets worse with cold and better with warmth. Median signs: Abdominal swelling, eating in the morning and vomiting in the evening, diarrhea, hiccups, cold limbs, stomachache getting better after vomiting. Minor signs: Belching, copious spitting, hands and feet feeling slightly cold, desire for hot drink, fondness for massage with heat, vomiting of clear saliva.

Applicable Western Diseases. Acute and chronic gastritis, gastric neurosis, gastroduodenal ulcer, phrenospasm, prolapse of gastric mucosa.

Treatment Symptoms. Stomachache, vomiting, diarrhea.

Clinical Cases. (1) A sixty-seven-year-old male patient named Liu had suffered from stomachaches for many years, with the stomachaches recurring on consuming cold foods or on exposure to cold weather. At the beginning, he was able to relieve the pain by drinking a mixture of white wine and brown sugar, but it gradually lost its effect. When he had a severe stomachache, he would experience a hard spot in the stomach area as big as the palm of his hand with a choking sensation in the stomach and profuse perspiration. A Chinese doctor diagnosed Liu's condition as Cold Stomach, mainly because the pain was induced by ingesting cold foods and tended to recur on exposure to cold temperatures. (2) One day a thirty-year-old male patient named Li gobbled down a lot of cold foods because he was very hungry, and he developed an intolerable stomachache afterward and was rushed to a hospital that evening. Groaning in agony, Li bent forward from the waist in pain, with his hands pressing against his stomach; he also had extremely cold hands, and his stomach was tense and hard and painful to the touch. Hearing about these symptoms later, a Chinese doctor diagnosed Li's condition as Cold Stomach, chiefly because the pain was induced by consuming cold foods and there was the presence of cold signs. (3) Xu, a forty-six-year-old male patient, had suffered from a duodenal bulbar ulcer for many years, but recently the pain had become more severe. He said that he liked using heat and massage to relieve the pain and that the pain got better after eating. Xu also occasionally vomited acid, and he had a fear of the cold, a poor complexion, fatigued limbs, and a pale tongue. A Chinese doctor diagnosed his condition as Cold Stomach, mainly because his duodenal ulcer and pain got better with warmth, and these are two important signs of this syndrome.

Treatment Principles. To warm the middle region, disperse cold, and relive vomiting.

Foods Chosen Based on Y-Scores. Asparagus (Stomach 1), bean curd (Stomach 0), beef (Stomach 2), bird's nest (Stomach 2), black and white pepper (Stomach 8), black fungus (Stomach 2), blood clam (Stomach 4), broad bean (Stomach 2), brome seed (Stomach 0), broomcorn (faxtail millet) (Stomach 2), brown sugar (Stomach 4), buckwheat (Stomach 0), catfish (Stomach 4), chestnut (Stomach 4), chicken (Stomach 4), Chinese cabbage (Stomach 2), coconut (L. intestine 2, Spleen 2, Stomach 2), common button mushroom (Stomach 0), corn (Stomach 2), cow's milk (Stomach

2), crown daisy (Stomach 8), cucumber (Stomach 0), eggplant (Stomach 0), fresh ginger (Stomach 6), freshwater shrimp (Stomach 4), garlic (Stomach 6), ginkgo (Stomach 6), goat's milk (L. intestine 4, Kidneys 4, Stomach 4), gold carp (Stomach 2), grass carp (Stomach 4), green-onion white head (Stomach 6), hawthorn fruit (Stomach 2), hyacinth bean (Stomach 2), lard (Spleen 0, Stomach 0), leaf or brown mustard (Stomach 6), ling (Stomach 0), mackerel (Spleen 2, Stomach 2), maltose (Spleen 4, Stomach 4), mandarin fish (Stomach 2), mung bean (Stomach 0), mutton (Stomach 4), olive (Stomach 0), onion (Stomach 6), papaya (Stomach 2), pea (Stomach 2), peach (Stomach 2), pineapple (Stomach 0), polished rice (Stomach 2), pomegranate (sour fruit) (Stomach 2), pork (Stomach -1), potato (Irish) (Stomach 2), radish (Stomach 1), red bayberry (Stomach 2), red date (Stomach 4), shiitake mushroom (Stomach 2), silver carp (Stomach 4), small white cabbage (Stomach 2), small-eyed carp (Stomach 4), sorghum (Stomach 4), squash (Stomach 4), sweet rice (or glutinous rice) (Stomach 4), sword bean (Stomach 4), taro (Stomach 3), towel gourd (Stomach 0), white fungus (Lungs 2, Kidneys 2, Stomach 2), whitebait (Stomach 2), wild cabbage (Stomach 2), wine (Stomach 3), yam bean (Stomach 0).

Generally Beneficial Foods and Other Foods to Be Chosen or Avoided. 1. Choose from the following warm foods: blood clam, caper, caraway seed, cassia bark (Japanese), cassia fruit (Japanese), chicken, chili-pepper leaf, chili rhizome, chive (Chinese), chive root and bulb (Chinese), chive seed (Chinese), cinnamon twig, clove, date, dill seed, fennel seed, fenugreek seed (Oriental), garlic (small), ginger (fresh), green-onion white head, mustard (white or yellow), mustard seed (white or yellow), nutmeg, pepper (black or white), prickly ash, rice (polished, long-grain), shallot (aromatic green onion), sorghum, star anise, sword bean (jack bean), and water chestnut. 2. Choose from these more easily digestible foods: areca nut (unripe), asafetida, bog bean (buck bean), buckwheat, cardamom seed, carrot, chicken gizzard, coriander (Chinese parsley), coriander seed, dill seed, distillers' grains, grapefruit (including peel), green-onion white head, hawthorn fruit, jackfruit, kiwifruit (Chinese gooseberry), lime (young trifoliate orange), lobster (sea prawn), longan seed, malt, millet sprouts, orange peel (sour or sweet), papaya, peach, quince, radish, red bayberry, sorghum, soybean (yellow), sweet basil, tomato, water chestnut, and whitefish.

3. Foods to be avoided in cases of indigestion are fried pea, goose, mango, raw chestnut, red date, sweet rice, taro, and yellow soybean.

Beneficial Herbs to Be Applied One Herb at a Time. Chen xiang (Lignum Aquilariae Resinatum), 4 g; fu zi (Radix Aconiti Praeparata), 11 g; gan jiang (Rhizoma Zingiberis), 7 g; gao liang (Jiangrhizoma Alpiniae Officinarum), 7 g; wu zhu yu (Fructus Euodiae), 7 g.

Beneficial Herbal Formulas to Be Applied One Formula at a Time. Fu Zi Li Zhong Wan, Li Zhong Wan, Liang Fu Wan, Wu Zhu Yu Tang.

8.4 Hot Stomach

When you are in good health, your y-score is Stomach 3; when you are ill, your y-score is Stomach 7.

Definition of the Syndrome. Hot Stomach is a syndrome in which there is excessive heat in the stomach that can be due to the consumption of too many hot foods, chronic Stomach Yin Deficiency, or energy congestion transforming into fire. The stomach is related to dry earth and is fond of dampness and dislikes dryness. It is also very susceptible to the attack of fire, and, because the stomach is related to dry earth, its energy can be easily transformed into heat or fire.

Clinical Signs and Symptoms. Major signs: Burning pain in the stomach, thirst with a desire for cold drink, acid swallowing, eating a lot but remaining hungry. Median signs: Periodic stomachache with burning sensation, bad breath, bitter taste in the mouth, bleeding from the gums and from the space between the teeth with pain, constipation. Minor signs: Depressed and quick tempered, insecure, dry sensation in the mouth, fever, headache, hiccups, hungry with good appetite, eating a lot but remaining thin, incapable of sound sleep in children, morning sickness, nosebleed, pain in the gums with swelling, pain in the throat, red and swollen throat, mouth ulcer, screaming during sleep in children, toothache, vomiting of blood, vomiting right after eating.

Applicable Western Diseases. Acute gastritis, acute pancreatitis, bleeding from upper digestive tract, chronic red nose, constipation, diabetes mellitus, diphtheria, diphtheritis, gastro duodenal ulcer, herpetic stomatitis, mastitis, perforation, periodontitis, phrenospasm, stomatitis, sty, summer fever in children, tonsillitis, ulcerative blepharitis.

Treatment Symptoms. Stomachache, vomiting, swelling of gums with pain.

Clinical Cases. (1) For three years, a male patient named Cai, age twenty-four, has suffered from a stomachache that has gradually worsened. Along with the stomachache, he has the following signs and symptoms: vomiting of acid, nausea and vomiting, stomach pain getting worse on consumption of hot foods or triggered by this, dry stools, and a fondness for cool foods. Cai was a habitual drinker of alcohol. A Chinese doctor diagnosed his condition as Hot Stomach, primarily because the pain he experiences becomes more severe with the consumption of hot foods or is provoked by this and because of his fondness for cool foods. (2) Suffering from a toothache for three consecutive days, Shen, a thirty-two-year-old female patient, went to a dentist, but was treated without effect. She also had a reddish complexion, constipation, short streams of urine, and thirst with a craving for cold drink. A Chinese doctor diagnosed Shen's condition as Hot Stomach mainly because of her thirst and craving for cold drink as well as her constipation. (3) A thirty-year-old male patient named Wan had recurrent ulcers in the mouth, on the tongue, and on the cheeks, which made eating very difficult for him. He experienced mild burning pain in those areas and also had a dry mouth, a yellowish coating on the tongue, dry stools, and mental depression. A Chinese doctor diagnosed his condition as Hot Stomach mostly on account of the burning ulcers in his mouth.

Treatment Principles. To clear and sedate stomach fire.

Foods Chosen Based on Y-Scores. Areca nut (Stomach -2), asparagus (Stomach 1), bamboo shoots (Stomach -2), banana (Stomach -2), barley (Stomach -3), bean curd (Stomach 0), beef (Stomach 2), bird's nest (Stomach 2), bitter gourd (balsam pear) (Stomach -8), black-bean seed (processed) (Stomach -8), black fungus (Stomach 2), broad bean (Stomach 2), brome seed (Stomach 0), broomcorn (faxtail millet) (Stomach 2), buckwheat (Stomach 0), celery (Stomach -1), Chinese cabbage (Stomach 2), Chinese toon leaf (Stomach -4), coconut (Stomach 2), common button mushroom (Stomach 0), corn (Stomach 2), cow's milk (Stomach 2), crab (Stomach -7), cucumber (Stomach 0), eggplant (Stomach 0), gold carp (Stomach 2), hami melon (Stomach -2), hawthorn fruit (Stomach 2), hyacinth bean (Stomach 2), kiwifruit (Kidneys -4, Stomach -4), lard (Spleen 0, Stomach 0), lettuce (Stomach -2), ling (Stomach 0), mackerel (Stomach 2), mandarin fish (Stomach 2), mandarin orange (Stomach -2), mango (Stomach -2), mung bean (Stomach 0), mung bean sprouts (Stomach -2), murrel (snakehead) (Stomach -2), muskmelon (cantaloupe) (Stomach -2), olive (Stomach 0), papaya (Stomach 2), pea (Stomach 2), peach (Stomach 2), pear (Stomach -2), pineapple (Stomach 0), polished rice (Stomach 2), pomegranate (sour fruit) (Stomach 2), pork (Stomach -1), potato (Irish) (Stomach 2), radish (Stomach 1), red bayberry (Stomach 2), seaweed (marine alga) (Stomach -8), shiitake mushroom (Stomach 2), small white cabbage (Stomach 2), soy sauce (Stomach -7), star fruit (carambola) (Spleen -4, Stomach -4), sugarcane (Stomach -2), sweet potato (Stomach -2), tangerine (Stomach -2), tea (Stomach -6), tea melon (Stomach -2), tomato (Stomach -4), towel gourd (Stomach 0), vinegar (Stomach -1), water chestnut (Stomach -2), white fungus (Stomach 2), whitebait (Stomach 2), wild cabbage (Stomach 2), yam bean (Stomach 0), yellow croaker (Stomach -1).

Generally Beneficial Foods and Other Foods to Be Chosen or Avoided. 1. Foods that are considered normally good for this syndrome are banana, bitter endive, black fungus, camellia, cattail, cucumber, licorice, lily flower, salt, spinach, and strawberry. 2. Choose from the following cold foods: adzuki bean, aloe vera, asparagus (lucid), bamboo shoots, banana, bitter endive, bitter gourd (balsam pear), brake (fern), burdock, camphor mint, cattail, Chinese wax gourd, crab, duck egg (preserved), endive (Chinese), fig, frog (pond), grapefruit, hair vegetable, honey, leaf beet (spinach beet, Swiss chard), lemon, lily flower, mung bean, mung-bean powder, mung bean sprouts, orchid leaf, peppermint, potato (Irish), pricking amaranth (amaranth, pigweed), purslane, rabbit, rambutan, romaine lettuce, Russian olive (oleaster), safflower fruit, salt, soybean paste, squash, star fruit (carambola), strawberry (Indian or mock), sweet basil, tofu, water spinach, and wheat. 3. Choose from these cool items: amaranth, bamboo shoots, bamboo shoots (bitter), barley, beer, bottle gourd, cantaloupe (muskmelon), Chinese wax gourd (pulp), crab, cucumber, eggplant (aubergine), flour, freshwater clam, gluten, jellyfish, Job's tears, kidney bean, kiwifruit (Chinese gooseberry), laver, lotus plumule, lotus sprouts, mare's milk, matrimony-vine leaf, millet, mulberry leaf, mung bean, peach leaf, pear, peppermint, peppermint oil, persimmon (including powder on its surface), pork brain, rice (polished), sea grass, seaweed, small white cabbage, star fruit (carambola), sugarcane, towel-gourd seed, towel-gourd sponge, watercress (water celery), watermelon (including white portion), wheat, wheat (floating), and wheat bran. 4. Avoid these hot and spicy items: alcohol, chili pepper (cayenne pepper), chive (Chinese), cinnamon bark (cassia), cinnamon twig, clove, coffee, garlic, ginger (fresh or dried), green onion (leaf and white head), mustard seed, nutmeg, onion, pepper (black or white), tea, and wine. They force yin energy to excrete through perspiration, which is harmful to both yin and energy. 5. Avoid these irritants: alcohol, coffee, tea, tobacco, and wine. They can irritate the stomach and produce damp heat, and fire is harmful to yin and energy. 6. Avoid greasy and fatty foods, such as animal fats (including lamb fat and oil), butter, chicken egg yolk, creams, fatty meats, fish-liver oils, fried foods, and lard. These foods can generate heat and produce phlegm, and they worsen indigestion, a poor appetite, jaundice, dysentery, and diarrhea.

Beneficial Herbs to Be Applied One Herb at a Time. Da huang (Radix Et Rhizoma Rhei), 15 g; huang lian (Rhizoma Coptidis), 12 g; huang qin (Radix Scutellariae), 15 g; lu gen (Rhizoma Phragmitis), 65 g; shi gao (Gypsum Fibrosum), 70 g; zhi mu (Rhizoma Anemarrhenae), 15 g; zhi zi (Fructus Gardeniae), 16 g.

Beneficial Herbal Formulas to Be Applied One Formula at a Time. Da Chai Hu Tang, Liang Ge San, Ma Zi Ren Wan, Qing Wei San.

9

Choosing Foods and Herbs to Boost the Liver and Cure Applicable Symptoms and Diseases

9.1 Liver Energy Congestion

When you are in good health, your y-score is Liver -3; when you are ill, your y-score is Liver -7.

Definition of the Syndrome. When excess energy affects the liver, this can lead to Liver Energy Congestion if the energy fails to circulate properly. The liver is situated in the lower hypochondrium region, and its meridian circles the genitals and passes through the lower abdomen up to the nipples. The liver is also conditioned to disperse energy, but emotional disturbance can cause energy congestion of the liver, which accounts for the discomfort in the chest as well as the abdominal swelling and pain. When liver energy upsurges to mix with phlegm in the throat, this will cause a subjective sensation of objects in the throat, which is called "plum pit" in Chinese medicine. Liver Energy Congestion can affect the spleen and the stomach, causing symptoms associated with these two organs.

Clinical Signs and Symptoms. Major signs: Swelling and pain in the breast, suppression of menses in women, running pain in the chest, the hypochondirum, and the lower abdomen. Median signs: Discomfort in the chest, jumpiness or sensations of something in the throat, abdominal obstructions, swelling of the liver and the spleen causing lumps, irregular menstruation, convulsions, morning sickness. Minor signs: Numbness, premature menstrual periods, shortage of milk secretion after childbirth, stomachache, subjective sensation of objects in the throat, vomiting of blood, whitish vaginal discharge.

Applicable Western Diseases and Conditions. Acute cholecystitis and cholecystolithiasis, acute epidemic icterohepatitis, acute pancreatitis, cancer of the esophagus, cancer of the uterine cervix, cholecystitis, cholecystolithiasis, chronic infectious hepatitis, cirrhosis, climacteric melancholia, epilepsy, herpes zoster, lymph-gland tuberculosis of the neck, mastitis, mastofibroma, menopause syndrome, neurosis, pelade, retinopathy, simple goiter, hyperthyroidism, ulcer, vaginal discharge, viral hepatitis (nonjaundice type).

Treatment Symptoms. Mental illness, menstrual disorders, pain in the hypochondrium, stomach, and abdomen.

Clinical Cases. (1) Lu, a twenty-one-year-old female patient, suddenly displayed the following symptoms during her first year of college, which were obviously due to her poor academic record and the strict discipline imposed by her father: insomnia, mental depression, meaningless speech, palpitations, and being easily in shock. A Chinese doctor diagnosed her condition as Liver Energy Congestion chiefly because of the emotional disturbance she was undergoing as a result of external pressure. (2) A fifty-year-old male patient named Ma had hepatitis for more than two years when he was diagnosed as being in the early stage of hepatic cirrhosis. His signs and symptoms included a poor complexion, abdominal distension, mild pain in the hypochondrium, a poor appetite, an occasional pricking sensation, fatigue, loose stools, and yellowish and meager urine. A Chinese doctor diagnosed his condition as Liver Energy Congestion, primarily because he suffered hepatic cirrhosis and mild pain in the hypochondrium.

Treatment Principles. To disperse the liver and regulate its energy.

Foods Chosen Based on Y-Scores. Black sesame seed (Liver 2), brown sugar (Liver 4), cherry (Liver 4), chicken liver (Liver 4), Chinese chive (Liver 6), corn silk (Liver 2), cuttlefish (Liver -3), day lily (Liver 0), eel (Liver 4), hairtail (Liver 4), hawthorn fruit (Liver 2), Japanese cassia bark (Liver 5), litchi nut (Liver 2), long-tailed anchovy (Liver 4), matrimony-vine fruit (Liver 2), perch (Liver 2), pine-nut kernel (Liver 4), plum (Liver 0), pork liver (Liver 1), rape (Liver 2), rape oil (Liver 6), shepherd's purse (Liver

6), star anise (Liver 5), towel gourd (Liver 0), variegated carp (big-head) (Liver 4), white eel (Liver 2), wine (Liver 3).

Generally Beneficial Foods and Other Foods to Be Chosen or Avoided. 1. Foods that are generally good for this syndrome are ambergris, beef, bird's nest, brown sugar, butterfish, caraway seed, cherry, chicken, coconut meat, common button mushroom, date (red or black), dill seed, garlic, goose meat, jackfruit, kumquat, mustard seed, mutton, oregano, red bean, rice, rock sugar, saffron, spearmint, squash, sweet basil, sweet potato, sweet rice, tofu, and turmeric. 2. Choose from these foods that promote energy circulation: ambergris, beef, black-eyed pea, camphor mint, caraway seed, cardamom seed, carrot, chicken egg, chive (Chinese leek), chive (Chinese), chive root and bulb (Chinese), chufa rhizome, chufa-stem leaf (earth almond, nut grass), clam (freshwater or saltwater), common button mushroom, dill seed, fennel seed, fingered citron (Buddha's hand), garlic, grapefruit, green onion (fibrous root and white head), hawthorn fruit, jasmine flower, kumquat, lemon leaf, lime (young trifoliate orange), litchi nut, litchi-nut seed, longan seed, loquat seed, lotus stem, malt, mango leaf, marjoram, muskmelon seed, mussel, mustard (leaf or brown), mustard seed, orange leaf, orange peel, oregano (wild), radish leaf, rapeseed, red bean, rose, saffron, scallion bulb, shiitake mushroom, spearmint, star anise, string bean, sweet basil, tangerine (including peel), trifoliate orange, trifoliate orange (near ripe), turmeric, and vinegar. 3. Avoid these hot and spicy foods and drinks: alcohol, chili pepper (cayenne pepper), chive (Chinese), cinnamon bark (cassia), cinnamon twig, clove, coffee, garlic, ginger (fresh or dried), green onion (leaf and white head), mustard seed, nutmeg, onion, pepper (black or white), tea, and wine. They force yin energy to excrete through perspiration, and this is harmful to heart yin and heart energy.

Beneficial Herbs to Be Applied One Herb at a Time. Bai shao yao (Radix Paeoniae Alba), 11 g; chai hu (Radix Bupleuri), 16 g; chuan lian zi (Fructus Meliae Toosendan), 11 g; hou po hua (Flos Magnoliae Officinalis), 7 g; qing pi (Pericarpium Citri Reticulatae Viride), 11 g; xiang fu (Rhizoma Cyperi), 11 g; zhi qiao (Fructus Aurantii), 11 g.

Beneficial Herbal Formulas to Be Applied One Formula at a Time. Chai Hu Shu Gan Tang, Xiao Yao San, Yi Guan Jian.

9.2 Liver Fire Flaming Upward

When you are in good health, your y-score is Liver 4; when you are ill, your y-score is Liver 8.

Definition of the Syndrome. When excess yang affects the liver, this can lead to Liver Fire Flaming Upward. This syndrome is primarily due to energy congestion in the liver that transforms into fire in the liver, because excessive energy means fire. Liver fire has a tendency to flame upward to attack the head, which accounts for the reddish complexion, pink eyes, headache, ringing in the ears, and deafness. Fire gets congested in the liver meridian, causing the burning pain in the hypochondrium. Liver fire can get mixed up with bile, which is why people with this syndrome have a bitter taste in the mouth and a dry mouth. Liver energy gets congested, causing the anger. Congested liver heat disturbs the spirits, and this gives rise to the insomnia and many dreams. Liver fire forces the blood to run wild, leading to the vomiting of blood and the nosebleed. Heat burns up body fluids, and this is the reason for the constipation and reddish urine.

Clinical Signs and Symptoms. Major signs: Reddish complexion, pink eyes, jumpiness, being prone to anger. Median signs: Headache on both sides of the head and around the eyes, headache that is severe, dizziness, ringing in the ears, deafness, jumpiness, burning pain in the ribs, dry sensation in the mouth, vomiting of blood or nosebleed in severe cases, yellowish urine, dry stools. Minor signs: Bleeding from the stomach.

Applicable Western Diseases. Acute conjunctivitis, acute pancreatitis, central retinal choroiditis, corneal opacity, enuresis, epilepsy, general infection, haematuria (discharge of urine containing blood), hemorrhage of retina, hypertension, hysteria, inflammation of auricular cartilage, intercostal neuritis, iridocyclitis, keratitis, papillary fibroma of lactiferous tubule, neurosis, phrenospasm, primary glaucoma, primary hepatoma, simple goiter (hyperthyroidism), zona.

Treatment Symptoms. Headache, ringing in the ears, deafness, bleeding, insomnia, acid regurgitation, maniac-type mental illness.

Clinical Cases. (1) A forty-seven-year-old male patient named Song suffered from a headache for an entire year, with these additional symptoms: dizziness, a reddish complexion, dry and hot sensations in the mouth, nosebleed, and a dark-purple coloring of the tongue. A Chinese doctor diagnosed his condition as Liver Fire Flaming Upward primarily because of his headache, dizziness, and reddish complexion. (2) Chai, a thirty-eight-year-old male patient, had a headache that was so severe that he felt as if his head was about to be blown off. He also had a reddish complexion, a dry mouth, a bitter taste in the mouth, and a red tongue with a yellowish coating, as well as anxiety and insomnia, and was shocked easily. A Chinese doctor diagnosed Chai's condition as Liver Fire Flaming Upward chiefly because of his severe headache, which can be caused only by fire in the liver. (3) Normally, Cao, a fifty-four-year-old female patient, had a bad temper. But one day she became sick after she lost her temper, with pink eyes, a headache, swelling in the ribs region, a bitter taste in the mouth, a dry mouth, a red tongue, and insomnia. A Chinese doctor diagnosed Cao's condition as Liver Fire Flaming Upward, mainly because a bad temper tends to be associated with liver fire.

Treatment Principles. To clear the liver and sedate the fire.

Foods Chosen Based on Y-Scores. Abalone (Liver -1), agar (Liver -5), arrowhead (Liver -6), beef liver (Liver 2), black sesame seed (Liver 2), celery (Liver -1), clam (freshwater) (Liver -5), corn silk (Liver 2), crab (Liver -7), cuttlefish (Liver -3), day lily (Liver 0), hawthorn fruit (Liver 2), jellyfish (Liver -3), litchi nut (Liver 2), loquat (Liver -2), mackerel (Liver -8), matrimony-vine fruit (Liver 2), mulberry (Liver -2), mussel (Liver -1), perch (Liver 2), plum (Liver 0), pork liver (Liver 1), purslane (Liver -6), rape (Liver 2), river clamshell (Liver -5), seaweed (marine alga) (Liver -7), tomato (Liver -4), towel gourd (Liver 0), vinegar (Liver -1), water spinach (Liver -2), white eel (Liver 2), wild rice gall (Liver -2).

Generally Beneficial Foods and Other Foods to Be Chosen or Avoided. 1. Foods that are normally good for this syndrome are abalone, asparagus, black fungus, chestnut, chicken egg, pork, royal jelly, rye, shepherd's purse, spinach, vinegar, and white fungus. 2. Avoid these yang-tonic foods for the kidneys: air bladder of shark, beef kidney, cassia fruit (Japanese), chestnut, chive seed (Chinese), cinnamon bark (cassia), clove, clove oil, deer kidney, dill seed, fennel root, fennel seed, fenugreek seed (Oriental), green-onion seed, lobster (sea prawn), mandarin-orange seed, oxtail, pistachio nut, pork testes, prickly ash root, raspberry, sheep or goat kidney, shrimp, sparrow egg, star anise, strawberry, and sword bean (jack bean). 3. Avoid hot and spicy items, such as alcohol, chili pepper (cayenne pepper), chive (Chinese), cinnamon bark (cassia), cinnamon twig, clove, coffee, garlic, ginger (fresh or dried), green onion (leaf and white head), mustard seed, nutmeg, onion, pepper (black or white), tea, and wine. They force yin energy to excrete through perspiration, which can contribute to the production of fire.

Beneficial Herbs to Be Applied One Herb at a Time. Huang lian (Rhizoma Coptidis), 2 g; huang qin (Radix Scutellariae), 15 g; jin qian cao (Herba Lysimachiae), 18 g; long dan (Radix Gentianae), 10 g; mu dan pi (Cortex Moutan Radicis), 11 g; zhi zi (Fructus Gardeniae), 16 g.

Beneficial Herbal Formulas to Be Applied One Formula at a Time. Da Ding Feng Zhu, Dan Zhi Xiao Yao San, Long Dan Xie Gan Tang.

9.3 *Liver Blood Deficiency*

When you are in good health, your y-score is Liver 1; when you are ill, your y-score is Liver 5.

Definition of the Syndrome. When there is an insufficient production of blood, a loss of blood, or a chronic illness, Liver Blood Deficiency can occur. The liver meridian is deficient as a result of poor nourishment, and this accounts for the mild pain in the hypochondrium. The blood cannot flow into the head and face in sufficient quantities to nourish the upper region, causing the pale complexion, dizziness, vertigo, and dry and obstructive sensations in the eyes. The blood cannot nourish the nails, which accounts for the nail disorders. The yin blood is incapable of controlling yang energy, with the latter transforming into wind, which brings about the twitching. The liver stores the blood and takes charge of dispersing its energy; but when liver energy becomes congested, one so afflicted is prone to shock and anger.

Clinical Signs and Symptoms. Major signs: Mild pain in the hypochondrium, dizziness and vertigo, dry and obstructive sensations in the eyes. Median signs: Nervousness, anger, blurred vision, numbness, meager menstrual flow or suppression of menses, yellowish and withered complexion, light or whitish color of lips. Minor signs: Dry and withered nails, nails' becoming thin, broken nails, prone to shock and fear, fatigue, many dreams, menstrual disorders, slightly insufficient menstrual flow, suppression of menses, jumping muscles that cannot be controlled, pale complexion, ringing in the ears like the sound of a cicada, insomnia, spasms.

Applicable Western Diseases. Anemia, night blindness, chronic hepatitis, hypertension, neurasthenia.

Treatment Symptoms. Chronic fatigue, dizziness, insomnia, numbness, night blindness, irregular menstrual periods, menstrual pain.

Clinical Cases. (1) In giving birth to her first child, a twenty-six-year-old female patient named Woo experienced excessive bleeding; then she gradually developed swelling in the eyes, sinus pain, blurred vision, headaches, dizziness, and congestion in the chest. A Chinese doctor diagnosed her condition as Liver Blood Deficiency, primarily because she lost so much blood, which affected her liver. (2) Song, a thirty-year-old male patient, suffered from trembling of the limbs for six months, with this becoming worse during the day and better at night. A Chinese doctor diagnosed his condition as Liver Blood Deficiency, chiefly because trembling is primarily due to this syndrome, which gives rise to another syndrome called Liver Wind.

Treatment Principles. To tone and nourish the blood in the liver.

Foods Chosen Based on Y-Scores. Abalone (Liver -1), agar (Liver -5), arrowhead (Liver-2), beef liver (Liver 2), black sesame seed (Liver 2), brown sugar (Liver 4), celery (Liver -1), cherry (Liver 4), chicken liver (Liver 4), corn silk (Liver 2), cuttlefish (Liver -3), day lily (Liver 0), hawthorn fruit (Liver 2), jellyfish (Liver -3), litchi nut (Liver 2), loquat (Liver -2), matrimony-vine fruit (Liver 2), mulberry (Liver -2), mussel (Liver -1), perch (Liver 2), pine-nut kernel (Liver 4), plum (Liver 0), pork liver (Liver 1), rape (Liver 2), tomato (Liver -4), towel gourd (Liver 0), variegated carp (bighead) (Liver 4), vinegar (Liver -1), water spinach (Liver -2), white eel (Liver 2), wild rice gall (Liver -2), wine (Liver 3).

Generally Beneficial Foods and Other Foods to Be Chosen or Avoided. 1. Choose from these tonic foods for the liver: beef liver, black sesame seed, chicken liver, chive seed (Chinese), matrimony-vine fruit, mulberry, mussel, perch, pork liver, rabbit liver, raspberry, royal jelly, sheep or goat liver, and strawberry. 2. Choose from the following blood-tonic foods: beef, beef liver, blood clam, chicken egg, cuttlefish, duck blood, grape, ham, litchi nut, liver, longan, mandarin fish, octopus, oxtail, oyster, pork liver, pork trotter, sea cucumber, soybean skin (black), and spinach.

Beneficial Herbs to Be Applied One Herb at a Time. Bai shao yao (Radix Paeoniae Alba), 11 g; bai zi ren (Semen Biotae), 11 g; dang gui (Radix Angelicae Sinensis), 11 g; gou qi zi (Fructus Lycii), 11 g; he shou wu (Radix Polygoni Multiflori), 15 g; nu zhen zi (Fructus Ligustri Lucidi), 11 g; shan zhu yu (Fructus Corni), 11 g; sheng di (Radix Rehmanniae), fresh, 35 g.

Beneficial Herbal Formulas to Be Applied One Formula at a Time. Bu Gan Tang, Si Wu Tang, Yi Guan Jian.

9.4 Liver Yin Deficiency.

When you are in good health, your y-score is Liver 3; when you are ill, your y-score is Liver 7.

Definition of the Syndrome. When yin deficiency affects the liver, this can lead to Liver Yin Deficiency. There are similarities between Liver Yin Deficiency and Liver Blood Deficiency, and the general rule to distinguish the two is this: If the patient displays a yellowish and withered complexion, light or white lips, and a fine pulse, then the condition is Liver Blood Deficiency; but if the patient exhibits hot sensations in the palms of the hands and the soles of the feet, a dry throat, night sweats, a red tongue with a light coating, and a fine, wiry, and rapid pulse, then it is Liver Yin Deficiency.

Clinical Signs and Symptoms. Major signs: Dizziness with blurred vision, headache that drags on and on, night blindness. Median signs: Ringing in the ears, insomnia, suppression of menses, twitching, both eyes' flickering, looking sideways, or looking upward. Minor signs: Clinching the teeth and grinding them, deafness, fainting after childbirth, mouth closed as if screwed up, blueness of the skin and continual twitching, numbness of the four limbs, overdue menstrual period, pain in the hypochondrium, pupils' looking upward, wind stroke, wriggling or numbness of muscles, wry mouth and eyes.

Applicable Western Diseases and Conditions. Alogia, aplastic anemia, cancer of the uterine cervix, cerebrovascular accidents, chronic active hepatitis, chronic infectious hepatitis, encephalitis B, epidemic encephalitis, gallbladder disease, hemiplegia, hypertension, hyperthyroidism, infectious hepatitis, Ménière's syndrome, menopause syndrome, neurosis in children, opisthotonos, optic neuritis, otogenic vertigo, preeclampsia and eclampsia, simple goiter (hyperthyroidism), trachoma, twisting spasmodic syndrome, vertigo.

Treatment Symptoms. Pain in the hypochondrium, dizziness, headache, chronic fatigue, fever due to an internal injury, excessive sweating, insomnia, sensations of obstruction and pain in the white of the eye, absent menstrual period, delayed menstrual period, vaginal bleeding.

Clinical Cases. (1) A fifty-one-year-old male patient named Sun exhibited the following symptoms: vertigo, a sensation of congestion and swelling in the back of head, jumpiness, poor sleep, many dreams, ringing in the ears, and a red tongue with a light coating. A Chinese doctor diagnosed his condition as Liver Yin Deficiency, chiefly because vertigo points to a liver disease and many of his symptoms, such as his jumpiness and red tongue, are signs of yin deficiency. (2) Guan, a forty-five-year-old male patient, had a history of hepatitis, and he was treated with Western medicine with good results. But he still experiences pain in the liver zone and also below the left ribs. Other symptoms include a dry mouth, a sore throat, a red tongue with tooth marks and a white coating, and insomnia. A Western physician diagnosed his condition as post-hepatitic syndrome. A Chinese doctor diagnosed it as Liver Yin Deficiency primarily because of the pain he has in the liver zone and his dry throat and red tongue.

Treatment Principles. To nourish the yin energy in the liver.

Foods Chosen Based on Y-Scores. Abalone (Liver -1), agar (Liver -5), arrowhead (Liver-2), beef liver (Liver 2), black sesame seed (Liver 2), celery (Liver -1), clam (freshwater) (Liver -5), corn silk (Liver 2), crab (Liver -7), cuttlefish (Liver -3), day lily (Liver 0), hawthorn fruit (Liver 2), jellyfish (Liver -3), litchi nut (Liver 2), loquat (Liver -2), mackerel (Liver -8), matrimony-vine fruit (Liver 2), mulberry (Liver -2), mussel (Liver -1), perch (Liver 2), plum (Liver 0), pork liver (Liver 1), purslane (Liver -6), rape (Liver 2), river clamshell (Liver -5), seaweed (marine alga) (Liver -8), tomato (Liver -4), towel gourd (Liver 0), vinegar (Liver -1), water spinach (Liver -2), white eel (Liver 2), wild rice gall (Liver -2), wine (Liver 3).

Generally Beneficial Foods and Other Foods to Be Chosen or Avoided. 1. Choose from the following yin-tonic foods: abalone, air bladder of shark, apple, apricot pit (sweet powder), asparagus (lucid), bean drink, bird's nest, bitter gourd (balsam pear), black-eyed pea, brown sugar, cantaloupe (muskmelon), cheeses, chicken egg, chicken eggshell (inner membrane), clam (saltwater or freshwater), coconut milk, crab, cuttlefish, date, duck, duck egg, fig, frog (river or pond), goose meat, grape, green turtle, honey, kidney bean, kumquat, lard, lemon, litchi nut, loquat (Japanese medlai), lotus rhizome, maltose, mandarin orange, mango, milk (cow's), mussel, oyster, pea, pear, pearl (powder), pineapple, pomegranate (sweet fruit), pork, rabbit, red bayberry, rice (polished), royal jelly, sea cucumber, shrimp, star fruit (carambola), string bean, sugarcane, tofu, tomato, turtle egg, walnut, watermelon, white fungus, white sugar, whitebait, and yam. 2. Choose from these liver-tonic foods: black sesame seed, beef liver, chicken liver, chive seed (Chinese), matrimony-vine fruit, mulberry, mussel, perch, pork liver, rabbit liver, raspberry, royal jelly, sheep or goat liver, and strawberry. 3. Avoid these hot and spicy items: alcohol, chili pepper (cayenne pepper), chive (Chinese), cinnamon bark (cassia), cinnamon twig, clove, coffee, garlic, ginger (fresh or dried), green onion (leaf and white head), mustard seed, nutmeg, onion, pepper (black or white), tea, and wine. They force yin energy to excrete through perspiration, and this is harmful to both yin and energy.

Beneficial Herbs to Be Applied One Herb at a Time. Bai shao yao (Radix Paeoniae Alba), 11 g; dang gui (Radix Angelicae Sinensis), 11 g; gou qi zi (Fructus Lycii), 11 g; he shou wu (Radix Polygoni Multiflori), 15 g; ju hua (Flos Chrysanthemi), 20 g; mo han lian (Herba Ecliptae), 11 g; mu li (Concha Ostrae), 35 g; nu zhen zi (Fructus Ligustri Lucidi), 11 g; sheng di (Radix Rehmanniae), fresh, 35 g; zhen zhu mu (Concha Margaritiferae Usta), 30 g.

Beneficial Herbal Formulas to Be Applied One Formula at a Time. Yi Guan Jian, Qi Ju Di Huang Wan, Dang Gui Liu Huang Tang, Liu Wei Di Huang Wan.

9.5 Liver Yang Upsurging (Yin Deficiency of the Liver and the Kidneys Affecting Liver Yang)

When you are in good health, your y-score is Liver 3; when you are ill, your y-score is Liver 7.

Definition of the Syndrome. In Liver Yang Upsurging, basically three things occur: First, liver yin becomes deficient with liver yang getting out of control. Second, liver energy elevates too much, causing floating yang; this is primarily due to excessive sex, disturbances of the seven emotions, and irregular eating. And third, liver yin becomes deficient as a result of too much fire in the liver meridian.

The nature of the liver is to disperse and store away blood. The liver is closely associated with the kidneys, which take charge of pure essence.

In this syndrome, liver yang gets out of control, and this accounts for the anger. Yang energy moves upward, giving rise to the reddish complexion, hot sensations, headache, and dizziness. Liver yang transforms into wind, which is the cause of the vertigo and fainting. And yin is unable to bring yang under control, which leads to the insomnia, many dreams, forgetfulness, and palpitations.

Clinical Signs and Symptoms. Major signs: Mental depression, jumpiness, prone to anger, reddish complexion, hot sensations in the body. Median signs: Vertigo, forgetfulness, palpitations, many dreams, headache in women, headache on the side of the head, headache with dizziness, burning sensation in the face, dry sensations in the mouth and throat, heavy sensation in the head with light sensation in the legs. Minor signs: Bitter taste in the mouth, dizziness, feeling insecure over sleep, heavy sensation in the head and light sensation in the feet, misty vision, numbness of fingers, pain and/or swelling in the ribs, red complexion, ringing in the ears and deafness.

Applicable Western Diseases and Conditions. Hypertension, hyperthyroidism, intestinal typhoid fever, menopause syndrome, otogenic vertigo, preeclampsia and eclampsia, primary hepatoma, senile cataract, trigeminal neuralgia, vertigo.

Treatment Symptoms. Headache, dizziness, ringing in the ears, deafness.

Clinical Cases. (1) Feeling as if he were living in the clouds, Chen, a fifty-eight-year-old male patient, suffered from vertigo. The attacks would occur three to six times every day, and he would close his eyes and try to stay calm. Other symptoms included frequent urination, a reddish complexion, hot sensations in the body, and cold feet. A Chinese doctor diagnosed Chen's condition as Liver Yang Upsurging primarily because of the vertigo he was experiencing along with his reddish complexion and hot sensations in the body. (2) A forty-six-year-old male patient named Zhuang exhibited the following symptoms: vertigo with ringing in the ears, flying spots in front of the eyes, a spinning sensation as if in a boat or on a train, stomach discomfort, nausea, palpitations, and poor sleep. He was diagnosed by a doctor of Western medicine as having Ménière's disease. A Chinese doctor diagnosed his condition as Liver Yang

Upsurging, mainly because vertigo with such intense spinning can be caused only by this syndrome. (3) Lim, a fifty-seven-year-old male patient, had a history of hypertension, accompanied by dizziness and spinning, swelling of the eyes, ringing in the ears, a dry mouth, weak loins, insecurity over sleep, and a thin, yellowish coating on the tongue. A Chinese doctor diagnosed his condition as Liver Yang Upsurging, chiefly because hypertension as well as dizziness and spinning are distinct signs of this syndrome.

Treatment Principles. To nourish yin, suppress yang, and sedate fire.

Foods Chosen Based on Y-Scores. Abalone (Liver -1), agar (Liver -5), arrowhead (Liver -2), beef liver (Liver 2), black sesame seed (Liver 2), celery (Liver -1), clam (freshwater) (Liver -5), corn silk (Liver 2), crab (Liver -7), cuttlefish (Liver -3), day lily (Liver 0), hawthorn fruit (Liver 2), jellyfish (Liver -3), litchi nut (Liver 2), loquat (Liver -2), mackerel (Liver -8), matrimony-vine fruit (Liver 2), mulberry (Liver -2), mussel (Liver -1), perch (Liver 2), plum (Liver 0), pork liver (Liver 1), purslane (Liver -6), rape (Liver 2), river clamshell (Liver -5), seaweed (marine alga) (Liver -8), tomato (Liver -4), towel gourd (Liver 0), vinegar (Liver -1), water spinach (Liver -2), white eel (Liver 2), wild rice gall (Liver -2), wine (Liver 3).

Generally Beneficial Foods and Other Foods to Be Chosen or Avoided. 1. Foods that are commonly good for this syndrome are abalone, celery, cheeses, chicken egg yolk, cuttlefish, duck, duck egg, kidney bean, oyster, pork, royal jelly, and white fungus. 2. Choose from among these nongreasy and bland foods: apple, banana, beef, brown sugar, cabbages, carrot, celery, chicken, chicken egg, Chinese cabbage, corn, cottage cheese, cow's milk, fish, fruit, honey, horse bean (broad bean), lean meats, lemon, lettuce, liver, lotus juice (fresh), millet, mung bean sprouts, mung bean, noodle, peach, pea, pear, polished rice, pork, orange, radish, rice, seaweed, skim milk, soybean sprouts, string bean, sweet potato, soybean, sword bean, taro, tofu, tomato, vegetables, watermelon, wheat, white fungus, white sugar, and yam. 3. Avoid the following hot and spicy items: alcohol, chili pepper (cayenne pepper), chive (Chinese), cinnamon bark (cassia), cinnamon twig, clove, coffee, garlic, ginger (fresh or dried), green onion (leaf and white head), mustard seed, nutmeg, onion, pepper (black or white), tea, and wine. They force yin energy to excrete through perspiration, and this is harmful to heart yin and heart energy.

Beneficial Herbs to Be Applied One Herb at a Time. Bai shao yao (Radix Paeoniae Alba), 11 g; dang gui (Radix Angelicae Sinensis), 11 g; gou qi zi (Fructus Lycii), 11 g; he shou wu (Radix Polygoni Multiflori), 15 g; ju hua (Flos Chrysanthemi), 20 g; mo han lian (Herba Ecliptae), 11 g; mu li (Concha Ostrae), 35 g; nu zhen zi (Fructus Ligustri Lucidi), 11 g; sheng di (Radix Rehmanniae), fresh, 35 g; zhen zhu mu (Concha Margaritifera Usta), 30 g.

Beneficial Herbal Formulas to Be Applied One Formula at a Time. Qi Ju Di Huang Wan, Tian Ma Gou Teng Yin, Zhen Zhu Mu Wan.

9.6 Internal Liver Wind Blowing

When you are in good health, your y-score is Liver 2; when you are ill, your y-score is Liver 6.

Definition of the Syndrome. When yin deficiency with yang excess affects the liver, this can lead to liver wind causing internal disturbance, which is characterized by shaking and tremors. This syndrome can take three forms: first, liver wind generated by extreme heat and characterized by high fever and twitching; second, liver wind induced by blood deficiency and distinguished by numbness, muscular jumping, and tremor of limbs; and third, liver yang transforming into wind and identified by symptoms of the head and hemiplegia (paralysis of one side of the body).

Clinical Signs and Symptoms. Both eyes flickering, both eyes looking sideways, both eyes looking upward, chronic convulsions in children, clinching the teeth and grinding them, dizziness with blurred vision, fainting, hemiplegia, mouth closed as if screwed up, blueness of the skin and continual twitching, opisthotonos, twitching, wriggling or numbness of muscles, wry mouth and eyes.

Applicable Western Diseases. Alogia, cerebrovascular accidents, Ménière's disease, neurosis in children, optic neuritis, otogenic vertigo, preeclampsia and eclampsia, simple goiter (hyperthyroidism), trachoma, twisting spasmodic syndrome, vertigo.

Treatment Symptoms. Dizziness, headache.

Clinical Cases. (1) For several years, a sixty-five-year-old male patient named Wang had suffered from headaches with vertigo. But recently he experienced a sudden worsening of both, triggered by emotional instability. Other symptoms included mental depression, a bitter taste in the mouth, blackouts, a red complexion as if intoxicated, his four limbs' gradually becoming numb, and sudden fainting. He was diagnosed in Western medicine as having hypertension. A Chinese doctor diagnosed Wang's condition as Internal Liver Wind Blowing mainly on account of the combination of headaches and vertigo, and the sudden fainting. (2) Yang, a thirty-three-year-old female patient, was afflicted with a strange condition: For six months, once a day, she suffered from locked hands and locked lips, with each attack lasting for more than an hour. She also had an aversion to being chilled, cold limbs, palpitations, and dry stools. A Chinese doctor diagnosed her condition as Internal Liver Wind Blowing, primarily because muscular spasms such as those occurring with locked hands and locked lips are distinct signs of this syndrome.

Treatment Principles. To calm down the liver and stop the wind.

Foods Chosen Based on Y-Scores. Abalone (Liver -1), agar (Liver -5), arrowhead (Liver -2), beef liver (Liver 2), black sesame seed (Liver 2), brown sugar (Liver 4), celery (Liver -1), cherry (Liver 4), chicken liver (Liver 4), corn silk (Liver 2), cuttlefish (Liver -3), day lily (Liver 0), hawthorn fruit (Liver 2), jellyfish (Liver -3), litchi nut (Liver 2), loquat (Liver -2), matrimony-vine fruit (Liver 2), mulberry (Liver -2), mussel (Liver -1), perch (Liver 2), pine-nut kernel (Liver 4), plum (Liver 0), pork liver (Liver 1), rape (Liver 2), tomato (Liver -4), towel gourd (Liver 0), variegated carp (bighead) (Liver 4), vinegar (Liver -1), water spinach (Liver -2), white eel (Liver 2), wild rice gall (Liver -2), wine (Liver 3).

Generally Beneficial Foods and Other Foods to Be Chosen or Avoided. 1. Choose from the following grease-free and bland foods: apple, banana, beef, brown sugar, cabbages, carrot, celery, chicken, chicken egg, Chinese cabbage, corn, cottage cheese, cow's milk, fish, fruit, honey, horse bean (broad bean), lean meats, lemon, lettuce, liver, lotus juice (fresh), millet, mung bean, mung bean sprouts, noodle, peach, pea, pear, polished rice, pork, orange, radish, rice, seaweed, skim milk, soybean sprouts, string bean, sweet potato, soybean, sword bean, taro, tofu, tomato, vegetables, watermelon, wheat, white fungus, white sugar, and yam. 2. Avoid these hot and spicy items: alcohol, chili pepper (cayenne pepper), chive (Chinese), cinnamon bark (cassia), cinnamon twig, clove, coffee, garlic, ginger (fresh or dried), green onion (leaf and white head), mustard seed, nutmeg, onion, pepper (black or white), tea, and wine. They force yin energy to excrete through perspiration, which is harmful to heart yin and heart energy. 3. Avoid foods that trigger a new or old disease, such as certain vegetables (common button mushroom, shiitake mushroom, winter bamboo shoots, spinach, and leaf or brown mustard) and meats (rooster, mutton, dog meat, gold carp, pork head, shrimp, crab, and lobster).

Beneficial Herbs to Be Applied One Herb at a Time. Ci ji li (Fructus Tribuli), 10 g; gou teng (Ramulus Uncariae Cum Uncis), 5 11 g; ju hua (Flos Chrysanthemi), 20 g; mu li (Concha Ostrae), 35 g; shi jue ming (Concha Haliotidis), 35 g; tian ma (Rhizoma Gastrodiae), 11 g; zhen zhu mu (Concha Margaritifera Usta), 30 g.

Beneficial Herbal Formulas to Be Applied One Formula at a Time. Da Ding Feng Zhu, Gou Teng Yin, Tian Ma Gou Teng Yin, Zhen Gan Xi Feng Tang.

9.7 Cold Obstructing the Liver Meridian

When you are in good health, your y-score is Liver -4; when you are ill, your y-score is Liver -8.

Definition of the Syndrome. This syndrome refers to the attack on the liver meridian by cold energy. It is most frequently seen in diseases affecting the testes and in hernia. The liver meridian circles the genitals to reach the lower abdomen, and this accounts for the cold pain in the genitals and the lower abdomen. The nature of cold is to contract, which accounts for the contractions of tendons and muscles. Yang is incapable of transforming water, which is the reason for the clear urine and the watery stools.

Clinical Signs and Symptoms. Major signs: Headache involving the top of the head, pain in the lower abdomen with swelling, scrotal hernia affecting the lower abdomen, stretching pain in the scrotum. Median signs: Pale complexion, chill, cold limbs, long and clear streams of urine, watery stools, vomiting of clear saliva, contractions of tendons and muscles.

Applicable Western Diseases. Chronic orchitis (testitis), disorders of testes and epididymis.

Treatment Symptoms. Abdominal pain, menstrual pain.

Clinical Cases. (1) A thirty-year-old male patient named Wang suddenly experienced an attack of acute pain in the lower abdomen, and with it came vomiting as well as frequent and weak urination. Two days later, the symptoms developed into intermittent pain and shrinking of the penis with numbness of the glans penis, in addition to pain in the lower abdomen and mental tension. A Chinese doctor diagnosed his condition as Cold Obstructing the Liver Meridian mainly because of the acute pain in the lower abdomen that affected the genitals. (2) Dong, a forty-year-old male patient, displayed the following symptoms: intolerable swelling and pain in the lower abdomen and passing of meager urine with difficulty. A Chinese doctor diagnosed his condition as Cold Obstructing the Liver Meridian, primarily because severe pain of this nature is usually caused by this syndrome.

Treatment Principles.   To warm the liver and disperse its cold energy.

Foods Chosen Based on Y-Scores.   Black sesame seed (Liver 2), brown sugar (Liver 4), cherry (Liver 4), chicken liver (Liver 4), Chinese chive (Liver 6), corn silk (Liver 2), cuttlefish (Liver -3), day lily (Liver 0), eel (Liver 4), hairtail (Liver 4), hawthorn fruit (Liver 2), Japanese cassia bark (Liver 5), litchi nut (Liver 2), long-tailed anchovy (Liver 4), matrimony-vine fruit (Liver 2), perch (Liver 2), pine-nut kernel (Liver 4), plum (Liver 0), pork liver (Liver 1), rape (Liver 2), rape oil (Liver 6), shepherd's purse (Liver 2), star anise (Liver 5), towel gourd (Liver 0), variegated carp (bighead) (Liver 4), white eel (Liver 2), wine (Liver 3).

Generally Beneficial Foods and Other Foods to Be Chosen or Avoided.   1. Choose from the following blood-tonic foods: beef, beef liver, blood clam, chicken egg, cuttlefish, duck blood, grape, ham, litchi nut, liver, longan, mandarin fish, octopus, oxtail, oyster, pork liver, pork trotter, sea cucumber, soybean skin (black), and spinach. 2. Choose from among these warm foods: blood clam, caper, caraway seed, cassia bark (Japanese), cassia fruit (Japanese), chicken, chili-pepper leaf, chili rhizome, chive (Chinese), chive root and bulb (Chinese), chive seed (Chinese), cinnamon twig, clove, date, dill seed, fennel seed, fenugreek seed (Oriental), fresh ginger, garlic (small), green-onion white head, mustard (white or yellow), mustard seed (white or yellow), nutmeg, pepper (black or white), prickly ash, rice (polished, long-grain), shallot (aromatic green onion), sorghum, star anise, sword bean (jack bean), and water chestnut. 3. Avoid the following cold foods: adzuki bean, aloe vera, asparagus (lucid), bamboo shoots, banana, bitter endive, bitter gourd (balsam pear), brake (fern), burdock, camphor mint, cattail, crab, endive (Chinese), fig, frog (pond), grapefruit, hair vegetable, honey, leaf beet (spinach beet, Swiss chard), lemon, lily flower, mung bean, mung-bean powder, mung bean sprouts, orchid leaf, peppermint, potato (Irish), preserved duck egg, pricking amaranth (amaranth, pigweed), purslane, rabbit, rambutan, romaine lettuce, Russian olive (oleaster), safflower fruit, salt, soybean paste, squash, star fruit (carambola), strawberry (Indian or mock), sweet basil, tofu, water spinach, wax gourd (Chinese), and wheat.

Beneficial Herbs to Be Applied One Herb at a Time. Chuan jiao (Pericarpium Zanthoxyli [Fructus Zanthoxyli]), 10 g; fu zi (Radix Aconiti Praeparata), 11 g; ju he (Semen Aurantii/Reticulata Blanco), 11 g; li zhi he (Semen Litchi), 11 g; rou gui (Cortex Cinnamomi), 5 g; wu yao (Radix Linderae), 10 g; wu zhu yu (Fructus Euodiae), 7 g; xiao hui xiang (Fructus Foeniculi), 11 g.

Beneficial Herbal Formulas to Be Applied One Formula at a Time. Dang Gui Si Ni Tang, Nuan Gan Jian, Shao Fu Zhu Yu Tang, Tian Tai Wu Yao San.

9.8 Damp Heat Attacking the Liver and Gallbladder

When you are in good health, your y-scores are Liver 2 and Gallbladder 2; when you are ill, your y-scores are Liver 6 and Gallbladder 6.

Definition of the Syndrome. When dampness and heat affect the liver and the gallbladder simultaneously, this can lead to Damp Heat Attacking the Liver and Gallbladder, which is characterized by symptoms associated with urination and the genitals.

Clinical Signs and Symptoms. Abdominal swelling, eating only a little, eczema in the scrotum, impotence, itch in the genitals, jaundice, nausea and vomiting, pain in the eyes, pain in the hypochondrium, meager urine, insomnia, thirst with no desire to drink, urination difficulty, vaginal discharge, yellowish-red urine.

Applicable Western Diseases. Acute cholecystitis, acute hepatitis, cholecystolithiasis, acute icterohepatitis, cervicitis, herpes zoster, pudendal eczema, purulent otitis media, vaginitis.

Treatment Symptoms. Pain in the hypochondrium, jaundice, testicular pain and swelling, itch in the female genitals, vaginal discharge, absent urination.

Clinical Cases. (1) For four years, Li, a thirty-one-year-old male patient, had a frequently recurring stomach condition that was controlled by drugs. But lately the attacks had become more severe, involving a range of diverse symptoms, such as pain in the right ribs and severe pain in the upper abdomen that worsen on massage, a bitter taste in the mouth, a dry throat, nausea and vomiting, a poor appetite, a yellowish appearance of the skin all over the body, meager yellowish-red urine, constipation, and a red tongue with a yellowish and greasy coating. A Chinese doctor diagnosed Li's condition as Damp Heat Attacking the Liver and Gallbladder, mainly on account of the fact that the ribs are the territory of the liver and the gallbladder, and many signs of damp heat were present, such as the bitter taste in the mouth and the yellowish-red urine. (2) A forty-two-year-old female patient named Hua exhibited a number of symptoms: Her skin, the sclera enclosing her eyeballs, and her nails turned the color of an orange, and she had pain in the right ribs, itching, chest congestion, no appetite, a slightly red tongue with a thin and yellowish coating, deep-red urine, and dry stools. She was diagnosed by a Western physician as having acute icteric hepatitis. A Chinese doctor diagnosed her condition as Damp Heat Attacking the Liver and Gallbladder, especially because a yellowish appearance is a sign of damp heat and the ribs are the territory of the liver and the gallbladder.

Treatment Principles. To clear heat in the liver and expel dampness in the liver and the gallbladder.

Foods Chosen Based on Y-Scores. Abalone (Liver -1), agar (Liver -5), arrowhead (Liver -2), beef liver (Liver 2), black sesame seed (Liver 2), brown sugar (Liver 4), celery (Liver -1), cherry (Liver 4), chicken liver (Liver 4), corn silk (Gallbladder 2, Liver 2), cuttlefish (Liver -3), day lily (Liver 0), hawthorn fruit (Liver 2), jellyfish (Liver -3), litchi nut (Liver 2), loquat (Liver -2), matrimony-vine fruit (Liver 2), mulberry (Liver -2), mussel (Liver -1), perch (Liver 2), pine-nut kernel (Liver 4), plum (Liver 0), pork liver (Liver 1), rape (Liver 2), tomato (Liver -4), towel gourd (Liver 0), variegated carp (bighead) (Liver 4), vinegar (Liver -1), water spinach (Liver -2), white eel (Liver 2), wild rice gall (Liver -2), wine (Liver 3).

Generally Beneficial Foods and Other Foods to Be Chosen or Avoided. 1. Choose from the following foods that are good for damp heat: adzuki bean sprouts, buckwheat, cantaloupe (muskmelon), carp (common), celery root, Chinese cabbage, coconut shell, corn silk, cucumber vine (stem), day lily, eggplant (aubergine), eggplant calyx, fig leaf, frog (river or pond), green turtle, hawthorn fruit, olive, pricking amaranth (amaranth, pigweed), soybean (yellow), soybean oil, soybean sprouts (dried, black), squash (flower and root), star fruit (carambola), sunflower (top of peduncle), turnip seed, water-rice root, wax gourd (Chinese), and wheat seedling. 2. Avoid items that are likely to trigger a chronic damp heat syndrome or intensify an existing one, such as alcohol, maltose, pork, and sweet rice. 3. Avoid these greasy and fatty foods: animal fats (including lamb fat and oil), butter, chicken egg yolk, creams, fatty meats, fish-liver oils, fried foods, and lard. They can generate heat and produce phlegm, and they worsen indigestion, a poor appetite, jaundice, dysentery, and diarrhea. 4. Choose from among the following grease-free, bland, and nonirritating foods: apple, banana, beef, brown sugar, cabbages, carrot, celery, chicken, chicken eggs, Chinese cabbage, corn, cottage cheese, cow's milk, fish, fruit, honey, horse bean (broad bean), lean meats, lemon, lettuce, liver, lotus juice (fresh), millet, mung bean, mung bean sprouts, noodle, peach, pea, pear, polished rice, pork, orange, radish, rice, seaweed, skim milk, soybean, soybean sprouts, string bean, sweet potato, sword bean, taro, tofu, tomato, vegetables, watermelon, wheat, white fungus, white sugar, and yam.

Beneficial Herbs to Be Applied One Herb at a Time. Ban xia (Rhizoma Pinelliae), 12 g; huang qin (Radix Scutellariae), 15 g; jin qian cao (Herba Lysimachiae), 18 g; long dan (Radix Gentianae), 10 g; qing hao (Herba Artemisiae Chinghao), 11 g; yin chen (Herba Artemisiae Scopariae), 21 g; yu jin (Radix Curcumae), 11 g.

Beneficial Herbal Formulas to Be Applied One Formula at a Time. Da Chai Hu Tang, Long Dan Xie Gan Tang, Qing Yi Tang, Yin Chen Hao Tang.

10

Choosing Foods and Herbs to Boost the Gallbladder and Cure Applicable Symptoms and Diseases

10.1 Gallbladder Excessive Heat

When you are in good health, your y-score is Gallbladder 3; when you are ill, your y-score is Gallbladder 7.

Definition of the Syndrome. With this syndrome, the congestion of gallbladder energy transforms into heat, which means congested heat gets accumulated in the gallbladder, with a bitter taste in the mouth and a dry throat as the primary symptoms.

Clinical Signs and Symptoms. Bitter taste in the mouth, cold sensations alternating with hot sensations, congested chest with discomfort in the stomach, vomiting, vomiting of bitter water, deafness, dizziness, feeling insecure over sleep, getting angry easily, jaundice, pain in the hypochondrium, insomnia with love of darkness, dislike of light, and mental depression.

Applicable Western Diseases. Accessory nasal sinusitis, acute cholycystitis, acute gastritis, chronic pancreatitis, otitis media, rhinitis, suppurative keratitis.

Treatment Symptoms. Dizziness, pain in the hypochondrium, jaundice, insomnia.

Clinical Cases. A female patient named Huang, age twenty-seven, displayed the following symptoms: continual pain in the upper-right abdomen that radiates toward the right scapula region, an aversion to being chilled, a fever of 38.6 degrees C (101.5 degrees F), no perspiration, nausea, vomiting, a loss of appetite, an

156

aversion to oil, and a pale-yellowish coating on the tongue. Huang was diagnosed by a doctor of Western medicine as having cholycystitis. A Chinese doctor diagnosed her condition as Gallbladder Excessive Heat, primarily because pain in the upper-right abdomen and an aversion to oil are closely associated with the gallbladder and a fever is a hot sign.

Treatment Principles. To clear heat and sedate the gallbladder.

Foods Chosen Based on Y-Scores. Corn silk (Gallbladder 2, Liver 2).

Generally Beneficial Foods and Other Foods to Be Chosen or Avoided. 1. Choose from among these grease-free, bland, and non-irritating foods: apple, banana, beef, brown sugar, cabbages, carrot, celery, chicken, chicken egg, Chinese cabbage, corn, cottage cheese, cow's milk, fish, fruit, honey, horse bean (broad bean), lean meats, lemon, lettuce, liver, lotus juice (fresh), millet, mung bean sprouts, mung bean, noodle, peach, pea, pear, polished rice, pork, orange, radish, rice, seaweed, skim milk, soybean sprouts, string bean, sweet potato, soybean, sword bean, taro, tofu, tomato, vegetables, watermelon, wheat, white fungus, white sugar, and yam. 2. Choose from the following more easily digestible foods: areca nut (unripe), asafetida, bog bean (buck bean), buckwheat, cardamom seed, carrot, chicken gizzard, coriander (Chinese parsley), coriander seed, dill seed, distillers' grains, grapefruit (including peel), green-onion white head, hawthorn fruit, jackfruit, kiwifruit (Chinese gooseberry), lime (young trifoliate orange), lobster (sea prawn), longan seed, malt, millet sprouts, orange peel (sweet or sour), papaya, peach, quince, radish, red bayberry, sorghum, soybean (yellow), sweet basil, tomato, water chestnut, and whitefish. 3. In cases of indigestion, these foods should be avoided: goose, fried pea, mango, raw chestnut, red date, sweet rice, taro, and yellow soybean. 4. Avoid these hot and spicy items: alcohol, chili pepper (cayenne pepper), chive (Chinese), cinnamon bark (cassia), cinnamon twig, clove, coffee, garlic, ginger (fresh or dried), green onion (leaf and white head), mustard seed, nutmeg, onion, pepper (black or white), tea, and wine. They force yin energy to excrete through perspiration, which is harmful to yin and energy. 5. Avoid the following irritants: alcohol, coffee, tea, tobacco, and wine. They can irritate the stomach and produce damp heat, and fire is harmful to yin and energy. 6. Avoid greasy and fatty foods, such as animal fats (including lamb fat and oil), butter, chicken egg yolk, creams, fatty meats, fish-liver oils, fried foods, and lard. They can generate heat and produce phlegm, and they aggravate indigestion, a poor appetite, jaundice, dysentery, and diarrhea.

Beneficial Herbs to Be Applied One Herb at a Time. Long dan cao (Radix Gentianae), 10 g; zhi zi (Fructus Gardeniae), 12 g; yin chen (Herba Artemisiae Capillaris), 30 g; qing-hao (Herba Artemisiae Chinghao), 6 g.

Beneficial Herbal Formulas to Be Applied One Formula at a Time. Dan Dao Pai Shi Tang, Xiao Chai Hu Tang.

10.2 Gallbladder Energy Deficiency

When you are in good health, your y-score is Gallbladder -2; when you are ill, your y-score is Gallbladder -6.

Definition of the Syndrome. When energy deficiency affects the gallbladder, it can lead to Gallbladder Energy Deficiency, which is characterized by timidity and palpitations.

Clinical Signs and Symptoms. Cowardice and getting scared easily, dizziness with a desire to lie down, love of sighing, misty vision.

Applicable Western Diseases. Neurasthenia.

Treatment Symptoms. Palpitations, insomnia, mental illness.

Clinical Cases. For more than ten years, a forty-five-year-old female patient named Zhang exhibited the following symptoms: a congested chest, vomiting of watery phlegm, palpitations, insomnia, perspiration, a greasy coating on the tongue, muscular spasms, forgetfulness, being suspicious, being easily in shock, becoming easily scared, no appetite, and low spirits. A Chinese doctor diagnosed her condition as Gallbladder Energy Deficiency, mainly because getting scared easily is a distinct sign of this syndrome.

Treatment Principles. To benefit energy and secure the spirits.

Foods Chosen Based on Y-Scores. Corn silk (Gallbladder 2, Liver 2).

Generally Beneficial Foods and Other Foods to Be Chosen or Avoided. 1. Choose from the following energy-tonic foods: beef, bird's nest, broomcorn, cherry, chicken, coconut meat, crane meat, date (red or black), eel, ginkgo (cooked), ginseng, goose meat, grape, herring, honey, jackfruit, loach, longan, mackerel, mandarin fish, octopus, pheasant, pigeon egg, pigeon meat, potato (Irish), rabbit, rice (fermented, glutinous), rice (glutinous or sweet), rice (polished), rice (polished, long-grain), rock sugar, shark's fin, sheep or goat meat, shiitake mushroom, snake melon, squash, sturgeon, sweet potato, tofu, turtledove, walnut root, and white string bean. 2. Avoid foods that exacerbate energy deficiency, such as scallion bulb and prickly ash. 3. Choose from among these grease-free, bland, and nonirritating foods: apple, banana, beef, brown sugar, cabbages, carrot, celery, chicken, chicken egg, Chinese cabbage, corn, cottage cheese, cow's milk, fish, fruit, honey, horse bean (broad bean), lean meats, lemon, lettuce, liver, lotus juice (fresh), millet, mung bean, mung bean sprouts, noodle, peach, pea, pear, polished rice, pork, orange, radish, seaweed, skim milk, soybean sprouts, string bean, soybean, sweet potato, sword bean, taro, tofu, tomato, vegetables, watermelon, wheat, white fungus, white sugar, and yam. 4. Avoid these irritants: alcohol, coffee, tea, tobacco, and wine. They can irritate the stomach and produce damp heat, and fire is harmful to yin and energy. 5. Avoid greasy and fatty foods, such as animal fats (including lamb fat and oil), butter, chicken egg yolk, creams, fatty meats, fish-liver oils, fried foods, and lard. They can generate heat and produce phlegm, and they exacerbate indigestion, a poor appetite, jaundice, dysentery, and diarrhea.

Beneficial Herbs to Be Applied One Herb at a Time. Ban xia (Rhizoma Pinelliae), 12 g; chen pi (Pericarpium Citri Reticulatae), 11 g; dang gui (Radix Angelicae Sinensis), 11 g; gan jiang (Rhizoma Zingiberis), 7 g; shan zhu yu (Fructus Corni), 11 g; sheng jiang (Rhizoma Zingiberis Recens), 10 g; shu di huang (Radix Rehmanniae), cooked, 18 g; suan zao ren (Semen Ziziphi Spinosae), 18 g; wu wei zi (Fructus Schisandrae), 4 g.

Beneficial Herbal Formulas to Be Applied One Formula at a Time. Suan Zao Ren Tang, Wen Dan Tang.

11

Choosing Foods and Herbs to Boost the Kidneys and Cure Applicable Symptoms and Diseases

11.1 Kidneys Yang Deficiency

When you are in good health, your y-score is Kidneys -4; when you are ill, your y-score is Kidneys -8.

Definition of the Syndrome. When yang deficiency affects the kidneys, this can lead to Kidneys Yang Deficiency, a syndrome mostly associated with chronic diseases involving the elderly and in chronic nephritis, hypothyroidism, neurasthenia, and so forth.

The waist is the palace of the kidneys, which accounts for the lumbago and weak legs. Kidneys yang is the source of yang energy throughout the whole body, leading to the fear of coldness and the cold limbs. Yang energy is unable to fill up brain marrow, causing the low spirits. The ears are the outlets of the kidneys, which is why there is the ringing in the ears and the deafness. The kidneys store pure essence that is essential to reproduction, which is the reason for the infertility, the impotence, and the ejaculation disorders. The kidneys are unable to warm the spleen and the stomach, causing the diarrhea.

Clinical Signs and Symptoms. Major signs: Lumbago, cold and weak lower limbs, fear of the cold. Median signs: Low spirits, dizziness, ringing in the ears and deafness, impotence, premature ejaculation, seminal emission, infertility in men and women, frequent urination at night, dribbling of urine. Minor signs: Abdominal swelling and fullness, chronic diarrhea, cold feet, cold loins and legs, cold sen-

160

sation in the genitals, cold sensation in the muscles, cough and panting, diarrhea, diarrhea before dawn, diarrhea with sticky and muddy
stools, difficult labor, discharge of watery and thin stools, dizziness,
edema, excessive perspiration, fatigue, foot weakness, frequent urination at night, hair falling out easily, hands and feet lacking warmth,
lack of appetite, loose teeth, neck swelling, pain and softness in the
loins and knees, palpitations, panting, perspiration on the forehead,
pleasant taste in the mouth, retention of urine, meager urine, shortness of breath, swelling of body, vaginal bleeding, wheezing.

Applicable Western Diseases and Conditions.   Amenorrhea,
angina pectoris, asthma, bronchial asthma, chronic bronchitis,
chronic enteritis, chronic nephritis, chronic prostatitis, chronic renal
failure, diabetes mellitus, endocrine disturbances, hepatic cirrhosis,
hyperaldosteronism (abnormally high levels of aldosterone in
blood), hypoadrenocorticism, hypothyroidism, menopause syndrome, nephrotic syndrome, neurasthenia, neurosis, otogenic vertigo, rheumatoid cardiopathy, sexual neurasthenia.

Treatment Symptoms.   Chronic fatigue, impotence, absent urination, edema, diarrhea, vaginal discharge.

Clinical Cases.   (1) For more than a month, a sixty-two-year-old
male patient named Zhang displayed dribbling of urine and difficult
urination. When he wanted to pass urine, the urine would not flow,
and each time it would take him half an hour and great effort to
pass his urine. He also had swelling and fullness in the lower
abdomen. A Chinese doctor diagnosed his condition as Kidneys
Yang Deficiency mainly due to the dribbling of the urine and his
older age. (2) A male patient named Chen, age forty-six, had
decreased sexual desire with a weak erection. He also had a backache and perspired profusely at work. In addition, he was highly
susceptible to an attack of the common cold, in which case he
would cough up whitish and sticky phlegm. A Chinese doctor diagnosed his condition as Kidneys Yang Deficiency primarily because
of his decreased sexual desire, backache, and profuse perspiration.
(3) A twenty-eight-year-old male patient by the name of Lee had a
history of neurasthenia with insecurity over sleep, seminal emission
with erotic dreams, dizziness, and weakness. Recently, he began to
display impotence, forgetfulness, palpitations, and a pale tongue. A
Chinese doctor diagnosed his condition as Kidneys Yang Deficiency,
especially because neurasthenia, seminal emission with erotic
dreams, and dizziness are signs of this syndrome.

Treatment Principles. To warm and tone the kidneys yang.

Foods Chosen Based on Y-Scores. Autumn bottle gourd (Kidneys 2), bird's nest (Kidneys 2), black sesame seed (Kidneys 2), black soybean (Kidneys 2), chestnut (Kidneys 4), chicken liver (Kidneys 4), Chinese chive (Kidneys 6), common carp (Kidneys 2), day lily (Liver 0, Kidneys 0), eel (Liver 4, Kidneys 4), goat's milk (Kidneys 4), gorgan fruit (Kidneys 2), grape (Kidneys 0), green onion (seed) (Kidneys 6), Japanese cassia bark (Kidneys 5), Job's tears (Kidneys 0), lobster (Kidneys 1), lotus (Kidneys 2), lotus seed (Kidneys 2), matrimony-vine fruit (Kidneys 2), mutton (Kidneys 4), perch (Kidneys 2), plum (Kidneys 0), prickly ash (Kidneys 6), star anise (Kidneys 5), string bean (Kidneys 2), tangerine (Kidneys -2), walnut (Kidneys 4), wheat (Kidneys 0), white eel (Kidneys 2), white fungus (Kidneys 2), yam (Kidneys 2).

Generally Beneficial Foods and Other Foods to Be Chosen or Avoided. 1. Foods that are generally good for this syndrome include clove, crabapple, dill seed, fennel, kidney, lobster, pistachio nut, raspberry, sardine, shrimp, sparrow, sparrow egg, and walnut. 2. Choose from among these yang-tonic foods for the kidneys: air bladder of shark, beef kidney, cassia fruit (Japanese), chestnut, chive seed (Chinese), cinnamon bark (cassia), clove, clove oil, deer kidney, dill seed, fennel root, fennel seed, fenugreek seed (Oriental), green-onion seed, lobster (sea prawn), mandarin-orange seed, oxtail, pistachio nut, pork testes, prickly ash root, raspberry, sheep or goat kidney, shrimp, sparrow egg, star anise, strawberry, and sword bean (jack bean). 3. Avoid the following cold foods: adzuki bean, aloe vera, asparagus (lucid), bamboo shoots, banana, bitter endive, bitter gourd (balsam pear), brake (fern), burdock, camphor mint, cattail, crab, endive (Chinese), fig, frog (pond), grapefruit, hair vegetable, honey, leaf beet (spinach beet, Swiss chard), lemon, lily flower, mung bean, mung-bean powder, mung bean sprouts, orchid leaf, peppermint, potato (Irish), preserved duck egg, pricking amaranth (amaranth, pigweed), purslane, rabbit, rambutan, romaine lettuce, Russian olive (oleaster), safflower fruit, salt, soybean paste, squash, star fruit (carambola), strawberry (Indian or mock), sweet basil, tofu, water spinach, wax gourd (Chinese), and wheat.

Beneficial Herbs to Be Applied One Herb at a Time. Ba ji tian (Radix Morindae Officinalis), 11 g; fu zi (Radix Aconiti Praeparata), 11 g; lu jiao jiao (Colla Cornus Cervi), 12 g; rou gui

(Cortex Cinnamomi), 5 g; shu di huang (Radix Rehmanniae), cooked, 18 g; tu si zi (Semen Cuscutae), 11 g; yin yang huo (Herba Epimedii), 11 g.

Beneficial Herbal Formulas to Be Applied One Formula at a Time. Ji Sheng Shen Qi Wan, Nei Bu Wan, Shen Qi Wan, You Gui Wan.

11.2 Kidneys Yin Deficiency

When you are in good health, your y-score is Kidneys 3; when you are ill, your y-score is Kidneys 7.

Definition of the Syndrome. When yin deficiency affects the kidneys, this can give rise to Kidneys Yin Deficiency. The kidneys are in charge of the bones, which is the reason for the lumbago and weak legs. Kidneys yin is the basis of yin energy throughout the entire body, which accounts for the skinniness. Kidneys Yin Deficiency can generate internal heat, causing the hot sensations, reddish appearance in the zygomatic regions, night sweats, and dry throat. Kidneys Yin Deficiency will lead to insufficient brain marrow, and this accounts for the dizziness and ringing in the ears. And it can generate fire to disturb the spirits, giving rise to the insomnia and many dreams. The kidneys store pure energy, and, when Kidneys Yin Deficiency generates fire, the fire can disturb the "room of pure essence" (this is the Chinese name for the place where sperm are stored and is similar to the epididymis in Western medicine); that accounts for the seminal emission and premature ejaculation.

Clinical Signs and Symptoms. Major signs: Lumbago with weak legs, dizziness, hot sensation in the "five hearts" (this refers to the five central places: two in the palms of the hands, two in the soles of the feet, and one in the chest, or heart; thus, we have five centers, which are called "five hearts"). Median signs: Visual whirling sensations, ringing in the ears and deafness, seminal emission, premature ejaculation, suppression of menses, infertility in women, night sweats, dry sensation in the mouth with no desire to drink, skinniness. Minor signs: Blurred vision, cold hands and feet, cough with phlegm containing blood or coughing up fresh blood, dry throat, fatigue, feeling miserable and hurried, fever, fever at night with burning sensations in the internal organs, blood in urine, hot sensations in the body and the center of hands and feet, warm skin and muscles, hot sensation in the body with solid stools, hot sensation in the center of palms, hot sensation in the soles of feet, irregular menstruation, night sweats, pain in the heels, pain in the loins (lumbago), pain in the tibia, retention of urine, ringing in the ears, seminal emission with dreams, insomnia, suppression of menses, thirst, toothache or shaky teeth, urinary strain.

Applicable Western Diseases and Conditions. Addison's disease, amenorrhea, anovulatory dysfunctional uterine bleeding, aplastic anemia, cancer of the uterine cervix, central retinal choroiditis, chronic glometrulonephritis, chronic nephritis, chronic pyelonephritis (chronic nephropyelitis), chronic weakness, diabetes insipidus, diabetes mellitus, general (disseminated) lupus erythematosus, haemoptysis, hepatic cirrhosis, hypertension, hyperthyroidism, lumbago, lupus erythematosus, menopause syndrome, neurothenia, otogenic vertigo, preeclampsia and eclampsia, primary hepatoma, prostatitis, pulmonary tuberculosis, renal tuberculosis, rheumatoid cardiopathy, sexual neurosis, tonsillitis, tuberculosis, tuberculosis of bones and joints, urinary infection, vaginal bleeding, vertigo, vertigo of the inner ear.

Treatment Symptoms. Seminal emission, insomnia, chronic fatigue, blood in urine, vaginal bleeding.

Clinical Cases. (1) Over the past six months, a thirty-nine-year-old male patient named Zhu displayed the following symptoms: dizziness, nervousness, a red tongue, hot sensations in the palms of the hands and the soles of the feet, insomnia, and night sweats. A Chinese doctor diagnosed his condition as Kidneys Yin Deficiency, in view of the fact that many of his symptoms are major signs of this syndrome. (2) Liu, a thirty-one-year-old male patient, exhibited these symptoms: dizziness, ringing in the ears, a dry throat, thirst, palpitations, insomnia, seminal emission with erotic dreams, and a poor memory. A Western physician diagnosed his condition as neurasthenia; a Chinese doctor diagnosed it as Kidneys Yin Deficiency, because many of his symptoms are important signs of this syndrome. (3) Over the course of several years, a thirty-two-year-old male patient named Yang suffered from recurrent chyluria (the presence of chyle in the urine due to an organic disease possibly of the kidneys), accompanied by hydrocele (an accumulation of serous fluid in the scrotum). One day when the disease attacked, he displayed other symptoms as well, including a dry mouth, a hot sensation in the palms of his hands, pain in the lower back, falling pain in the lower abdomen, discharge of urine that looks like ointment and oil, and a light-red tongue. A Chinese doctor diagnosed his condition as Kidneys Yin Deficiency, primarily because symptoms of damp heat are due to this syndrome.

Treatment Principles. To water and tone yin energy in the kidneys.

Foods Chosen Based on Y-Scores. Autumn bottle gourd (Kidneys 2), bird's nest (Kidneys 2), black sesame seed (Kidneys 2), black soybean (Kidneys 2), clam (freshwater) (Kidneys -5), common carp (Kidneys 2), cuttlefish (Kidneys -3), day lily (Kidneys 0), frog (Kidneys -5), gorgan fruit (Kidneys 2), grapefruit (Kidneys -4), grape (Kidneys 0), jellyfish (Kidneys -3), Job's tears (Kidneys 0), kiwifruit (Kidneys -4), lobster (Kidneys 1), lotus (Kidneys 2), lotus seed (Kidneys 2), matrimony-vine fruit (Kidneys 2), matrimony-vine leaf (Kidneys -4), mulberry (Kidneys -2), mussel (Kidneys -1), perch (Kidneys 2), plum (Kidneys 0), pork (Kidneys -1), pork kidney (Kidneys -3), river clamshell (Kidneys -5), salt (Kidneys -7), sea cucumber (Kidneys -1), seaweed (marine alga) (Kidneys -8), soy sauce (Kidneys -7), string bean (Kidneys 2), tangerine (Kidneys -2), wheat (Kidneys 0), white eel (Kidneys 2), white fungus (Kidneys 2), yam (Kidneys 2).

Generally Beneficial Foods and Other Foods to Be Chosen or Avoided. 1. Foods that are normally good for this syndrome are abalone, asparagus, chestnut, chicken egg, chicken liver, cuttlefish, duck, duck egg, oyster, pork, pork kidney, royal jelly, and white fungus. 2. Choose from these yin-tonic foods: abalone, air bladder of shark, apple, apricot pit (sweet powder), asparagus (lucid), bean drink, bird's nest, bitter gourd (balsam pear), black-eyed pea, brown sugar, cantaloupe (muskmelon), cheeses, chicken egg, chicken eggshell (inner membrane), clam (freshwater or saltwater), coconut milk, crab, cuttlefish, date, duck, duck egg, fig, frog (river or pond), goose meat, grape, green turtle, honey, kidney bean, kumquat, lard, lemon, litchi nut, loquat (Japanese medlai), lotus rhizome, maltose, mandarin orange, mango, milk (cow's), mussel, oyster, pea, pear, pearl (powder), pineapple, pomegranate (sweet fruit), pork, rabbit, red bayberry, rice (polished), royal jelly, sea cucumber, shrimp, star fruit (carambola), string bean, sugarcane, tofu, tomato, turtle egg, walnut, watermelon, white sugar, whitebait, white fungus, and yam. 3. Items to be avoided in cases of deficiency heat are alcohol, cayenne pepper, Chinese chive, dog meat, eel, and fresh ginger. 4. Items to be avoided in cases of fire deficiency are garlic, Japanese cassia bark, litchi nut, prickly ash, star anise, and walnut.

Beneficial Herbs to Be Applied One Herb at a Time. Gou qi zi (Fructus Lycii), 11 g; gui ban (Plastrum Testudinis), 30 g; he shou wu (Radix Polygoni Multiflori), 15 g; shan yao (Rhizoma Dioscoreae), 20 g; shan zhu yu (Fructus Corni), 11 g; shu di huang (Radix Rehmanniae), cooked, 18 g.

Beneficial Herbal Formulas to Be Applied One Formula at a Time. Da Bu Yin Wan, Liu Wei Di Huang Wan, Zuo Gui Wan.

11.3 Insufficient Kidneys Pure Essence (Kidneys Yin Deficiency Affecting Reproduction)

When you are in good health, your y-score is Kidneys 3; when you are ill, your y-score is Kidneys 7.

Definition of the Syndrome. Insufficient Kidneys Pure Essence refers to a deprivation of kidneys essence, so that the sea of marrow becomes empty, resulting in slow growth, premature aging, and weak limbs. The kidneys are the innate source of life, taking charge of growth and reproduction, which accounts for the slow growth in children and the premature aging. The kidneys take charge of the bones, and this has to do with the fontanel's not being closed on time and the weak legs. The teeth are extensions of bone, which accounts for the loose teeth. Because pure essence is in short supply, it cannot fill up brain marrow, giving rise to the lower intelligence, forgetfulness, dizziness, and idiotic look. The ears are the outlets of the kidneys, and this is why there is the ringing in the ears and deafness. The kidneys produce semen, which is the reason for the low sex drive and the infertility in both men and women.

Clinical Signs and Symptoms. Major signs: Slow growth in children, sexual decline in adults, premature aging. Median signs: Deafness, decreased hearing, dizziness, fontanel's not closed on time, infertility, ringing in the ears, loose teeth. Minor signs: Idiotic look, weak bones, forgetfulness.

Applicable Western Diseases. Arteriosclerosis, infertility, innate malnutrition in children, rickets, senile dementia.

Treatment Symptoms. Slow development in children, dizziness, chronic fatigue, impotence.

Clinical Cases. (1) Having been married for five years without children, a thirty-three-year-old male patient named Yao underwent a physical examination at a Chinese medicine clinic that showed an insufficient sperm count. Yao also displayed lumbago as well as hot sensations in the palms of the hands and the soles of the feet. A doctor at the clinic diagnosed his condition as Insufficient Kidneys Pure Essence, primarily because pure essence of the kidneys is responsible for sperm production. (2) Wong, a five-year-old girl, exhibited paralysis of the lower limbs, skinniness, slow movements, a yellowish complexion, and slow growth. A Chinese doctor diagnosed her condition as Insufficient Kidneys Pure Essence, mainly in view of the fact that pure essence of the kidneys is responsible for growth in the early years of life.

Treatment Principles. To tone the kidneys and fill up the kidneys essence.

Foods Chosen Based on Y-Scores. Autumn bottle gourd (Kidneys 2, Spleen 2), bird's nest (Kidneys 2), black sesame seed (Kidneys 2), black soybean (Kidneys 2), clam (freshwater) (Kidneys -5), common carp (Kidneys 2), cuttlefish (Kidneys -3), day lily (Kidneys 0), frog (Kidneys -5), gorgan fruit (Kidneys 2), grapefruit (Kidneys -4), grape (Kidneys 0), jellyfish (Kidneys -3), Job's tears (Kidneys 0), kiwifruit (Kidneys -4), lobster (Kidneys 1), lotus (Kidneys 2), lotus seed (Kidneys 2), matrimony-vine fruit (Kidneys 2), matrimony-vine leaf (Kidneys -4), mulberry (Kidneys -2), mussel (Kidneys -1), perch (Kidneys 2), plum (Kidneys 0), pork (Kidneys -1), pork kidney (Kidneys -3), river clamshell (Kidneys -5), salt (Kidneys -7), sea cucumber (Kidneys -1), seaweed (marine alga) (Kidneys -8), soy sauce (Kidneys -7), string bean (Kidneys 2), tangerine (Kidneys -2), wheat (Kidneys 0), white eel (Kidneys 2), white fungus (Kidneys 2), yam (Kidneys 2).

Generally Beneficial Foods and Other Foods to Be Chosen or Avoided. 1. Choose from the following yang-tonic foods for the kidneys: air bladder of shark, beef kidney, cassia fruit (Japanese), chestnut, chive seed (Chinese), cinnamon bark (cassia), clove, clove oil, deer kidney, dill seed, fennel root, fennel seed, fenugreek seed (Oriental), green-onion seed, lobster (sea prawn), mandarin-orange seed, oxtail, pistachio nut, pork testes, prickly ash root, raspberry, sheep or goat kidney, shrimp, sparrow egg, star anise, strawberry, and sword bean (jack bean). 2. Choose from these yin-tonic foods for the kidneys: black-eyed pea, black sesame seed, chicken liver, fish air bladder, frog (forest), lotus (fruit and seed), matrimony-vine fruit, millet, mulberry, mullet (black or striped), mussel, perch, pigeon egg, pigeon meat, pork kidney, scallop (dried), sea cucumber, string bean, walnut, wheat, and wild cabbage. 3. According to the *Yellow Emperor's Clas-*

sics of Internal Medicine, published in the third century, B.C., "Patients with lung diseases should eat sweet rice, chicken, peach, and onions; they should eat pungent foods and avoid bitter foods. Other foods also good for the lungs include wheat and barley, mutton, almond, and scallion bulb. The lungs are most vulnerable to upsurging energy; when this occurs, eat bitter foods right away in order to sedate the lungs. When the lungs start to constrict energy, eat sour foods right away in order to constrict and tone up the energy of the lungs. Eat pungent foods to sedate the lungs when necessary."

Beneficial Herbs to Be Applied One Herb at a Time. Shu di (Radix Rehmanniae), steamed, 25 g; shan zhu yu (Fructus Corni), 10 g; gou qi zi (Fructus Lycii), 10 g.

Beneficial Herbal Formulas to Be Applied One Formula at a Time. He Che Wan, Zuo Gui Wan.

11.4 Loosening of Kidneys Energy (Kidneys Energy Deficiency Affecting the Bladder)

When you are in good health, your y-score is Kidneys -2; when you are ill, your y-score is Kidneys -6.

Definition of the Syndrome. Loosening of Kidneys Energy refers to the bladder's being out of control or a relaxation of the semen gate due to an energy deficiency of the kidneys.

The kidneys and the bladder have a relationship with each other; when the kidneys are deficient, the bladder will lose its power of controlling urine, which accounts for the many disorders in urination. The kidneys are in control of the semen gate; when the kidneys are deficient, the semen gate will become loose, causing ejaculation disorders. The ears are the outlets of the kidneys, giving rise to the ringing in the ears and deafness. The kidneys are in control of the waist region, which is the reason for the lumbago.

Clinical Signs and Symptoms. Major signs: Inability to retain urine and to control ejaculation, premature ejaculation, sliding ejaculation, frequent urination at night in particular, incontinence of urination with dribbling, prone to miscarriage in women. Median signs: Lumbago, weak legs, pale complexion, fatigue, ringing in the ears and deafness. Minor signs: Bed-wetting in children, clear and long streams of urine, clear and white vaginal discharge, dizziness, dribbling of urine, fetus motion, seminal emission without erotic dreams, vaginal discharge, vaginal bleeding.

Applicable Western Diseases.   Adnexitis, diabetes insipidus, enuresis neurasthenia, nocturia, prostatitis, senile prostatic hyperplasia.

Treatment Symptoms.   Seminal emission, urination disorders, vaginal discharge, miscarriage.

Clinical Cases.   (1) Lim, a thirty-three-year-old male patient, displayed the following symptoms: seminal emission without dreams, dizziness, ringing in the ears, a poor complexion, an aversion to the cold, and lumbago. A Chinese doctor diagnosed his condition as Loosening of Kidneys Energy, mainly on account of the fact that ejaculation disorders are due to this syndrome and many of his other symptoms support this diagnosis. (2) Even though she is sixteen years old, Chang, a female patient, has been wetting her bed one or two times almost every night for many years. She also urinates frequently during the daytime, has a pale complexion, and grinds her teeth at night. A Chinese doctor diagnosed her condition as Loosening of Kidneys Energy, especially because an inability to control urination is primarily due to this syndrome and other symptoms displayed by the patient coincide with this diagnosis. (3) For two years, a forty-five-year-old male patient named Zhou has suffered from incontinence of urination. His inability to control his urination occurs particularly in winter, when he wets his pants constantly, but even in the hot summer months he still needs to change clothes a few times a day. Other symptoms include his four limbs' staying cold all the time, weak loins, fatigue, and a pale tongue. A Chinese doctor diagnosed his condition as Loosening of Kidneys Energy, chiefly because incontinence of urination is a major sign of this syndrome and weak loins, fatigue, and a pale complexion are other symptoms associated with this syndrome.

Treatment Principles.   To fix and constrict the energy of the kidneys, to tone the kidneys and benefit energy, to solidify and constrict kidneys essence.

Foods Chosen Based on Y-Scores.   Autumn bottle gourd (Kidneys 2), bird's nest (Kidneys 2), black sesame seed (Kidneys 2), black soybean (Kidneys 2), chestnut (Kidneys 4), chicken liver (Kidneys 4), Chinese chive (Kidneys 6), common carp (Kidneys 2), day lily (Kidneys 0), eel (Kidneys 4), goat's milk (Kidneys 4), gorgan fruit (Kidneys 2), grape (Kidneys 0), green onion (seed) (Kidneys 6), Japanese cassia bark (Kidneys 5), Job's tears (Kidneys 0), lobster (Kidneys 1), lotus (Kidneys 2), lotus seed (Kidneys 2), matrimony-vine fruit (Kidneys 2), mutton (Kidneys 4), perch (Kidneys 2), plum (Kidneys 0), prickly ash (Kidneys 6), star anise (Kidneys 5), string bean (Kidneys 2), tangerine (Kidneys -2), walnut (Kidneys 4), wheat (Kidneys 0), white fungus (Kidneys 2), yam (Kidneys 2).

Generally Beneficial Foods and Other Foods to Be Chosen or Avoided. 1. Foods that are normally good for this syndrome are chicken, crabapple, gorgan fruit, raspberry, stamens, strawberry, walnut, and yam. 2. Choose from these foods that can control seminal ejaculation: black-eyed pea, chive (Chinese), chive root and bulb (Chinese), chive seed (Chinese), crabapple, fenugreek seed (Oriental), fish air bladder, ginkgo (cooked), gorgan fruit, kelp, lotus (fruit, seed, leaf, rhizome joint, and stem), magnolia-vine fruit (Chinese), matrimony-vine fruit, mussel, peach (dried, unripe), oyster shell, palm (root and seed), plantain, pomegranate peel, pork kidney, pork marrow, prickly ash, rapeseed, raspberry, reed rhizome, rose root (Chinese), Russian olive (oleaster), sago-cycas flower, sea cucumber, string bean, walnut, and yam. 3. Foods to be avoided in cases of seminal emission are clam (river, shelled), oyster, and wild rice gall. 4. Choose from these foods that can control diarrhea: bayberry (red skin), bitter gourd (flower, root, and vine), black-eyed pea, broad bean (stem), broomcorn, buckwheat sprouts, common button mushroom, crabapple, cucumber (leaf and root), eggplant root, fig, flour, ginkgo leaf, gorgan fruit, green prune, guava (green and dried), guava leaf, hyacinth bean (lablab bean), hyacinth-bean leaf, Job's tears, kudzu seed, kudzu-vine root, lotus (fruit and seed), lotus (leaf and leaf base), mung-bean leaf, palm (flower and seed), peach-tree resin, persimmon, persimmon cake, pistachio nut, pomegranate (sour fruit), pomegranate (peel and root bark), pork skin, prune, prune (leaf and root), quail, rabbit liver, rambutan, rice (glutinous or sweet), rice (polished), rice sprouts, Russian olive (oleaster), shepherd's purse flower, sorghum, squash leaf, string bean, sweet potato (vine leaf), taro (leaf and stalk), turtle egg, walnut-tree bark, wax-gourd leaf (Chinese), and yellow croaker. 5. Foods to be avoided in cases of diarrhea include amaranth, black sesame seed, duck, eggplant, eel, honey, lard, lily (bulb and leaf), purslane, sea cucumber, sesame oil, water spinach, white eel, and wild cabbage.

Beneficial Herbs to Be Applied One Herb at a Time. Jin ying zi (Fructus Rosae Laevigatae), 11 g; lian xu (Stamen Nelumbinis), 7 g; mu li (Concha Ostrae), 35 g; sang piao xiao (Ootheca Mantidis), 11 g; shan yao (Rhizoma Dioscoreae), 20 g; tu si zi (Semen Cuscutae), 11 g; wu wei zi (Fructus Schisandrae), 4 g; yi zhi ren (Fructus Zigiberis Nigri), 11 g.

Beneficial Herbal Formulas to Be Applied One Formula at a Time. Ji Sheng Bi Jing Wan, Tu Si Zi Wan, Shen Qi Wan, Sang Piao Xiao San.

11.5 Kidneys Unable to Absorb Inspiration (Kidneys Deficiency Affecting the Lungs)

When you are in good health, your y-score is Kidneys -3; when you are ill, your y-score is Kidneys -7.

Definition of the Syndrome. When the kidneys are deficient, they may become incapable of absorbing inspiration, which results in poor inspiration. The lungs control respiration, and the kidneys take charge of absorbing inspiration. Chronic cough and asthma can cause a deficiency of the lungs, which can in turn contribute to a deficiency of the kidneys, with the kidneys unable to absorb inspiration so that the air returns to the lungs before it reaches the kidneys; this accounts for the panting, shortness of breath, and tendency to expire more than inspire particularly when one is moving. Yang deficiency of the kidneys gives rise to the fatigue, excessive perspiration, low and weak voice, bluish complexion, and cold limbs; yin deficiency of the kidneys accounts for the red complexion with mental depression and for the dry mouth and throat.

Clinical Signs and Symptoms. Major signs: Panting, shortness of breath, more expiration than inspiration particularly on movement, weak loins and knees. Median signs: Fatigue, excessive perspiration, low and weak voice, greenish complexion, cold limbs, red complexion with depression, dry mouth and throat. Minor signs: Breathing difficulty, fear of the cold, frequent fear of coldness in both hands and feet, perspiration due to hot weather or putting on warm clothes, swelling of the lungs, wheezing.

Applicable Western Diseases. Asthma, bronchial asthma, cardiac asthma, chronic asthmatic bronchitis, dropsy (edema) of the face, emphysema.

Treatment Symptoms. Chronic shortness of breath.

Clinical Cases. (1) A male patient named Wong, age eighty-two, had a chronic cough, and even the slightest movements would cause shortness of breath and panting, particularly in cold weather. Other symptoms he exhibited were a slightly yellowish complexion, skinniness, a choking sensation in the chest, more expiration than inspiration, puffiness in the lower limbs, and sleepiness. A Chinese doctor diagnosed his condition as Kidneys Unable to Absorb Inspiration, chiefly because a chronic cough and breathing difficulty often involve both the lungs and the kidneys. (2) Having a history of a chronic cough for more than ten years, Liu, a fifty-nine-year-old male patient, experienced a worsening of symptoms over the past month, with shortness of breath and with desperation for air in addition to the cough. He was diagnosed in a Western hospital as having a recurrent infection of chronic bronchitis and emphysema. A Chinese doctor diagnosed his condition as Kidneys Unable to Absorb Inspiration, mainly on account of the fact that desperation for air is due to the inability of the kidneys to absorb air, so that the patient has to inhale more air by means of breathing deeply. (3) Every winter, a forty-three-year-old male patient by the name of Sing came under the attack of asthma, with more expiration than inspiration, shortness of breath, panting, coughing up watery phlegm, a pale tongue, cold limbs, and a weak pulse. A Chinese doctor diagnosed his condition as Kidneys Unable to Absorb Inspiration, primarily because more expiration than inspiration is a major sign of this syndrome.

Treatment Principles. To tone the kidneys and improve the kidneys' capacity for absorbing inspiration.

Foods Chosen Based on Y-Scores. Autumn bottle gourd (Kidneys 2), bird's nest (Kidneys 2), black sesame seed (Kidneys 2), black soybean (Kidneys 2), chestnut (Kidneys 4), chicken liver (Kidneys 4), Chinese chive (Kidneys 6), common carp (Kidneys 2), day lily (Kidneys 0), eel (Liver 4, Kidneys 4), goat's milk (Kidneys 4), gorgan fruit (Kidneys 2), grape (Kidneys 0), green onion (seed) (Kidneys 6), Japanese cassia bark (Kidneys 5), Job's tears (Kidneys 0), lobster (Kidneys 1), lotus (Kidneys 2), lotus seed (Kidneys 2), matrimony-vine fruit (Kidneys 2), mutton (Kidneys 4), perch (Kidneys 2), plum (Kidneys 0), prickly ash (Kidneys 6), star anise (Kidneys 5), string bean (Kidneys 2), tangerine (Kidneys -2), walnut (Kidneys 4), wheat (Kidneys 0), white eel (Kidneys 2), white fungus (Kidneys 2), yam (Kidneys 2).

Generally Beneficial Foods and Other Foods to Be Chosen or Avoided. 1. Foods that are normally beneficial for this syndrome are abalone, asparagus, chestnut, chicken egg, chicken liver, clove, crabapple, cuttlefish, dill seed, duck, duck egg, fennel, lobster, milk, oyster, pistachio nut, pork, pork kidney, raspberry, royal jelly, sardine, shrimp, sparrow, sparrow egg, walnut, and white fungus. 2. Foods to be avoided in cases of kidney disease are monosodium glutamate and green onion.

Beneficial Herbs to Be Applied One Herb at a Time. Dang shen (Radix Codonopsis Pilosulae), 15 g; hu tao ren (Semen Juglandis Regiae), 11 g; ren shen (Radix Ginseng), 35 g; shan zhu yu (Fructus Corni), 11 g; shu di huang (Radix Rehmanniae), cooked, 18 g; wu wei zi (Fructus Schisandrae), 4 g; zi he che (Placenta Hominis), 5 g; zi shi ying (Fluoritum), 15 g.

Beneficial Herbal Formulas to Be Applied One Formula at a Time. Du Qi Wan, Ren Shen Ge Jie San, Ren Shen Hu Tao Tang, Qi Wei Du Qi Wan.

12

Choosing Foods and Herbs to Boost the Bladder and Cure Applicable Symptoms and Diseases

12.1 Bladder Damp Heat

When you are in good health, your y-score is Bladder 1; when you are ill, your y-score is Bladder 5.

Definition of the Syndrome. Bladder Damp Heat refers to an accumulation of dampness and heat in the bladder that obstructs normal energy transformation in the bladder and is characterized by burning sensations and urination disorders.

When damp heat invades the bladder, this will cause a malfunction of the bladder in transforming water, which accounts for the many urination disorders. When dampness and heat affect the kidneys, this causes the lumbago.

Clinical Signs and Symptoms. Major signs: Frequent urination, urinary strain, pain on urination, difficulty in urination, sudden interruption during urination, burning sensation on urination. Median signs: Blood in urine, short and red streams of urine, turbid urine. Minor signs: Pain on urination, urine like water from washing rice in children, red and damp and sticky surface of genitals in girls.

Applicable Western Diseases. Acute cystitis, acute urethritis, chyluria, haematuria, prostatitis, pyelonephritis, urinary calculus, urinary infection, urine retention, urodialysis.

Treatment Symptoms. Absent urination, difficult urination.

Clinical Cases. (1) Three days before being examined by a doctor of Chinese medicine, a forty-two-year-old female patient named

Cao displayed the following symptoms: shivering with chills, a high fever, frequent urination, an urgent desire to urinate, and a burning sensation and pain in the urethra. A Western physician had diagnosed her condition as acute cystitis. The Chinese doctor diagnosed it as Bladder Damp Heat primarily because of the difficult urination and the burning sensation she had been experiencing. (2) Having a history of acute cystitis, Yao, a thirty-year-old female patient, complained of the recurrence of it four or five times in recent months. Her current symptoms include frequent urination with short streams of urine, a burning sensation in the urethra, and lumbago. A Chinese doctor diagnosed her condition as Bladder Damp Heat mainly on account of the frequent urination with short streams of urine and the burning sensation. (3) Zhang, a thirty-two-year-old male patient, suffered from lumbago and had blood in his urine. He was diagnosed by a Western doctor as having urinary calculus and treated with some good results. He also experienced a burning sensation on urination, passed urine with difficulty, and had a yellowish and greasy coating on his tongue. A Chinese doctor diagnosed his condition as Bladder Damp Heat, chiefly because urinary calculus with urination disorders and a yellowish and greasy coating on the tongue are distinct signs of this syndrome.

Treatment Principles. To clear heat and benefit dampness.

Foods Chosen Based on Y-Scores. Hops (Bladder -6), kohlrabi (Bladder 1), long-kissing sturgeon (Bladder 2), river snail (Bladder -5), spiral-shelled snail (Bladder -2), watermelon (Bladder -2), winter melon (Bladder -1).

Generally Beneficial Foods and Other Foods to Be Chosen or Avoided. 1. Choose from among the following grease-free, bland, and nonirritating foods: apple, banana, beef, brown sugar, cabbages, carrot, celery, chicken, chicken egg (especially the white part), Chinese cabbage, corn, cottage cheese, cow's milk, fish, fruit, honey, horse bean (broad bean), lean meats, lemon, lettuce, liver, lotus juice (fresh), millet, mung bean, mung bean sprouts, noodle, orange, peach, pea, pear, polished rice, pork, radish, rice, seaweed, skim milk, soybean, soybean sprouts, string bean, sweet potato, sword bean, taro, tofu, tomato, vegetables, watermelon, wheat, white fungus, white sugar, and yam. 2. Choose from these foods that can promote urination: adzuki bean sprouts, air bladder of shark, ambergris, apple, areca nut, asparagus, bitter bamboo shoots, bottle gourd, bottle gourd (autumn), cantaloupe (muskmelon), carp (common), carrot, cattail (including pollen), Chinese cabbage, Chinese wax gourd (pulp), cinnamon twig, clam (saltwater), clamshell (sea) powder, coffee, corn (sweet or Indian), crown daisy, cucumber, cuttlefish egg, dace, eggplant (aubergine), grape, green-onion white head, kidney bean, kiwifruit root (Chinese gooseberry), kohlrabi, ladle gourd, laver, lettuce (stalk and leaf), licorice, loach, mandarin orange, mango, marjoram, mulberry, mung bean, onion, papaya, pea, pineapple, plum, radish (leaf and seed), rice (polished), Russian olive (oleaster), shepherd's purse, snail (river), sorghum, soybean (black), soybean (yellow), rice soup, taro, tea, tofu, water spinach, watermelon (including white portion), wax cell of honeycomb, wheat (floating), whitebait, whitefish, wild cabbage, and wild rice gall (water-oat gall).

Beneficial Herbs to Be Applied One Herb at a Time. Bian xu (Herba Polygoni Avicularis), 11 g; hai jin sha (Spora Lygodii), 11 g; hua shi (Talcum), 15 g; huang bai (Cortex Phellodendri), 15 g; jin qian cao (Herba Lysimachiae), 18 g; mu tong (Caulis Aristolochiae), 8 g; qu mai (Herba Dianthi), 11 g; zhi mu (Rhizoma Anemarrhenae), 15 g.

Beneficial Herbal Formulas to Be Applied One Formula at a Time. Ba Zheng San, Bei Xie Fen Qing Yin, Xiao Ji Yin Zi.

12.2 Bladder Cold and Deficiency

When you are in good health, your y-score is Bladder -4; when you are ill, your y-score is Bladder -8.

Definition of the Syndrome. Bladder Cold and Deficiency refers to a deficient and cold bladder due to a yang deficiency of the kidneys, with the kidneys unable to warm the bladder so that the bladder becomes incapable of controlling urination.

When the bladder is cold and deficient, it will lose its power of controlling urination, which is why urination disorders occur. This syndrome generally arises from two other syndromes: Kidneys Yang Deficiency and Loosening of Kidneys Energy.

Clinical Signs and Symptoms. Major signs: Frequent urination with clear and long stream of urine. Median signs: Suppression of urination with dribbling of urine, diminished urination. Minor signs: Blackish complexion, edema, incontinence of urine.

Applicable Western Diseases. Enuresis, retention of urine due to prostatic hyperplasia.

Treatment Symptoms. Incontinence of urination, absent urination.

Clinical Cases. (1) Hong, a thirteen-year-old female patient, displayed the following symptoms: puffiness in the face and especially around the eyes, bed-wetting at night, frequent urination once in a while, and a poor complexion. A Chinese doctor diagnosed her condition as Bladder Cold and Deficiency primarily as a result of the urination disorders and the puffiness in the face and around the eyes. (2) A sixteen-year-old male patient named Zhang suffered from malnutrition, skinniness, and bed-wetting at night that increases in frequency when he is extremely tired. A Chinese doctor diagnosed his condition as Bladder Cold and Deficiency, mainly because the bladder is colder at night than during the daytime, which accounts for the bed-wetting at night.

Treatment Principles. To warm the kidneys and the bladder.

Foods Chosen Based on Y-Scores. Catfish (Bladder 4), hops (Bladder -6), kohlrabi (Bladder 1), long-kissing sturgeon (Bladder 2), spiral-shelled snail (Bladder -2), watermelon (Bladder -2), winter melon (Bladder -1).

Generally Beneficial Foods and Other Foods to Be Chosen or Avoided. 1. Choose from among these hot and spicy items: alcohol, chili pepper (cayenne pepper), chive (Chinese), cinnamon bark (cassia), cinnamon twig, clove, coffee, garlic, ginger (fresh or dried), green onion (leaf and white head), mustard seed, nutmeg, onion, pepper (black or white), tea, and wine. They force yin energy to excrete through perspiration, which is harmful to yin and energy. 2. Choose from the following warm foods: blood clam, caper, caraway seed, cassia bark (Japanese), cassia fruit (Japanese), chicken, chili-pepper leaf, chili rhizome, chive (Chinese), chive root and bulb (Chinese), chive seed (Chinese), cinnamon twig, clove, date, dill seed, fennel seed, fenugreek seed (Oriental), fresh ginger, green-onion white head, mustard (white or yellow), mustard seed (white or yellow), nutmeg, pepper (black or white), prickly ash, rice (polished, long-grain), shallot (aromatic green onion), small garlic, sorghum, star anise, sword bean (jack bean), and water chestnut. 3. Avoid these cold foods: adzuki bean, aloe vera, asparagus (lucid), bamboo shoots, banana, bitter endive, bitter gourd (balsam pear), brake (fern), burdock, camphor mint, cattail, crab, endive (Chinese), fig, frog (pond), grapefruit, hair vegetable, honey, leaf beet (spinach beet, Swiss chard), lemon, lily flower, mung bean, mung-bean powder, mung bean sprouts, orchid leaf, peppermint, potato (Irish), preserved duck egg, pricking amaranth (amaranth, pig-weed), purslane, rabbit, rambutan, romaine lettuce, Russian olive (oleaster), safflower fruit, salt, soybean paste, squash, star fruit (carambola), strawberry (Indian or mock), sweet basil, tofu, water spinach, wax gourd (Chinese), and wheat.

Beneficial Herbs to Be Applied One Herb at a Time. Fu pen zi (Fructus Rubi), 11 g; jin ying zi (Fructus Rosae Laevigatae), 11 g; long gu (Os Draconis), 18 g; sang piao xiao (Ootheca Mantidis), 11 g; shan yao (Rhizoma Dioscoreae), 20 g; tu si zi (Semen Cuscutae), 11 g; wu yao (Radix Linderae), 10 g; yi zhi ren (Fructus Zigiberis Nigri), 11 g.

Beneficial Herbal Formulas to Be Applied One Formula at a Time. Ji Sheng Shen Qi Wan, Sang Piao Xiao San, Suo Niao Wan, Tu Si Zi San.

13

Choosing Foods and Herbs to Boost the Heart and Cure Applicable Symptoms and Diseases

13.1 Heart Energy Deficiency

When you are in good health, your y-score is Heart -2; when you are ill, your y-score is Heart -6.

Definition of the Syndrome. Heart Energy Deficiency refers to the hypofunctioning of the heart that results in insecure spirits, poor energy circulation, and poor blood circulation. This is generally due to internal injuries, fatigue, or abuse of drug therapy, such as an excessive application of drugs to induce perspiration. Heart Energy Deficiency can affect the lungs, the spleen, and the kidneys in particular as time goes on, and it can also lead to blood coagulation and the production of phlegm.

With this syndrome, the heart energy is in short supply, so the heart has insufficient pushing power, which accounts for the palpitations, nervousness, weak pulse, chest discomfort, and shortness of breath. When people are involved in strenuous labor, they will consume heart energy, which intensifies the symptoms. When people have a shortage of heart energy, they will not wish to talk. A shortage of heart energy will also reduce the efficiency of defense energy, which gives rise to the excessive perspiration. The body does not have sufficient energy to nourish the heart, causing the sleepiness. Nor does the body have sufficient energy for securing the spirits, which results in the insomnia, forgetfulness, and palpitations, as well as being easily in shock and being prone to sadness and crying.

179

Energy deficiency produces phlegm, which accounts for the twitching. When energy is in deficiency, it cannot push the blood efficiently, and this is why there is the chest pain.

Clinical Signs and Symptoms. Major signs: Palpitations, nervousness, chest discomfort, shortness of breath that worsens on labor. Median signs: Mentally fatigued, meager energy, too lazy to talk, pale complexion, excessive perspiration, insomnia, forgetfulness, sleepiness, prone to sadness and crying, chest pain, twitching, mentally confused, easily in shock. Minor signs: Pain in the heart, panting, shortness of breath, perspiration, white complexion.

Applicable Western Diseases. Anemia, arrhythmia (arrhythmia cordia), cardiomyopathy, epilepsy, myopia (hypometropia, nearsightedness), neurasthenia, neurosis.

Treatment Symptoms.   Palpitations, insomnia, chest pain, epilepsy, chronic fatigue.

Clinical Cases. (1) Wang, a twenty-year-old female patient, displayed symptoms similar to those of insanity: She kept moving her limbs as if she were dancing, sung and laughed, and felt sudden sadness and joy, with a slight sensation of heat in the skin and a dribbling of urine. A Chinese doctor diagnosed Wang's condition as Heart Energy Deficiency, especially because she was prone to sadness and crying and was mentally confused, which arose from an inability of her heart to nourish her spirits. (2) At five years of age, a little boy named Xu displayed a pale complexion, low spirits, poor sleep, shortness of breath, a choking sensation in the chest, a poor appetite, fatigue, and sixty pulse beats per minute. A Chinese doctor diagnosed his condition as Heart Energy Deficiency, primarily because many signs of this syndrome were present.

Treatment Principles.   To tone and benefit the energy in the heart.

Foods Chosen Based on Y-Scores.   Adzuki bean (Heart 0), arrowhead (Heart -2), brome seed (Heart 0), chili pepper (cayenne pepper) (Heart 8), coffee (Heart 1), cow's milk (Heart 2), hami melon (Heart -2), Japanese cassia bark (Heart 5), lily (bulb and leaf) (Heart -2), longan nut (Heart 4), lotus (Heart 2), lotus seed (Heart 2), mung bean (Heart 0), muskmelon (cantaloupe) (Heart -2), oyster (Heart -1), persimmon (Heart -2), scallion bulb (Heart 2), sea cucumber (Heart -1), watermelon (Heart -2), wheat (Heart 0).

Generally Beneficial Foods and Other Foods to Be Chosen or Avoided.   1. Choose from the following grease-free and bland foods: apple, banana, beef, brown sugar, cabbages, carrot, celery, chicken, chicken egg white, Chinese cabbage, corn, cottage cheese, cow's milk, fish, fruit, honey, horse bean (broad bean), lean meats, lemon, lettuce, liver, lotus juice (fresh), millet, mung bean, mung bean sprouts, noodle, orange, peach, pea, pear, polished rice, pork, radish, rice, seaweed, skim milk, soybean, soybean sprouts, string bean, sweet potato, sword bean, taro, tofu, tomato, vegetables, watermelon, wheat, white fungus, white sugar, and yam. 2. Avoid these hot and spicy items: alcohol, chili pepper (cayenne pepper), chive (Chinese), cinnamon bark (cassia), cinnamon twig, clove, coffee, garlic, ginger (fresh or dried), green onion (leaf and white head), mustard seed, nutmeg, onion, pepper (black or white), tea, and wine. They force yin energy to excrete through perspiration, which is harmful to heart yin and heart energy. 3. Cold foods are harmful to spleen yang, so avoid these cold foods: adzuki bean, aloe vera, asparagus (lucid), bamboo shoots, banana, bitter endive, bitter gourd (balsam pear), brake (fern), burdock, camphor mint, cattail, crab, endive (Chinese), fig, frog (pond), grapefruit, hair vegetable, honey, leaf beet (spinach beet, Swiss chard), lemon, lily flower, mung bean, mung-bean powder, mung bean sprouts, orchid leaf, peppermint, potato (Irish), preserved duck egg, pricking amaranth (amaranth, pigweed), purslane, rabbit, rambutan, romaine lettuce, Russian olive (oleaster), safflower fruit, salt, soybean paste, squash, star fruit (carambola), strawberry (Indian or mock), sweet basil, tofu, water spinach, wax gourd (Chinese), and wheat.

Beneficial Herbs to Be Applied One Herb at a Time. Dang shen (Radix Codonopsis Pilosulae), 15 g; huang qi (Radix Astragali Seu Hedysari), 40 g; ren shen (Radix Ginseng), 35 g; tai zi shen (Radix Pseudostellariae), 11 g.

Beneficial Herbal Formulas to Be Applied One Formula at a Time. An Shen Wan, Du Shen Wan, Gan Mai Da Zao Tang, Shen Fu Tang.

13.2 Heart Yang Deficiency

When you are in good health, your y-score is Heart -4; when you are ill, your y-score is Heart -8.

Definition of the Syndrome. When yang deficiency affects the heart, this becomes Heart Yang Deficiency, which is characterized by palpitations, chest pain, and fatigue. Heart Yang Deficiency is frequently an extension of Heart Energy Deficiency. When heart yang is deficient, the heart loses its pushing power, which accounts for the palpitations and nervousness. When blood circulation slows down, the blood can coagulate, causing the chest pain. Deficient yang energy is responsible for the sleepiness, cold limbs, excessive perspiration, and feeling too lazy to talk, and there is insufficient yang energy for it to move upward to the face, which is the reason for the pale complexion.

Clinical Signs and Symptoms. Major signs: Palpitations, shortness of breath, choking sensation in the chest, chest pain intensified by labor, aversion to the cold, cold limbs. Median signs: Fatigued, too lazy to talk, meager energy, excessive perspiration, pale complexion or slightly dark complexion, sleepiness. Minor signs: Getting scared easily with rapid heartbeat, unconsciousness.

Applicable Western Diseases. Angina pectoris, cardiac neurosis, cardiopathy, circulatory failure due to chronic illness or heart failure, coronary heart disease, diphtheria, heart disease, myocarditis, neurosis, rheumatoid cardiopathy.

Treatment Symptoms. Palpitations, chest pain, chronic fatigue.

Clinical Cases. (1) After having a common cold, Chung, a thirty-seven-year-old female patient, displayed these three symptoms: chest discomfort, mild pain in the heart region, and more than 110 pulse beats per minute. She was diagnosed in a Western hospital as having myocarditis. A Chinese doctor diagnosed her condition as Heart Yang Deficiency, primarily because she had heart symptoms triggered by a common cold and she had a rapid pulse rate. (2) A forty-year-old male patient named Hong had a pulse of only fifty beats per minute, with chest discomfort, shortness of breath, acute panting on climbing stairs, an aversion to the cold, and cold limbs. He also had a history of vertigo. A Chinese doctor diagnosed his condition as Heart Yang Deficiency chiefly because of his respiratory symptoms, low pulse rate, aversion to the cold, and cold limbs.

Treatment Principles. To tone yang energy in the heart.

Foods Chosen Based on Y-Scores. Adzuki bean (Heart 0), arrowhead (Heart-2), brome seed (Heart 0), chili pepper (cayenne pepper) (Heart 8), coffee (Heart 1), cow's milk (Heart 2), hami melon (Heart -2), Japanese cassia bark (Heart 5), lily (bulb and leaf) (Heart -2), longan nut (Heart 4), lotus (Heart 2), lotus seed (Heart 2), mung bean (Heart 0), muskmelon (cantaloupe) (Heart -2), oyster (Heart -1), persimmon (Heart -2), scallion bulb (Heart 2), sea cucumber (Heart -1), watermelon (Heart -2), wheat (Heart 0).

Generally Beneficial Foods and Other Foods to Be Chosen or Avoided. 1. Foods that are usually good for this syndrome are cinnamon, date (red or black), dried ginger, kidney, lobster, sardine, shrimp, star anise, water spinach, and wheat. 2. Choose from the following protein-rich foods: beans, cereal grains, cheeses, chicken egg (especially the white part), corn (Indian), fish, green leafy vegetables, lean meats, liver, milk, millet, nuts, peanut, sea cucumber, sesame seed, sorghum, soybean, sunflower seed, tofu, walnut, and wheat. 3. Choose from these low-salt foods in cases of edema: apple, beef, brown sugar, chicken, chicken egg, Chinese cabbage, coffee, corn, cow's milk, fruit, honey, lamb, lemon, lettuce, liver, millet, oils, peach, polished rice, pork, orange, soybean, tea, tofu, and white sugar. 4. Choose from the following foods that are low in cholesterol: beans, breads, cereal grains, cottage cheese, egg white, fat-free milk, fish, lean meats, oils, pea, poultry, sea cucumber, veal, and vegetable oils. 5. Avoid the following foods that are high in cholesterol: beef, beef brain, butter, chicken liver, duck egg, duck liver, goose egg, hairtail, ham, lamb brain, lard, pork, pork brain, pork kidney, pork liver, rabbit, river crab, sausages, and shrimp.

Beneficial Herbs to Be Applied One Herb at a Time. Dang shen (Radix Codonopsis Pilosulae), 15 g; fu zi (Radix Aconiti Praeparata), 11 g; gan cao (Radix Glycyrrhizae), 11 g; huang qi (Radix Astragali Seu Hedysari), 40 g; rou gui (Cortex Cinnamomi), 5 g; xie bai (Bulbus Allii Macrostemi), 11 g.

Beneficial Herbal Formulas to Be Applied One Formula at a Time. Dan Shen Yin, Ding Zhi Wan, Gui Zhi Gan Cao Tang, Si Ni Tang.

13.3 Heart Yin Deficiency

When you are in good health, your y-score is Heart 3; when you are ill, your y-score is Heart 7.

Definition of the Syndrome. When yin deficiency affects the heart, this becomes Heart Yin Deficiency, which is characterized by a red tip of the tongue or an ulcer on the tongue, in addition to the symptoms observed in Heart Blood Deficiency.

When the heart is in short supply of yin energy, there will be insufficient heart yin to nourish the heart, which accounts for the palpitations. Yin deficiency can cause fire to disturb the spirits, bringing about the mental depression, forgetfulness, insomnia, and many dreams. Yin deficiency is responsible for the dry mouth and throat, and it can produce fire deficiency, which gives rise to the tidal fever, night sweats, hot sensations, and reddish zygomatic regions.

Clinical Signs and Symptoms. Major signs: Palpitations, mental depression, insomnia, many dreams. Median signs: Hot sensations of the five hearts (the centers in the palms of the hands, the soles of the feet, and the chest), tidal fever in the afternoon, reddish appearance of the zygomatic regions, night sweats, dry mouth and throat, forgetfulness. Minor signs: Discharge of dry stools, dry tongue, forgetfulness, hiccups, low fever.

Applicable Western Diseases. Anemia, arrhythmia (arrhythmia cordia), diphtheria, functional low fever, heart disease, hyperthyroidism, myocarditis, neurosis, paroxysmal tachycardia, rheumatoid cardiopathy.

Treatment Symptoms. Palpitations, nervousness, chronic fatigue, insomnia.

Clinical Cases. (1) Chen, a thirty-four-year-old female patient, has suffered paroxysmal tachycardia for seven years, and she tends to come under attack when she is fatigued. Her symptoms include palpitations, nervousness, a congested chest, many dreams, red cheeks, and a red tongue. A Chinese doctor diagnosed her condition as Heart Yin Deficiency primarily because of her palpitations and many dreams. (2) A thirty-eight-year-old male patient named Woo suffered palpitations for almost ten years, with irregular heartbeats often triggered by external events, a rapid pulse, constantly feeling tense, and a red tongue. A Chinese doctor diagnosed his condition as Heart Yin Deficiency mainly on account of his palpitations and red tongue.

Treatment Principles. To tone the yin energy in the heart.

Foods Chosen Based on Y-Scores. Adzuki bean (Heart 0), arrowhead (Heart-2), bitter gourd (balsam pear) (Heart -8), brome seed (Heart 0), coffee (Heart 1), cow's milk (Heart 2), hami melon (Heart -2), lily (bulb and leaf) (Heart -2), lotus (Heart 2), lotus seed (Heart 2), matrimony-vine leaf (Heart -4), mung bean (Heart 0), muskmelon (cantaloupe) (Heart -2), oyster (Heart -1), persimmon (Heart -2), scallion bulb (Heart 2), sea cucumber (Heart -1), tea (Heart -6), watermelon (Heart -2), wheat (Heart 0).

Generally Beneficial Foods and Other Foods to Be Chosen or Avoided. 1. Choose from these blood-tonic foods: beef, beef liver, blood clam, chicken egg (especially the yolk), cuttlefish, duck blood, grape, ham, litchi nut, liver, longan, mandarin fish, octopus, oxtail, oyster, pork liver, pork trotter, sea cucumber, soybean skin (black), and spinach. 2. Hot and spicy foods and drinks can harm yin energy and transform into fire, so avoid alcohol, chili pepper (cayenne pepper), chive (Chinese), cinnamon bark (cassia), cinnamon twig, clove, coffee, garlic, ginger (fresh or dried), green onion (leaf and white head), mustard seed, nutmeg, onion, pepper (black or white), tea, and wine. They force yin energy to excrete through perspiration, which is harmful to heart yin and heart energy.

Beneficial Herbs to Be Applied One Herb at a Time. Bai he (Bulbus Lilii), 11 g; bai shao yao (Radix Paeoniae Alba), 11 g; bai zi ren (Semen Biotae), 11 g; dan shen (Radix Salviae Miltiorrhizae), 10 g; dang gui (Radix Angelicae Sinensis), 11 g; E jiao (Colla Corii Asini [Gelatina Nigra]), 11 g; mai men dong (Radix Ophiopogonis), 11 g; sheng di (Radix Rehmanniae), fresh, 35 g; shu di huang (Radix Rehmanniae), cooked, 18 g; yu zhu (Rhizoma Polygonati Odorati), 11 g.

Beneficial Herbal Formulas to Be Applied One Formula at a Time. Bai Zi Yang Xin Tang, Bu Xin Dan, Gui Pi Tang, Suan Zao Ren Tang.

13.4 Heart Blood Deficiency

When you are in good health, your y-score is Heart 1; when you are ill, your y-score is Heart 5.

Definition of the Syndrome. Heart Blood Deficiency refers to a shortage of blood in the heart that causes anxiety and insecure spirits. This syndrome is generally due to a chronic illness in which the body is unable to produce blood, a chronic loss of blood, or excessive fatigue.

The heart is the organ that stores the spirits, and it is also the master of the blood vessels. When Heart Blood Deficiency occurs, there will be insufficient blood in the heart, so the heart will not be properly nourished and the spirits will have no place to stay, which accounts for the palpitations and nervousness. There is insufficient blood to nourish the heart, and the spirits have no regular residence, leading to insomnia and many dreams. Deficient blood is incapable of nurturing and nourishing the brain, which is the reason for the dizziness and forgetfulness. There is insufficient blood to flow upward to nourish the tongue and the face; this is why there is the withered and yellowish complexion, the pale lips, and the pale tongue.

Clinical Signs and Symptoms. Major signs: Palpitations, nervousness, insomnia, many dreams, forgetfulness. Median signs: Dizziness, withered and yellowish complexion, pale complexion, pale lips, night sweats. Minor signs: Anemia, fainting after childbirth, fatigue, irregular menstruation, menstrual bleeding

Applicable Western Diseases. Chronic leukemia, heart disease, hemorrhage, hyperthyroidism, mental illness, neurosis.

Treatment Symptoms. Palpitations, nervousness, insomnia, chronic fatigue.

Clinical Cases. (1) Zhang, a fifty-eight-year-old male patient, displayed these symptoms: insomnia, nervousness, headaches, a dry mouth, dizziness, and dry stools. A Chinese doctor diagnosed his condition as Heart Blood Deficiency, because many of his symptoms are signs of this syndrome. (2) A month after having a baby, a twenty-eight-year-old patient named Ding exhibited the following symptoms: dizziness, palpitations, sleeping problems with many dreams, excessive perspiration, being easily in shock, dry stools, and yellowish urine. She thought she was just overtired, but a Chinese doctor diagnosed her condition as Heart Blood Deficiency, mainly because she had lost so much blood during the delivery.

Treatment Principles. To nourish the blood and tone the heart.

Foods Chosen Based on Y-Scores. Adzuki bean (Heart 0), arrowhead (Heart -2), bitter gourd (balsam pear) (Heart -8), brome seed (Heart 0), coffee (Heart 1), cow's milk (Heart 2), hami melon (Heart -2), lily (bulb and leaf) (Heart -2), lotus (Heart 2), lotus seed (Heart 2), matrimony-vine leaf (Heart -4), mung bean (Heart 0), muskmelon (cantaloupe) (Heart -2), oyster (Heart -1), persimmon (Heart -2), scallion bulb (Heart 2), sea cucumber (Heart -1), tea (Heart -6), watermelon (Heart -2), wheat (Heart 0).

Generally Beneficial Foods and Other Foods to Be Chosen or Avoided. 1. It is important to eat on a regular basis, because Heart Blood Deficiency is often due to a weak stomach and spleen. You should also avoid excessive eating, for it can cause harm to the spleen and the stomach, which are the sources of the blood. 2. Choose protein-source foods and easily digestible foods, and avoid greasy foods that can produce damp phlegm and obstruct the free passage of blood vessels, causing heart pain. 3. Other foods that are recommended include black fungus, chicken, pork liver, red date, rice, rock sugar, and spinach.

Beneficial Herbs to Be Applied One Herb at a Time. Bai shao yao (Radix Paeoniae Alba), 11 g; bai zi ren (Semen Biotae), 11 g; dan shen (Radix Salviae Miltiorrhizae), 10 g; dang gui (Radix Angelicae Sinensis), 11 g; E jiao (Colla Corii Asini [Gelatina Nigra]), 11 g; long yan rou (Arillus Longan), 11 g; mai men dong (Radix Ophiopogonis), 11 g; sheng di (Radix Rehmanniae), fresh, 35 g; shu di huang (Radix Rehmanniae), cooked, 18 g; yu zhu (Rhizoma Polygonati Odorati), 11 g.

Beneficial Herbal Formulas to Be Applied One Formula at a Time. Bu Xin Dan, Dang Gui Bu Xue Tang, Tian Wang Bu Xin Dan, Zhi Gan Cao Tang.

13.5 Heart Fire Flaming

When you are in good health, your y-score is Heart 4; when you are ill, your y-score is Heart 8.

Definition of the Syndrome. Too much yang energy in the heart can produce heart fire that flames upward. This excessive yang energy can be brought on by the transformation of five excessive emotions into fire, the transformation of six pathogens into fire, or an excessive consumption of hot and pungent foods that transform into fire.

The heart is the organ that stores the spirits; it has the tongue as its outlet, and its glory is manifested in the face. When heart fire is present, this will disturb the spirits of the heart, causing the spirits to be insecure, which accounts for the mental depression and insomnia in milder cases and the insanity and delirium in severe cases. Heart fire flames upward, causing the red complexion, red tongue, and canker sore in the mouth and on the tongue with decomposition and pain. Fire harms fluids, which brings about the thirst, yellowish urine, and dry stools. Heat coagulates blood, leading to the ulcer. Heat harms blood vessels and forces blood to run wild, giving rise to the vomiting of blood, nosebleed, yellowish coating on the tongue, and rapid pulse.

Clinical Signs and Symptoms. Major signs: Ulcer on the tongue, mental depression, insomnia. Median signs: Red complexion, thirst, yellowish urine, dry stools, vomiting of blood, nosebleed, insanity, delirium, skin ulcer with redness and pain, fever. Minor signs: Bleeding from gums, cold hands and feet, dribbling after urination, feeling miserable, hot sensation in the center of the palms, morning sickness, mouth canker sores, not being alert, pain on urination, palpitations, pulpy and decayed tongue and mouth, seminal emission.

Applicable Western Diseases. Acute cholecystitis, acute urinary infection, central retinal choroiditis, general infection, glossitis (glottitis), haematuria (discharge of urine containing blood), hemorrhage of upper digestive tract, muguet, neurosis, recurrent canker sores, schizophrenia.

Treatment Symptoms. Blood in urine, insomnia, palpitations.

Clinical Cases. (1) Hong, a thirty-year-old male patient, displayed ulcers on the tongue for three days, with the following additional symptoms: thirst, a red tongue with a yellowish coating, a burning sensation on urination, yellowish urine, and stress. A Chinese doctor diagnosed his condition as Heart Fire Flaming especially because of the ulcers on his tongue and his hot symptoms. (2) For as long as fifteen years, a thirty-one-year-old male patient named Li has suffered from recurrent ulcers on the tongue. Lately, he has had more frequent attacks and an increasing number of ulcers, which now cover the entire tongue and are red, full of pus, and painful, affecting his speech and eating. A Chinese doctor diagnosed his condition as Heart Fire Flaming primarily because of the red ulcers on his tongue. (3) Liu, a little boy, age two, had a fever for four days, with erosive ulcers on the tongue, saliva overflowing from the mouth, bad breath, swollen gums with pain, dry stools, short and red streams of urine, jumpiness, and a loss of appetite. A Chinese doctor diagnosed his condition as Heart Fire Flaming, in view of the fact that ulcers on the tongue are a major sign of this syndrome and other symptoms such as swollen and painful gums and dry stools point to it too.

Treatment Principles. To clear heat in the heart and sedate fire, to nourish yin energy in the heart.

Foods Chosen Based on Y-Scores. Adzuki bean (Heart 0), arrowhead (Heart -2), bitter gourd (balsam pear) (Heart -8), brome seed (Heart 0), coffee (Heart 1), cow's milk (Heart 2), hami melon (Heart -2), lily (bulb and leaf) (Heart -2), lotus (Heart 2), lotus seed (Heart 2), matrimony-vine leaf (Heart -4), mung bean (Heart 0), muskmelon (cantaloupe) (Heart -2), oyster (Heart -1), persimmon

(Heart -2), scallion bulb (Heart 2), sea cucumber (Heart -1), tea (Heart -6), watermelon (Heart -2), wheat (Heart 0).

Generally Beneficial Foods and Other Foods to Be Chosen or Avoided. 1. Foods that are considered normally good for this syndrome are asparagus, bamboo shoots, banana, bitter endive, black fungus, cattail, cucumber, Job's tears, leaf beet, lily flower, liver, mung bean, pear peel, peppermint, purslane, salt, spinach, and strawberry. 2. Choose from the following grease-free and bland foods: apple, banana, beef, brown sugar, cabbages, carrot, celery, chicken, chicken egg (especially the white part), Chinese cabbage, corn, cottage cheese, cow's milk, fish, fruit, honey, horse bean (broad bean), lean meats, lemon, lettuce, liver, lotus juice (fresh), millet, mung bean, mung bean sprouts, noodle, peach, pea, pear, polished rice, pork, orange, radish, rice, seaweed, skim milk, soybean, soybean sprouts, string bean, sweet potato, sword bean, taro, tofu, tomato, vegetables, watermelon, wheat, white fungus, white sugar, and yam. 3. Avoid these hot and spicy items: alcohol, chili pepper (cayenne pepper), chive (Chinese), cinnamon bark (cassia), cinnamon twig, clove, coffee, garlic, ginger (fresh or dried), green onion (leaf and white head), mustard seed, nutmeg, onion, pepper (black or white), tea, and wine. They force yin energy to excrete through perspiration, and this is harmful to heart yin and heart energy, contributing to the production of fire.

Beneficial Herbs to Be Applied One Herb at a Time. Fu ling (Poria), 14 g; huang lian (Rhizoma Coptidis), 12 g; lian zi xin (Plumula Nelumbinis), 4 g; mu tong (Caulis Aristolochiae), 8 g; sheng di (Radix Rehmanniae), fresh, 35 g; zhi zi (Fructus Gardeniae), 16 g.

Beneficial Herbal Formulas to Be Applied One Formula at a Time. Dao Chi San, Xiao Ji Yin Zi, Zhi Bai Di Huang Wan.

13.6 Phlegm Fire Disturbing the Heart

When you are in good health, your y-score is Heart 4; when you are ill, your y-score is Heart 8.

Definition of the Syndrome. Phlegm Fire Disturbing the Heart indicates that there is phlegm in the heart that has transformed into fire due to the presence of heat. This can be attributed to an excessive consumption of foods with a tendency to produce phlegm, or to emotional disturbances that cause energy congestion to turn into fire, thereby transforming body fluids into phlegm.

When phlegm fire affects the heart, this can give rise to the insanity, insomnia, and stroke. Fire and phlegm come together to disturb the spirits, which accounts for the palpitations, mental depression, insomnia, and many dreams. Fire can become wild, causing the insanity and violent behavior. The nature of fire is to flame upward, which brings about the red complexion.

Clinical Signs and Symptoms. Major signs: Palpitations, mental depression, insomnia, emotional disturbances, maniac behavior, loss of consciousness, delirium, high fever, sound of phlegm in the throat. Median signs: Red complexion, rough breath, fondness for cold drink, chest discomfort, copious phlegm, coughing up yellowish and sticky phlegm, red urine, constipation, incoherent speech, irregular laughter and crying, violent behavior, use of abusive language, dizziness, many dreams. Minor signs: Discharge of white and watery phlegm, love of laughter and being happy, not being alert, phlegm rumbling in the throat, swollen sensation in tip of tongue causing a desire to stick it out.

Applicable Western Diseases. Acute cerebrovascular disease, arrhythmia (arrhythmia cordia), cerebrovascular accidents, chronic cor pulmonale, epilepsy, insanity, neurosis, schizophrenia (schizophrenosis), stroke.

Treatment Symptoms. Mental illness, insomnia, stroke.

Clinical Cases. (1) Over the course of fifteen years, a twenty-three-year-old female patient named Gong had suffered from mania, which had initially been triggered by a sudden frenzy. She had been treated with some good results, and the symptoms were basically under control. But in the past month, her symptoms took a turn for the worse, and she exhibited violent behavior, destroying property and attacking people. She also displayed a red tongue with a yellowish and greasy coating. A Chinese doctor diagnosed Gong's condition as Phlegm Fire Disturbing the Heart primarily because of her maniac behavior and the greasy coating on her tongue. (2) Eight years ago, a twenty-eight-year-old male patient named Yang was in shock and subsequently became sick. At first he talked a lot, and then he cried or laughed constantly or remained silent. He was diagnosed by a psychiatrist as having schizophrenia and treated for it in a mental hospital. Yang has a strong physical constitution, and he coughs up copious phlegm normally. A Chinese doctor diagnosed his condition as Phlegm Fire Disturbing the Heart, mainly because his illness was triggered by shock, which affects the heart, and he coughs up copious phlegm.

Treatment Principles. To sedate fire and expel phlegm in the heart.

Foods Chosen Based on Y-Scores. Adzuki bean (Heart 0), arrowhead (Heart -2), bitter gourd (balsam pear) (Heart -8), brome seed (Heart 0), coffee (Heart 1), cow's milk (Heart 2), hami melon (Heart -2), lily (bulb and leaf) (Heart -2), lotus (Heart 2), lotus seed (Heart 2), matrimony-vine leaf (Heart -4), mung bean (Heart 0), muskmelon (cantaloupe) (Heart -2), oyster (Heart -1), persimmon (Heart -2), scallion bulb (Heart 2), sea cucumber (Heart -1), tea (Heart -6), watermelon (Heart -2), wheat (Heart 0).

Generally Beneficial Foods and Other Foods to Be Chosen or Avoided. 1. Choose from these soft and bland foods: breads, cakes, cheeses, cooked fruit, cookies, corn (Indian), custards, fine wheat, fish, fowl, fried egg, fruit juices, gelatin, ice cream, milk, puddings, ripe banana, soft egg, soft rice, tapioca, and tofu. 2. Fatty foods can produce phlegm, so avoid apricot pit (powder), butter, chicken egg yolk, corn oil, cottonseed, creams, fatty meats, fish-liver oils, lamb fat, lamb oil, lard, nuts, peanut, peanut oil, pine-nut kernel, rape-seed oil, sesame seed, soybean oil, sunflower oil, sunflower seed, tea oil, vegetable oils, and walnut. 3. Avoid these hot and spicy items: alcohol, chili pepper (cayenne pepper), chive (Chinese), cinnamon bark (cassia), cinnamon twig, clove, coffee, garlic, ginger (fresh or dried), green onion (leaf and white head), mustard seed, nutmeg, onion, pepper (black or white), tea, and wine. They force yin energy to excrete through perspiration, which can transform into fire. 4. Avoid these foods that can trigger a new or old disease: certain vegetables (common button mushroom, shiitake mushroom, winter bamboo shoots, spinach, and leaf or brown mustard) and meats (rooster, mutton, dog meat, gold carp, pork head, shrimp, crab, and lobster).

Beneficial Herbs to Be Applied One Herb at a Time. Ban xia (Rhizoma Pinelliae), 12 g; dan nan xing (Arisaema Cum Bile), 8 g; fu ling (Poria), 14 g; ju hong (Exocarpium Citri Grandis), 7 g; shi chang pu (Rhizoma Acori Graminei), 5 g; yu jin (Radix Curcumae), 11 g; yuan zhi (Radix Polygalae), 11 g; zhu huang (Concretio Silicea Bambusae), 5 g; zhu li (Bamboo liquid), 50 g.

Beneficial Herbal Formulas to Be Applied One Formula at a time. Meng Shi Gun Tan Tang, Qing Qi Hua Tan Wan, Su He Xiang Wan, Xie Xin Tang.

14

Choosing Foods and Herbs to Boost the Small Intestine and Cure Applicable Symptoms and Diseases

14.1 Excessive Heat in the Small Intestine

When you are in good health, your y-score is S. intestine 3; when you are ill, your y-score is S. intestine 7.

Definition of the Syndrome. When there is excessive heat in the heart, the heat can flow downward to the small intestine, giving rise to this syndrome. And when foods are accumulated in the stomach or in the spleen for a prolonged period of time, this can generate heat that flows downward to the small intestine, also causing this syndrome.

If the excessive heat in the small intestine comes from the heart, there will be mental depression, thirst, and an ulcer on the tongue. If the heat comes from the stomach and the spleen, this can cause soft stools, a heavy sensation in the body, and a yellowish and greasy coating on the tongue.

The small intestine distinguishes between clear and turbid substances. It sends the clear substance to the spleen to nourish the whole body, and divides the turbid substance into waste matter and liquids. Then the waste matter is transported to the large intestine and the liquids to the bladder. Therefore, urination disorders can originate from the bladder or the small intestine, and the two types should be distinguished from each other.

Clinical Signs and Symptoms. Major signs: Sore throat, mental depression, ulcer on the tongue, reddish urine or blood in urine,

192

pain in the penis. Median signs: Urination difficulty, deafness, soreness on the tongue. Minor signs: Abdominal swelling around the navel that gets relieved on the passing of gas, pain in the lower abdomen affecting the lumbar spine and testicles.

Applicable Western Diseases. Aphtha.

Treatment Symptoms. Burning pain on urination, ulcer on the tongue, pain in the penis, blood in urine.

Clinical Cases. A thirty-year-old male patient by the name of Ding displayed the following symptoms: blood in urine, low spirits, a rapid pulse rate, and a thick, yellowish, and dry coating on the tongue. A Chinese doctor diagnosed his condition as Excessive Heat in the Small Intestine, primarily because certain symptoms like the blood in his urine, the coating on his tongue, and his mental depression point to this syndrome.

Treatment Principles. To clear heat and promote energy flow in the small intestine.

Foods Chosen Based on Y-Scores. Adzuki bean (S. intestine 0), bottle gourd (S. intestine -2), common button mushroom (S. intestine 0), ling (S. intestine 0), river snail (S. intestine -5), salt (S. intestine -7), small white cabbage (S. intestine 2), spinach (S. intestine 0), tea melon (S. intestine -2), water spinach (S. intestine -2), winter melon (S. intestine -1).

Generally Beneficial Foods and Other Foods to Be Chosen or Avoided. 1. Choose from the following cold foods: adzuki bean, aloe vera, asparagus (lucid), bamboo shoots, banana, bitter endive, bitter gourd (balsam pear), brake (fern), burdock, camphor mint, cattail, crab, endive (Chinese), fig, frog (pond), grapefruit, hair vegetable, honey, leaf beet (spinach beet, Swiss chard), lemon, lily flower, mung bean, mung-bean powder, mung bean sprouts, orchid leaf, peppermint, potato (Irish), preserved duck egg, pricking amaranth (amaranth, pigweed), purslane, rabbit, rambutan, romaine lettuce, Russian olive (oleaster), safflower fruit, salt, soybean paste, squash, star fruit (carambola), strawberry (Indian or mock), sweet basil, tofu, water spinach, wax gourd (Chinese), and wheat. 2. Choose from these foods that are beneficial for a hot syndrome: banana, bitter endive, black fungus, salt, spinach, strawberry, bamboo shoots, cucumber, Job's tears, laver, leaf beet, mung bean, peppermint, and purslane. However, certain foods are likely to trigger a chronic hot syndrome or intensify an existing one, such as chili pepper (cayenne pepper), dog meat, ginger, Japanese cassia bark, matrimony-vine fruit, mutton, and pepper (black or white). 3. Avoid these hot and spicy items: alcohol, chili pepper (cayenne pepper), chive (Chinese), cinnamon bark (cassia), cinnamon twig, clove, coffee, garlic, ginger (fresh or dried), green onion (leaf and white head), mustard seed, nutmeg, onion, pepper (black or white), tea, and wine. They force yin energy to excrete through perspiration, which is harmful to yin and energy.

Beneficial Herbs to Be Applied One Herb at a Time. Sheng di (Radix Rehmanniae), 30 g; mu tong (Caulis Arstolochiae Manshuriensis), 10 g; zhu ye (Folium Bambusae In Taeniam), 12 g; zhi zi (Fructus Gardeniae), 12 g; huang lian (Rhizoma Coptidis), 10 g; huang bai (Cortex Phellodendri), 10 g; da huang (Radix et Rhizoma Rhei), 12 g.

Beneficial Herbal Formulas to Be Applied One Formula at a Time. Dao Chi San, Liang Ge San.

14.2 Small Intestine Energy Congestion (Small Intestine Energy Pain)

When you are in good health, your y-score is S. intestine -3: when you are ill, your y-score is S. intestine -7.

Definition of the Syndrome. Small Intestine Energy Congestion refers to an accumulation of external cold pathogens in the small intestine, which is primarily seen in intestinal spasms and hernia. Although this syndrome occurs in the small intestine, it is closely related to a cold liver. Emotional disturbances or an invasion of cold pathogens can cause energy congestion of the liver, and this accounts for the pain in the distribution of the liver meridian, which is close to the small intestine.

Clinical Signs and Symptoms. Major signs: Acute pain in the lower abdomen below the navel affecting the back, lower-abdomen pain affecting the lumbar spine and testicles, scrotal hernia affecting the lower abdomen, abdominal swelling, intestinal rumbling. Median signs: Comfort following bowel movement or passing of gas, hernia pain in the scrotum, pain affecting the testicles or vagina. Minor signs: Falling of testicle on one side, causing walking difficulty.

Applicable Western Diseases. Enterocele, enterospasm (intestinal spasms), gastrointestinal spasm, hernia, incarcerated hernia at early stage.

Treatment Symptoms. Pain in the lower abdomen.

Clinical Cases. Wang, a three-year-old boy, had a hernia with paroxysmal abdominal pain surrounding the navel, and he would press the region with both hands to try to relieve the pain. But the pain seemed unbearable, and the little boy kept bending forward apparently to try to control it. He did find that the pain would be relieved somewhat when the region was warmed. A Chinese doctor diagnosed his condition as Small Intestine Energy Pain primarily because of the hernia with acute pain in the lower abdomen below the navel.

Treatment Principles. To regulate energy, warm the liver, disperse cold, and relieve pain.

Foods Chosen Based on Y-Scores. Adzuki bean (S. intestine 0), bottle gourd (S. intestine -2), common button mushroom (S. intestine 0), ling (S. intestine 0), small white cabbage (S. intestine 2), spinach (S. intestine 0), tea melon (S. intestine -2), water spinach (S. intestine -2), winter melon (S. intestine -1).

Generally Beneficial Foods and Other Foods to Be Chosen or Avoided. 1. Choose from the following foods that promote energy circulation: ambergris, black-eyed pea, beef, camphor mint, caraway seed, cardamom seed, carrot, chicken egg, chive (Chinese leek), chive (Chinese), chive root and bulb (Chinese), chufa rhizome, chufa stem and leaf (earth almond, nut grass), citron (fingered), clam (freshwater and saltwater), common button mushroom, dill seed, fennel seed, fingered citron (Buddha's hand), garlic, grapefruit, green onion (fibrous root and white head), hawthorn fruit, jasmine flower, kumquat, leaf or brown mustard, lemon leaf, lime (young trifoliate orange), litchi nut (including seed), longan seed, loquat seed, lotus stem, malt, mango leaf, marjoram, muskmelon seed, mussel, mustard seed, orange (peel and leaf), oregano (wild), radish leaf, rapeseed, red bean, rose, saffron, scallion bulb, shiitake mushroom, spearmint, star anise, string bean, sweet basil, sweet green, tangerine (including peel), trifoliate orange, trifoliate orange (near ripe), turmeric, and vinegar. 2. Avoid these cold foods: adzuki bean, aloe vera, asparagus (lucid), bamboo shoots, banana, bitter endive, bitter gourd (balsam pear), brake (fern), burdock, camphor mint, cattail, crab, endive (Chinese), fig, frog (pond), grapefruit, hair vegetable, honey, leaf beet (spinach beet, Swiss chard), lemon, lily flower, mung bean, mung bean-powder, mung bean sprouts, orchid leaf, peppermint, potato (Irish), preserved duck egg, pricking amaranth (amaranth, pigweed), purslane, rabbit, rambutan, romaine lettuce, Russian olive (oleaster), safflower fruit, salt, soybean paste, squash, star fruit (carambola), strawberry (Indian or mock), sweet basil, tofu, water spinach, wax gourd (Chinese), and wheat. 3. Avoid these greasy and fatty foods: animal fats (including lamb fat and oil), butter, chicken egg yolk, creams, fatty meats, fish-liver oils, fried foods, and lard. Such foods can generate heat and produce phlegm, and they are bad for indigestion, a poor appetite, jaundice, dysentery, and diarrhea.

Beneficial Herbs to Be Applied One Herb at a Time. Chen pi (Pericarpium Citri Reticulatae), 11 g; chuan lian zi (Fructus Meliae Toosendan), 11 g; hou po (Cortex Magnoliae Officinalis), 11 g; mu xiang (Radix Aucklandiae/Radix Saussureae), 6 g; qing pi (Pericarpium Citri Reticulatae Viride), 11 g; wu yao (Radix Linderae), 10 g; xiang fu (Rhizoma Cyperi), 11 g; yan hu suo (Rhizoma Corydalis), 11 g; zhi qiao (Fructus Aurantii), 11 g.

Beneficial Herbal Formulas to Be Applied One Formula at a Time. Hui Xiang Ju He Wan, Tian Tai Wu Yao San.

15

Choosing Foods and Herbs to Boost Two Internal Organs Simultaneously and Cure Applicable Symptoms and Diseases

15.1 No Communication between the Kidneys and Heart (Heart Fire Flaming with Kidneys Yin Deficiency)

When you are in good health, your y-scores are Kidneys 3 and Heart 4; when you are ill, your y-scores are Kidneys 7 and Heart 8.

Definition of the Syndrome. The kidneys are water in the lower region, and the heart is fire in the upper region. Under normal circumstances, kidneys water and heart fire adjust to each other to maintain a balance, but deficient kidneys water can fail to control heart fire and excessive heart fire can fail to move downward to control kidneys water. This syndrome involves the symptoms due to both Kidneys Yin Deficiency and Heart Fire Flaming in excess.

In this syndrome, kidneys water is in decline in the lower region and heart fire is in abundance in the upper region. Heart Fire Flaming gives rise to the mental depression, insomnia, palpitations, and nervousness. Kidneys Yin Deficiency causes the dizziness, ringing in the ears, forgetfulness, and lumbago. And because Heart Fire Flaming fails to travel downward to warm the kidneys, this accounts for the cold limbs.

Clinical Signs and Symptoms. Major signs: Weak lower back, insomnia. Median signs: Lumbago, weak legs, dizziness, ringing in the ears, palpitations, seminal emission in men, night sweats. Minor signs: Deafness, dizziness, face becoming red when fatigued or working hard, feeling miserable with love of darkness and dislike of light, forgetfulness, light tidal fever, nervousness, seminal emission with dreams.

Applicable Western Diseases.   Arrhythmia, hyperthyroidism, insomnia, menopause syndrome, neurosis, recurrent canker sores, prostatitis.

Treatment Symptoms.   Palpitations with nervousness, insomnia, seminal emission, forgetfulness.

Clinical Cases.   (1) Zheng, a thirty-nine-year-old male patient, exhibited the following chronic signs and symptoms: insomnia, many dreams, palpitations, dizziness, fatigue, excessive perspiration, skinniness, a pale complexion, a red tongue, and a light coating on the tongue. A Chinese doctor diagnosed his condition as No Communication between the Kidneys and Heart primarily because of the insomnia and the several supporting signs of this syndrome, such as the many dreams and dizziness. (2) A thirty-five-year-old male patient named Gu had insomnia for many years, along with other symptoms such as a bitter taste in the mouth, numbness in the tongue, and a hot sensation in the back of the head with an occasional headache. A Chinese doctor diagnosed Gu's condition as No Communication between the Kidneys and Heart, as chronic insomnia is the major sign of this syndrome.

Treatment Principles.   To water kidneys yin and subdue heart fire, to promote communication between the kidneys and the heart.

Foods Chosen Based on Y-Scores.   Chicken egg yolk (Kidneys 2, Heart 2), lotus (fruit, seed, and root) (Kidneys 2, Heart 2), lotus plumule (Kidneys -8, Heart -8), matrimony-vine leaf (Kidneys -4, Heart -4), sea cucumber (Kidneys -1, Heart -1), shark air bladder (Kidneys -1, Heart -1), wheat (Kidneys 0, Heart 0). In addition, foods can be chosen under the individual organs involved.

Generally Beneficial Foods and Other Foods to Be Chosen or Avoided.   1. Foods that are considered generally good for this syndrome are abalone, asparagus, bamboo shoots, banana, bitter endive, bog bean, chicken egg, oyster, pork, royal jelly, wheat, and white fungus. 2. Choose from these yin-tonic foods for the kidneys: black-eyed pea, black sesame seed, chicken liver, fish air bladder, frog (forest), lotus (fruit and seed), matrimony-vine fruit, millet, mulberry, mullet (black or striped), mussel, perch, pigeon (egg and meat), pork kidney, scallop (dried), sea cucumber, string bean, walnut, wheat, and wild cabbage. 3. Choose from these foods that are good for fire deficiency: asparagus, bamboo shoots, banana, bitter endive, black fungus, cattail, chicken egg, cucumber, duck egg, Job's tears, leaf beet, lily flower, liver, mung bean, oyster, peppermint, purslane, pork, royal jelly, salt, spinach, and strawberry. 4. Foods to be avoided in cases of fire deficiency are garlic, Japanese cassia bark, lichi nut, prickly ash, star anise, and walnut.

Beneficial Herbs to Be Applied One Herb at a Time. Huang lian (Rhizoma Coptidis), 12 g; mai men dong (Radix Ophiopogonis), 11 g; rou gui (Cortex Cinnamomi), 5 g; sheng di (Radix Rehmanniae), fresh, 35 g; wu wei zi (Fructus Schisandrae), 4 g; xuan shen (Radix Scrophulariae), 35 g.

Beneficial Herbal Formulas to Be Applied One Formula at a Time. An Shen Ding Zhi Wan, Huang Lian E Jiao Tang, Jiao Tai Wan, Xin Shen Liang Jiao Tang.

15.2 Simultaneous Deficiency of the Heart and Spleen

When you are in good health, your y-scores are Heart 5 and Spleen 6; when you are ill, your y-scores are Heart 5 and Spleen 6.

Definition of the Syndrome. Simultaneous Deficiency of the Heart and Spleen indicates the presence of Heart Blood Deficiency that causes Spleen Energy Deficiency, so that the spleen becomes incapable of governing the blood to control bleeding.

There is a close relationship between the heart and the spleen. The spleen is the source of energy and of blood production and transformation; it also governs the blood. When spleen energy is deficient, there will be an insufficient production of blood, and, when the spleen fails to govern the blood, the blood will overflow from the blood vessels. All of this will lead to Heart Blood Deficiency, which will intensify the extent of Spleen Energy Deficiency.

Clinical Signs and Symptoms. Major signs: Palpitations, insomnia, abdominal swelling, watery stools. Median signs: Mental depression, many dreams, forgetfulness, decreased appetite, fatigue, weakness, withered and yellowish complexion. Minor signs: Eating only a little, fatigue, forgetfulness, impotence, irregularity of periods or extended menstruation, nervousness, night sweats, shortness of breath, withered and yellowish complexion.

Applicable Western Diseases. Angina pectoris, aplastic anemia, arrhythmia (arrhythmia cordia), chronic enteritis, chronic nephritis, climacteric melancholia, congestive cardiac failure, corneal opacity, dysfunctional uterine bleeding (metropathia hemorrhagica), hysteria, insomnia, neurasthenia, neurosis, rheumatoid cardiopathy, thrombocytopenia purpura.

Treatment Symptoms.   Chronic fatigue, palpitations with nervousness, insomnia, forgetfulness, dizziness, bleeding.

Clinical Cases.   (1) A thirty-eight-year-old female patient by the name of Wang experienced a choking sensation in the chest, and she also displayed palpitations, fatigue, and a love of sighing. She was diagnosed in a Western hospital as having bradycardia, with forty-eight pulse beats per minute. In addition, her menstruation continued nonstop for five months and she had a pale complexion and tongue. A Chinese doctor diagnosed Wang's condition as Simultaneous Deficiency of the Heart and Spleen mainly because of the palpitations and extended menstruation. (2). Sun, a female patient, age thirty, suffered from neurasthenia for two years, followed by toxemia of pregnancy. After a cesarean section, she reported having stomach discomfort, a poor appetite, insomnia, palpitations, shortness of breath, a love of sighing, dizziness, forgetfulness, and a pale tongue; she also complained of generally being too weak to talk. A Chinese doctor diagnosed Sun's condition as Simultaneous Deficiency of the Heart and Spleen, because many of her symptoms are signs of this syndrome.

Treatment Principles.   To tone and benefit both the heart and the spleen, to benefit energy and produce blood.

Foods Chosen Based on Y-Scores.   Danggui (Spleen 1, Heart 1), lotus (fruit, seed, and root) (Spleen 2, Heart 2), matrimony-vine leaf (Spleen,-4, Heart -4), pheasant (Spleen 2, Heart 2), red-vine spinach (Spleen -4, Heart -4), sour date (Spleen 0, Heart 0), wheat (Spleen 0, Heart 0). Foods can also be chosen under the individual organs involved.

Generally Beneficial Foods and Other Foods to Be Chosen or Avoided.   1. Foods that are generally beneficial for this syndrome are apple cucumber, beef liver, chestnut, chicken egg, cuttlefish, horse bean, Irish potato, Job's tears, longan nut, mandarin fish, oyster, pork liver, rice, royal jelly, sea cucumber, water spinach, and yam. 2. Choose from the following blood-tonic foods: beef, beef liver, blood clam, chicken egg (especially the yolk), cuttlefish, date (red or black), duck blood, grape, ham, litchi nut, liver, longan, mandarin fish, octopus, oxtail, oyster, pork liver, pork trotter, sea cucumber, soybean skin (black), and spinach. 3. Choose from these energy-tonic foods: beef, bird's nest, broomcorn, cherry, chicken, coconut meat, crane meat, date, eel, ginkgo (cooked), ginseng, goose meat, grape, herring, honey, jackfruit, loach, longan, mackerel, mandarin fish, octopus, pheasant, pigeon (egg and meat), potato (Irish), rabbit, rice (fermented, glutinous), rice (glutinous or sweet), rice (polished), rice (polished, long-grain), rock sugar, shark's fin, sheep or goat meat, shiitake mushroom, snake melon, squash, sturgeon, sweet potato, tofu, turtledove, walnut root, and white string bean. 4. Choose from these heart tonics: air bladder of shark, ambergris, beer, chicory, coffee, ginkgo leaf, ginseng, longan, lotus (fruit and seed), rock sugar, tea, and wheat. 5. Choose from these tonic foods for the spleen and pancreas: apple cucumber, beef, bird's nest, black-eyed pea, broomcorn, caraway seed, carp gall (grass), carrot, cassia bark (Japanese), cherry leaf, chestnut, cinnamon bark (cassia), corn cob, crown daisy, date (red or black), dill seed, frog (pond), garlic, ham, horse bean (broad bean, fava bean), hyacinth bean (lablab bean), hyacinth-bean flower, Job's tears root, longan, lotus (fruit and seed), mullet (black or striped), pearl sago, perch, pheasant, pineapple, pistachio nut, pork pancreas, rice (glutinous or sweet), rice (polished), rice sprouts, royal jelly, string bean, white string bean, whitefish, and yam.

Beneficial Herbs to Be Applied One Herb at a Time. Bai zhu (Rhizoma Atractylodis Macrocephalae), 11 g; da zao (Fructus Ziziphi Jujubae), 18 g; dang gui (Radix Angelicae Sinensis), 11 g; dang shen (Radix Codonopsis Pilosulae), 15 g; gan cao (Radix Glycyrrhizae), 11 g; huang qi (Radix Astragali Seu Hedysari), 40 g; shu di huang (Radix Rehmanniae), cooked, 18 g.

Beneficial Herbal Formulas to Be Applied One Formula at a Time. Gui Pi Tang, Si Wu Tang, Xin Pi Shuang Bu Tang, Yang Xin Tang.

15.3 Yang Deficiency of the Heart and Kidneys

When you are in good health, your y-scores are Heart 4 and Kidneys -4; when you are ill, your y-scores are Heart -8 and Kidneys -8.

Definition of the Syndrome. Yang energy in the heart and yang energy in the kidneys work together to warm the internal organs, promote blood circulation, and transform body fluids. When yang deficiency affects both the heart and the kidneys, this can lead to

Yang Deficiency of the Heart and Kidneys, which is characterized by internal coldness, poor blood circulation, and water stoppage.

Heart Yang Deficiency leads to poor blood circulation, which accounts for the palpitations, the feeling of oppression in the heart and chest, and the bluish-purple nails and lips. Kidneys Yang Deficiency gives rise to poor water transformation, causing the diminished urination and puffy limbs. Water stoppage with the inability of clear yang to elevate is the reason for the dizziness. Yang deficiency leads to internal coldness, which accounts for the fear of the cold and the cold limbs. And poor nourishment of tendons and muscles brings about the muscular twitching and cramps.

Clinical Signs and Symptoms. Major signs: Palpitations, meager urine. Median signs: Cold limbs, edema, chest pain, feeling oppressed in the heart and chest, bluish-purple nails and lips, fear of the cold, muscular twitching and cramps. Minor signs: Discharge of blood from the anus before menstrual periods, discharge of watery and thin stools, frequent urination, pain in the chest, nervousness, shock, phlegm.

Applicable Western Diseases. Arrhythmia (arrhythmia cordia), chronic nephritis, coronary heart disease, cor pulmonale, hyperaldosteronism, hypothyroidism, myocarditis, nephrotic syndrome, rheumatic cardiopathy, viral myocarditis.

Treatment Symptoms. Edema, palpitations, nervousness, chest pain.

Clinical Cases. For close to a decade, a thirty-year-old female patient named Zhang suffered from heart disease without treatment. Over the past month, she also began to display the following symptoms: puffiness particularly in the lower limbs, shortness of breath, nervousness, meager urine, white and greasy coating on the tongue, and slow pulse rates. A Chinese doctor diagnosed her condition as Yang Deficiency of the Heart and Kidneys, in view of the fact that puffiness in the lower limbs is a strong sign of Kidneys Yang Deficiency and meager urine and nervousness are signs of the overall syndrome.

Treatment Principles. To warm and tone the heart and the kidneys.

Foods Chosen Based on Y-Scores. Chicken egg yolk (Kidneys 2, Heart 2), Japanese cassia bark (Kidneys 6, Heart 6), Japanese cassia fruit (Kidneys 5, Heart 5), lotus (fruit, seed, and root) (Kidneys 2, Heart 2), sea cucumber (Kidneys -1, Heart -1), shark air bladder

(Kidneys -1, Heart -1), wheat (Kidneys 0, Heart 0). Foods can also be chosen under the individual organs involved.

Generally Beneficial Foods and Other Foods to Be Chosen or Avoided. 1. Foods that are generally good for this syndrome are cinnamon, clove, crabapple, date (red or black), dill seed, dried ginger, fennel, kidney, lobster, pistachio nut, raspberry, sardine, shrimp, sparrow (including egg), star anise, walnut, water spinach, and wheat. 2. Choose from the following yang-tonic foods for the kidneys: air bladder of shark, beef kidney, cassia fruit (Japanese), chestnut, chive seed (Chinese), cinnamon bark (cassia), clove (including oil), deer kidney, dill seed, fennel (root and seed), fenugreek seed (Oriental), green-onion seed, lobster (sea prawn), mandarin-orange seed, oxtail, pistachio nut, pork testes, prickly ash root, raspberry, sheep or goat kidney, shrimp, sparrow egg, star anise, strawberry, and sword bean (jack bean). 3. Choose from these heart tonics: air bladder of shark, ambergris, beer, chicory, coffee, ginkgo leaf, ginseng, longan, lotus (fruit and seed), rock sugar, tea, and wheat.

Beneficial Herbs to Be Applied One Herb at a Time. As this syndrome involves two organs simultaneously, it is normally treated by an herbal formula that deals with both organs.

Beneficial Herbal Formulas to Be Applied One Formula at a Time. Bao Yuan Tang, Zhen Wu Tang.

15.4 Energy Deficiency of the Spleen and Lungs

When you are in good health, your y-scores are Spleen -2 and Lungs -2; when you are ill, your y-scores are Spleen -6 and Lungs -6.

Definition of the Syndrome. A chronic cough can take a heavy toll on the lungs, causing Lungs Energy Deficiency. When the lungs are deficient, the spleen can be affected so that Spleen Energy Deficiency occurs as well. On the other hand, poor nourishment of the spleen can lead to Spleen Energy Deficiency, which affects the lungs so that Lungs Energy Deficiency takes place too. Or when energy deficiency affects the spleen and the lungs simultaneously, this can lead to Energy Deficiency of the Spleen and Lungs.

Clinical Signs and Symptoms. Major signs: Chronic cough, shortness of breath, copious white phlegm. Median signs: Abdominal swelling, coughing up and spitting phlegm and saliva, loss of appetite, diarrhea with sticky and muddy stools. Minor signs: Poor appetite with indigestion, fatigue of the four limbs, skinniness, skinniness with weakness.

Applicable Western Diseases. Asthma, chronic bronchitis, pertussis (whooping cough), pulmonary emphysema, pulmonary tuberculosis.

Treatment Symptoms. Common cold, cough.

Clinical Cases. Since he was six years old, Wang, a male patient, now age sixteen, has suffered from asthma. He loves eating greasy and fatty foods, and coughs up copious phlegm during an asthma attack. A recent attack lasted for one week, with acute breathing difficulty, the sound of phlegm in the throat, copious whitish phlegm, a congested chest, a loss of appetite, a puffy face, palpitations, and weakness. A Chinese doctor diagnosed his condition as Energy Deficiency of the Spleen and Lungs, chiefly because asthma is a major sign of this syndrome and copious white phlegm and a loss of appetite point to it as well.

Treatment Principles. To benefit energy and strengthen the spleen, to nourish the lungs and transform phlegm.

Foods Chosen Based on Y-Scores. Royal jelly (Lungs 2, Spleen 2), Strawberry (Lungs -2, Spleen -2). Foods can also be chosen under the individual organs involved.

Generally Beneficial Foods and Other Foods to Be Chosen or Avoided. 1. Foods that are considered to be generally good for this syndrome are apple cucumber, beans, bog bean, carrot, cheeses, chestnut, chicken egg yolk, date (red or black), gold carp, grape, ham, horse bean, hyacinth bean, Job's tears, Irish potato, longan nut, maltose, mandarin fish, mutton, rock sugar, royal jelly, squash, string bean, sweet rice, whitefish, and yam. 2. Choose from the following energy-tonic foods: beef, bird's nest, broomcorn, cherry, chicken, coconut meat, crane meat, date (red or black), eel, ginkgo (cooked), ginseng, goose meat, grape, herring, honey, jackfruit, loach, longan, mackerel, mandarin fish, octopus, pheasant, pigeon (egg and meat), potato (Irish), rabbit, rice (fermented, glutinous), rice (glutinous or sweet), rice (polished), rice (polished, long-grain), rock sugar, shark's fin, sheep or goat meat, shiitake mushroom, snake melon, squash, sturgeon, sweet potato, tofu, turtledove, walnut root, and white string bean. 3. Avoid foods that are unfavorable for energy deficiency, such as scallion bulb and prickly ash. 4. Choose from among these tonic foods for the spleen and pancreas: apple cucumber, beef, bird's nest, black-eyed pea, broomcorn, caraway seed, carp gall (grass), carrot, cassia bark (Japanese), cherry leaf, chestnut, cinnamon bark (cassia), corn cob, crown daisy, date (red or black), dill seed, frog (pond), garlic, ham, horse bean (broad bean, fava bean), hyacinth bean (lablab bean), hyacinth-bean flower, Job's tears root, longan, lotus (fruit and seed), mullet (black or striped), pearl sago, perch, pheasant, pineapple, pistachio nut, pork pancreas, rice (glutinous or sweet), rice (polished), rice sprouts, royal jelly, string bean, white string bean, whitefish, and yam. 5. Choose from these tonic foods for the lungs: air bladder of shark, cheeses, garlic, ginkgo (cooked), ginseng (Western), Job's tears, milk (cow's), pork lung, pork pancreas, rice (glutinous or sweet), walnut, whitebait, and yam.

Beneficial Herbs to Be Applied One Herb at a Time. Bai zhu (Rhizoma Atractylodis Macrocephalae), 11 g; bian dou (Semen Lalab), 22 g; dang shen (Radix Codonopsis Pilosulae), 15 g; huang qi (Radix Astragali Seu Hedysari), 40 g; shan yao (Rhizoma Dioscoreae), 20 g; yi yi ren (Semen Coicis), 22 g.

Beneficial Herbal Formulas to Be Applied One Formula at a Time. Bu Zhong Yi Qi Tang, Liu Jun Zi Tang, Shen Ling Bai Zhu San, Shen Su Yin.

15.5 Yang Deficiency of the Spleen and Kidneys

When you are in good health, your y-scores are Spleen -4 and Kidneys -4; when you are ill, your y-scores are Spleen -8 and Kidneys -8.

Definition of the Syndrome. When yang deficiency affects both the spleen and the kidneys, this can lead to Yang Deficiency of the Spleen and Kidneys, or Spleen Yang Deficiency can cause Kidneys Yang Deficiency and vice versa. However, in clinical practice, most of the time Spleen Yang Deficiency occurs first, causing Kidneys Yang Deficiency.

With this syndrome, there is a shortage of yang energy in the kidneys, so that kidneys yang cannot warm the lower back and the knees, which accounts for the cold pain in the lower back and the knees. There is a shortage of yang energy in the spleen, so that spleen yang fails to mobilize and absorb the pure substance of water and grains, which is the reason for the chronic diarrhea. Spleen yang fails to warm the body; this is why there are the cold sensations and the cold limbs as well as the pale complexion. Kidneys Yang Deficiency with internal stoppage of water is responsible for the diminished urination. Water overflowing into the skin causes the puffy face and limbs. And the spleen fails to control water with water flowing into the abdominal cavity, giving rise to the abdominal swelling that is as big as a drum.

Clinical Signs and Symptoms.   Major signs: Cold pain in the lower back and knees, diarrhea at dawn, chronic diarrhea, puffy face and limbs. Median signs: Shivering with cold sensations in the limbs, fatigue, weakness, lack of energy, feeling too lazy to talk, stools' containing undigested foods, poor appetite, abdominal swelling, meager urine with puffy skin, pale complexion. Minor signs: Feeling physically weak and too lazy to talk, cold hands and feet, diarrhea with sticky and muddy stools, eating only a little, edema that occurs all over the body, frequent urination with clear and white urine, phlegm rumbling with panting.

Applicable Western Diseases.   Anemia, aplastic anemia, ascites due to cirrhosis, cancer of the uterine cervix, cervical cancer, chronic cor pulmonale, chronic dysentery, chronic enteritis, chronic glometrulonephritis, chronic nephritis, chronic nonspecific ulcerative colitis, dysentery, hepatic cirrhosis, menopause syndrome, prostatitis, pulmonary tuberculosis, tympanites, uremia.

Treatment Symptoms.   Chronic fatigue, diarrhea, edema, paralysis, discharge of blood from the anus.

Clinical Cases.   (1) After undergoing a gastrectomy to treat a gastric ulcer, a forty-two-year-old male patient named Li displayed the following symptoms: indigestion, abdominal swelling, soft stools and diarrhea, blood in stools, a pale complexion, and fatigue. A Chinese doctor diagnosed his condition as Yang Deficiency of the Spleen and Kidneys, primarily because a loss of blood in surgery leads to many symptoms that are signs of this syndrome. (2) A forty-six-year-old male patient named Lim had his entire left kidney removed a decade ago because of a kidney stone. His right kidney deteriorated after he underwent recent surgery to remove a kidney tumor. Lim caught a common cold a few months ago and reported having diminished urination afterward. At that time, he was diagnosed in a Western hospital as having chronic nephritic uremia. Later, he also developed the following symptoms: nausea and vomiting, dislike of food, diarrhea, a poor complexion, a puffy face, fatigue, dizziness, lower-back pain, puffiness in the lower limbs particularly in the afternoon, and a pale and fat tongue. A

Chinese doctor diagnosed Lim's condition as Yang Deficiency of the Spleen and Kidneys mainly on account of the kidney operation and the puffiness in the face and lower limbs.

Treatment Principles. To warm up and tone both the spleen and the kidneys.

Foods Chosen Based on Y-Scores. Autumn bottle gourd (Kidneys 2, Spleen 2), carp (common) (Kidneys 2, Spleen 2), chestnut (Kidneys 4, Spleen 4), cinnamon bark (Kidneys 7, Spleen 7), clove (Kidneys 6, Spleen 6), clove oil (Kidneys 7, Spleen 7), day lily (Kidneys 0, Spleen 0), dill seed (Kidneys 6, Spleen 6), eel (Kidneys 4, Spleen 4), gorgan fruit (Kidneys 2, Spleen 2), grapefruit peel (Kidneys 3, Spleen 3), grape (Kidneys 0, Spleen 0), Japanese cassia bark (Kidneys 6, Spleen 6), Job's tears (Kidneys 0, Spleen 0), mutton (Kidneys 4, Spleen 4), oxtail (Kidneys 1, Spleen 1), perch (Kidneys 2, Spleen 2), pistachio nut (Kidneys 7, Spleen 7), pork (Kidneys -1, Spleen -1), prickly ash (Kidneys 6, Spleen 6), shark's fin (Kidneys -1, Spleen -1), soybean (black) (Kidneys 2, Spleen 2), star anise (Kidneys 5, Spleen 5), string bean (Kidneys 2, Spleen 2), wheat (Kidneys 0, Spleen 0), white eel (Kidneys 2, Spleen 2), yam (Kidneys 2, Spleen 2). Foods can also be chosen under the individual organs involved.

Generally Beneficial Foods and Other Foods to Be Chosen or Avoided. 1. Foods that are generally beneficial for this syndrome are air bladder of shark, cayenne pepper, chicken, clove, crabapple, dill seed, fennel, kidney, lobster, mustard (white or yellow), mutton, nutmeg, pepper (black or white), pistachio nut, prickly ash, raspberry, sardine, shrimp, sparrow (including egg), sword bean, and walnut. 2. Choose from these yang-tonic foods for the kidneys: air bladder of shark, beef kidney, cassia fruit (Japanese), chestnut, chive seed (Chinese), cinnamon bark (cassia), clove, clove oil, deer kidney, dill seed, fennel (root and seed), fenugreek seed (Oriental), green-onion seed, lobster (sea prawn), mandarin-orange seed, oxtail, pistachio nut, pork testes, prickly ash root, raspberry, sheep or goat kidney, shrimp, sparrow egg, star anise, strawberry, and sword bean (jack bean). 3. Choose from these tonic foods for the spleen and pancreas: apple cucumber, beef, bird's nest, black-eyed pea, broomcorn, caraway seed, carp gall (grass), carrot, cassia bark (Japanese), cherry leaf, chestnut, cinnamon bark (cassia), corn cob, crown daisy, date (red or black), dill seed, frog (pond), garlic, ham, horse bean (broad bean, fava bean), hyacinth bean (lablab bean), hyacinth-bean flower, Job's tears root, longan, lotus (fruits and seed), mullet (black or striped), pearl sago, perch, pheasant, pineapple, pistachio nut, pork pancreas, rice (glutinous or sweet), rice (polished), rice sprouts, royal jelly, string bean, white string bean, whitefish, and yam. 4. Choose from the following warm foods: blood clam, caper, caraway seed, cassia bark and fruit (Japanese), chicken, chili-pepper leaf, chili rhizome, chive (Chinese), chive root and bulb (Chinese), chive seed (Chinese), cinnamon twig, clove, date, dill seed, fennel seed, fenugreek seed (Oriental), fresh ginger, green-onion white head, mustard (white or yellow), mustard seed (white or yellow), nutmeg, pepper (black or white), prickly ash, rice (polished, long-grain), shallot (aromatic green onion), small garlic, sorghum, star anise, sword bean (jack bean), and water chestnut. 5. Avoid these cold foods: adzuki bean, aloe vera, asparagus (lucid), bamboo shoots, banana, bitter endive, bitter gourd (balsam pear), brake (fern), burdock, camphor mint, cattail, crab, endive (Chinese), fig, frog (pond), grapefruit, hair vegetable, honey, leaf beet (spinach beet, Swiss chard), lemon, lily flower, mung bean, mung-bean powder, mung bean sprouts, orchid leaf, peppermint, potato (Irish), preserved duck egg, pricking amaranth (amaranth, pigweed), purslane, rabbit, rambutan, romaine lettuce, Russian olive (oleaster), safflower fruit, salt, soybean paste, squash, star fruit (carambola), strawberry (Indian or mock), sweet basil, tofu, water spinach, wax gourd (Chinese), and wheat.

Beneficial Herbs to Be Applied One Herb at a Time. Bai zhu (Rhizoma Atractylodis Macrocephalae), 11 g; dang shen (Radix Codonopsis Pilosulae), 15 g; fu ling (Poria), 14 g; fu zi (Radix Aconiti Praeparata), 11 g; gan jiang (Rhizoma Zingiberis), 7 g; huang qi (Radix Astragali Seu Hedysari), 40 g; lu jiao jiao (Colla Cornus Cervi), 12 g; rou dou kou (Semen Myristicae), 8 g; rou gui (Cortex Cinnamomi), 5 g.

Beneficial Herbal Formulas to Be Applied One Formula at a Time. Bu Qi Yun Pi Tang, Fu Zi Li Zhong Tang, Shi Pi Yin, Zhen Wu Tang.

15.6 Yin Deficiency of the Lungs and Kidneys

When you are in good health, your y-scores are Lungs 3 and Kidneys 3; when you are ill, your y-scores are Lungs 7 and Kidneys 7.

Definition of the Syndrome. When yin deficiency affects the lungs and the kidneys simultaneously, this can lead to Yin Deficiency of the Lungs and Kidneys. However, in the majority of cases, Lungs Yin Deficiency occurs first, causing Kidneys Yin Deficiency.

Yin Deficiency of the Lungs and Kidneys normally arises from a chronic cough that has caused Lungs Yin Deficiency to affect the kidneys. In some cases, Kidneys Yin Deficiency may occur first, as a result of excessive sex, for example. But most clinical signs and symptoms of this syndrome are those of Lungs Yin Deficiency, with the additional signs and symptoms of Kidneys Yin Deficiency.

Clinical Signs and Symptoms. Major signs: Cough without phlegm or with little phlegm, steaming bones (*gu zheng*), tidal fever. Median signs: Phlegm containing blood, sore loins and weak legs, hot sensations, red zygomatic regions, dry sensation in the mouth but drinking only a little, seminal emission, night sweats, skinniness. Minor signs: Diminished urination, dry sensation in the mouth at night, fatigue, morbid hunger, shortness of breath on movement, insomnia, urgent panting, wheezing, white complexion.

Applicable Western Diseases. Asthma, bronchial asthma, chronic bronchitis, chronic cor pulmonale, chronic nephritis, diabetes insipidus, diabetes mellitus, emphysema, lung cancer, nasopharyngeal cancer, pulmonary tuberculosis.

Treatment Symptoms. Cough, loss of voice, chronic fatigue.

Clinical Cases. (1) For many years, a thirty-six-year-old male patient named Guo had suffered from pulmonary tuberculosis and had been treated without results. He presently displays the following signs and symptoms: skinniness, red cheeks, a frequent cough, coughing up a mixture of phlegm and blood, a low-sounding cough, a congested chest, palpitations, shortness of breath, dizziness, ringing in the ears, night sweats, dry and hot skin, hot sensations in the palms of the hands and the soles of the feet, a dry mouth with no desire to drink, abdominal swelling, a poor appetite, diarrhea with four to five bowel movements every day, a red and dry tongue, and tooth marks on the sides of the tongue. A Chinese doctor diagnosed Guo's condition as Yin Deficiency of the Lungs and Kidneys, primarily because there are many signs of yin deficiency involving the lungs and the kidneys. (2) A year before, a twenty-nine-year-old female patient by the name of Wong came down with a hoarse voice as a result of excessive sadness, and she was treated without effect. Subsequently, her hoarseness worsened to the point that she would completely lose her voice after talking only a little while.

Other symptoms she exhibited were dizziness, vertigo, lumbago, sore loins and weak legs, fatigue, a dry throat and mouth, and a pale tongue. A Chinese doctor diagnosed her condition as Yin Deficiency of the Lungs and Kidneys, mainly because the throat is the door to the lungs and because sore loins and weak legs are signs of Kidneys Yin Deficiency.

Treatment Principles. To water yin, lubricate the lungs, and benefit the kidneys.

Foods Chosen Based on Y-Scores. White fungus (Lungs 2, Kidneys 2). In addition, foods can be chosen under the individual organs involved.

Generally Beneficial Foods and Other Foods to Be Chosen or Avoided. 1. Choose from among these yin-tonic foods: abalone, air bladder of shark, apple, apricot pit (sweet powder), asparagus (lucid), bean drink, bird's nest, bitter gourd (balsam pear), black-eyed pea, brown sugar, cantaloupe (muskmelon), cheeses, chicken egg (especially the yolk), chicken eggshell (inner membrane), clam (freshwater or saltwater), coconut milk, crab, cuttlefish, date, duck, duck egg, fig, frog (river or pond), goose meat, grape, green turtle, honey, kidney bean, kumquat, lard, lemon, litchi nut, loquat (Japanese medlai), lotus rhizome, maltose, mandarin orange, mango, milk (cow's), mussel, oyster, pea, pear, pearl (powder), pineapple, pomegranate (sweet fruit), pork, rabbit, red bayberry, rice (polished), royal jelly, sea cucumber, shrimp, star fruit (carambola), string bean, sugarcane, tofu, tomato, turtle egg, walnut, watermelon, white fungus, white sugar, whitebait, and yam. 2. Choose from these foods that are good for fire deficiency: asparagus, bamboo shoots, banana, bitter endive, black fungus, cattail, chicken egg, cucumber, duck egg, Job's tears, leaf beet, lily flower, liver, mung bean, oyster, peppermint, pork, purslane, royal jelly, salt, spinach, and strawberry. 3. Avoid the following foods that can intensify fire: garlic, Japanese cassia bark, lichi nut, prickly ash, star anise, and walnut. 4. Avoid the following foods and drinks that can cause heat deficiency: alcohol, cayenne pepper, Chinese chive, dog meat, eel, and fresh ginger. 5. Choose from these yin-tonic foods for the kidneys: black-eyed pea, black sesame seed, chicken liver, fish air bladder, frog (forest), lotus (fruit and seed), matrimony-vine fruit, millet, mulberry, mullet (black or striped), mussel, perch, pigeon (meat and egg), pork kidney, scallop (dried), sea cucumber, string bean, walnut, wheat, and wild cabbage. 6. Choose from these food tonics for the lungs: air bladder of shark, cheeses, garlic, ginkgo (cooked), ginseng (Western), Job's tears, milk (cow's), pork lung, pork pancreas, rice (glutinous or sweet), walnut, whitebait, and yam.

Beneficial Herbs to Be Applied One Herb at a Time. Bei sha shen (Radix Glehniae), 11 g; mai men dong (Radix Ophiopogonis), 11 g; sheng di (Radix Rehmanniae), fresh, 35 g; tian dong (Radix Asparagi), 14 g; wu wei zi (Fructus Schisandrae), 4 g; xuan shen (Radix Scrophulariae), 35 g.

Beneficial Herbal Formulas to Be Applied One Formula at a Time. Bai He Gu Jin Tang, Da Bu Yin Wan, Ren Shen Gu Ben Wan, Ren Shen Hu Tao Tang.

15.7 Yin Deficiency of the Liver and Kidneys

When you are in good health, your y-scores are Liver 3 and Kidneys 3; when you are ill, your y-scores are Liver 7 and Kidneys 7.

Definition of the Syndrome. When yin deficiency affects the liver and the kidneys at the same time, this can lead to Yin Deficiency of the Liver and Kidneys, in which Liver Yin Deficiency causes Kidneys Yin Deficiency or vice versa.

The liver stores blood, the kidneys store pure essence, and the two organs depend on each other for the production of blood and pure essence, respectively; in Chinese medicine, this is called "the liver and kidneys' originating from the same source." This syndrome displays the clinical signs and symptoms of Liver Yin Deficiency and Kidneys Yin Deficiency simultaneously.

Clinical Signs and Symptoms. Major signs: Pain in the hypochondrium, dizziness, weak loins and tibia. Median signs: Insomnia with forgetfulness, zygomatic regions on both sides' appearing tender and red, night sweats, many dreams, hot sensations in the five hearts (five centers in palms of hands, soles of feet, and chest), seminal emission, meager menstrual flow or suppression of menstruation, dizziness, ringing in the ears, numbness of limbs, difficulty in flexing and extending, jumpy muscles. Minor signs: Difficulty in both defecating and urinating, dry eyes and throat, fatigue, headache with pain in the bony ridge forming the eyebrow, irregularity of menstrual periods, menstrual pain, lumbago, night blindness, paralysis, strong penis with easy erection, vaginal discharge, pale complexion.

Applicable Western Diseases. Anemia, angina pectoris, auditory vertigo, cervical cancer, chronic hepatitis, chronic nephritis, cirrhosis, consumptive diseases, corneal opacity, epilepsy, flaccid paralysis, hypertension, iridocyclitis, menopause syndrome, menoxenia, neurosis, optic nerve disease, pulmonary tuberculosis, retinopathy, senile cataract, tympanites, tumors, uremia, viral hepatitis (nonjaundice type).

Treatment Symptoms. Pain in the hypochondrium, lumbago, chronic fatigue, bleeding, dizziness, premature menstrual period, menstrual pain, absent period.

Clinical Cases. (1) Chen, a fifty-eight-year-old male patient, suffered from vertigo and headaches for several years. He also complained of ringing in the ears, lower-back pain, numbness in the left half of the body, a poor memory, and insomnia, as well as being scared easily. A Chinese doctor diagnosed his condition as Yin Deficiency of the Liver and Kidneys, because vertigo is a sign of Liver Yin Deficiency and ringing in the ears and lower-back pain are primarily signs of Kidneys Yin Deficiency. (2) A male patient named Li, age thirty-five, suffered from insomnia with severe headaches at night. He also felt painful pressure in the shoulders and the upper arms as if being tightly bandaged, with pain below the right ribs. When he was at work, he experienced pain throughout his entire body, and he usually had a red and dry tongue. A Chinese doctor diagnosed Li's condition as Yin Deficiency of the Liver and Kidneys, on account of the fact that the liver is supposed to nourish the tendons, but when liver yin is deficient it becomes incapable of doing so.

Treatment Principles. To water and tone the liver and the kidneys.

Foods Chosen Based on Y-Scores. Black sesame seed (Liver 2, Kidneys 2), chive seed (Liver 3, Kidneys 3), clam (freshwater) (Liver -5, Kidneys -5), clamshell (river) (Liver -5, Kidneys -5), cuttlebone (Liver -2, Kidneys -2), cuttlefish (Liver -3, Kidneys -3), eel blood (Liver -3, Kidneys -3), jellyfish (Liver -3, Kidneys -3), kelp (Liver -7, Kidneys -7), kidney (deer) (Liver 2, Kidneys 2), matrimony-vine fruit (Liver 2, Kidneys 2), mulberry (Liver -2, Kidneys -2), mussel (Liver -1, Kidneys -1), oyster shell (Liver -5, Kidneys -5), perch (Liver 2, Kidneys 2), plum (Liver 0, Kidneys 0), raspberry (Liver 2, Kidneys 2), seaweed (marine alga) (Liver -8, Kidneys -8), white eel (Liver 2, Kidneys 2). Foods can also be chosen under the individual organs involved.

Generally Beneficial Foods and Other Foods to Be Chosen or Avoided. 1. Foods that are normally beneficial for this syndrome are abalone, asparagus, bird's nest, brown sugar, cheeses, chestnut, chicken egg, chicken liver, cuttlefish, duck, duck egg, kidney bean, mussel, oyster, pork, pork kidney, royal jelly, and white fungus. 2. Choose from among the following yin-tonic foods: abalone, air bladder of shark, apple, apricot pit (sweet powder), asparagus (lucid), bean drink, bird's nest, bitter gourd (balsam pear), black-eyed pea, brown sugar, cantaloupe (muskmelon), cheeses, chicken egg (especially the yolk), chicken eggshell (inner membrane), clam (freshwater or saltwater), coconut milk, crab, cuttlefish, date, duck, duck egg, fig, frog (river or pond), goose meat, grape, green turtle, honey, kidney bean, kumquat, lard, lemon, litchi nut, loquat (Japanese medlai), lotus rhizome, maltose, mandarin orange, mango, milk (cow's), mussel, oyster, pea, pear, pearl (powder), pineapple, pomegranate (sweet fruit), pork, rabbit, red bayberry, rice (polished), royal jelly, sea cucumber, shrimp, star fruit (carambola), string bean, sugarcane, tofu, tomato, turtle egg, walnut, watermelon, white fungus, white sugar, whitebait, and yam. 3. Choose from these yin-tonic foods for the kidneys: black-eyed pea, black sesame seed, chicken liver, fish air bladder, frog (forest), lotus (fruit and seed), matrimony-vine fruit, millet, mulberry, mullet (black or striped), mussel, perch, pigeon (egg and meat), pork kidney, scallop (dried), sea cucumber, string bean, walnut, wheat, and wild cabbage. 4. Choose from these food tonics for the blood: beef, beef liver, blood clam, chicken egg (especially the yolk), cuttlefish, duck blood, grape, ham, litchi nut, liver, longan, mandarin fish, octopus, oxtail, oyster, pork liver, pork trotter, sea cucumber, soybean skin (black), and spinach. 5. Foods and drinks to be avoided in cases of heat deficiency include alcohol, cayenne pepper, Chinese chive, dog meat, eel, and fresh ginger.

Beneficial Herbs to Be Applied One Herb at a Time. Gou qi zi (Fructus Lycii), 11 g; gui ban (Plastrum Testudinis), 30 g; huang bai (Cortex Phellodendri), 15 g; sang shen (Fructus Mori), 18 g; shan zhu yu (Fructus Corni), 11 g; sheng di (Radix Rehmanniae), fresh, 35 g; shu di huang (Radix Rehmanniae), cooked, 18 g; xuan shen (Radix Scrophulariae), 35 g; zhi mu (Rhizoma Anemarrhenae), 15 g.

Beneficial Herbal Formulas to Be Applied One Formula at a Time. Bie Jia Yang Yin Jian, Da Bu Yin Wan, Gu Yin Jian, Hu Qian Wan, Zuo Gui Wan.

15.8 Disharmony between the Liver and Spleen (Liver Excess with Spleen Deficiency)

When you are in good health, your Y-scores are Liver -3 and Spleen -2; when you are ill, your y-scores are Liver -7 and Spleen -6.

Definition of the Syndrome. Disharmony between the Liver and Spleen is a syndrome that refers to the following two patterns. First, energy congestion in the liver gives rise to pent-up energy in the liver, and the liver can overreact to its own congested energy by drastically dispersing it, which causes harm to the spleen. Second, the liver is the master of the spleen, and a deficient spleen can be easily harmed by the liver.

Clinical Signs and Symptoms. Major signs: Abdominal pain preceding diarrhea, less abdominal pain following diarrhea. Median signs: Swelling of rib region, poor appetite, congested sensations in the stomach, stomachache, belching, acid swallowing, nausea, vomiting, abdominal swelling, intestinal rumbling, discharge of watery stools, flatulence. Minor signs: Chronic diarrhea, jumpiness and being prone to anger, fatigued spirits, hungry with no appetite, thirst with no desire to drink, vaginal discharge.

Applicable Western Diseases. Chronic enteritis, chronic hepatitis, cirrhosis, primary hepatoma, schistosomial liver disease, schistosomiasis, viral hepatitis (nonjaundice type).

Treatment Symptoms. Diarrhea, pain in the hypochondrium, abdominal pain, irregular menstrual periods, vaginal discharge.

Clinical Cases. (1) A male patient named Chen, age thirty-three, had chronic enteritis; he exhibited diarrhea with four to five bowel movements every day, abdominal rumbling and pain before a bowel movement, and discharge of bubbly stools. A Chinese doctor diagnosed his condition as Disharmony between the Liver and Spleen, especially because abdominal pain before a bowel movement is a distinct sign of this syndrome. (2) For more than two years, a twenty-eight-year-old male patient named Sun has suffered from abdominal pain and diarrhea, in which case he would have four to five bowel movements a day. He always experiences pain before the diarrhea and a lessening of the pain following it. He was diagnosed by a Western doctor as having irritable bowel syndrome. A Chinese doctor diagnosed his condition as Disharmony between the Liver and Spleen, on account of the fact that abdominal pain preceding diarrhea and less pain after it are major signs of this syndrome.

Treatment Principles. To disperse energy congestion in the liver, to strengthen the spleen, to harmonize the stomach.

Foods Chosen Based on Y-Scores. Brown sugar (Liver 4, Spleen 4), cherry (Liver 4, Spleen 4), danggui (Liver 1, Spleen 1), day lily (Liver 0, Spleen 0), eel (Liver 4, Spleen 4), hairtail (Liver 4, Spleen 4), hawthorn fruit (Liver 2, Spleen 2), Japanese cassia bark (Liver 6, Spleen 6), litchi nut (Liver 2, Spleen 2), long-tailed anchovy (Liver 4, Spleen 4), loquat (Liver -2, Spleen -2), perch (Liver 2, Spleen 2), rape (Liver 2, Spleen 2), sour date (Liver 0, Spleen 0), star anise (Liver 5, Spleen 5), white eel (Liver 2, Spleen 2), wild rice gall (Liver -2, Spleen -2). Foods can also be chosen under the individual organs involved.

Generally Beneficial Foods and Other Foods to Be Chosen or Avoided. 1. Foods that are generally good for this syndrome are apple cucumber, bog bean, brown sugar, carrot, chestnut, corn cob, gold carp, horse bean, hyacinth bean, Job's tears, kumquat, mandarin orange, potato (Irish), royal jelly, string bean, whitefish, and yam. 2. Choose from these foods that can tranquilize the liver: brown sugar, carp (grass), cassia fruit (Japanese), citron seed, fingered citron flower, kumquat leaf, loquat seed, mandarin-orange leaf, orange leaf, pine-nut kernel, rose (steamed extract), and trifoliate orange. 3. Avoid these hot and spicy items: alcohol, chili pepper (cayenne pepper), chive (Chinese), cinnamon bark (cassia), cinnamon twig, clove, coffee, garlic, ginger (dried or fresh), green onion (leaf and white head), mustard seed, nutmeg, onion, pepper (black or white), tea, and wine. They force yin energy to excrete through perspiration, which is harmful to yin and energy. 4. Avoid the following irritants: alcohol, coffee, tea, tobacco, and wine. They can irritate the stomach and produce damp heat, and fire is harmful to yin and energy.

Beneficial Herbs to Be Applied One Herb at a Time. Bai shao yao (Radix Paeoniae Alba), 11 g; bai zhu (Rhizoma Atractylodis Macrocephalae), 11 g; chai hu (Radix Bupleuri), 16 g; chen pi (Pericarpium Citri Reticulatae), 11 g; fang feng (Radix Ledebouriellae), 10 g; gan cao (Radix Glycyrrhizae), 11 g; zhi qiao (Fructus Aurantii), 11 g.

Beneficial Herbal Formulas to Be Applied One Formula at a Time. Chai Hu Shu Gan San, Huang Qin Tang, Long Dan Xie Gan Tang, Xie Huang San.

15.9 Disharmony between the Liver and Stomach (Liver Energy Congestion with Stomach Deficiency)

When you are in good health, your y-scores are Liver -3 and Stomach -2; when you are ill, your y-scores are Liver -7 and Stomach -6.

Definition of the Syndrome. Disharmony between the Liver and Stomach is a syndrome involving the following two patterns. First, energy congestion in the liver leads to pent-up energy in the liver, with the liver's possibly overreacting to its own congested energy by drastically dispersing it, which causes harm to the stomach; second, the liver is the master of the stomach, and a deficient stomach can be easily harmed by the liver.

When energy congestion in the liver affects the stomach, this causes the pain and swelling in the chest and hypochondrium regions as well as the belching and the hiccups. Energy congestion in the liver transforms into fire, affecting the stomach, which accounts for the vomiting of acid. Energy congestion in the liver is also responsible for the jumpiness and anger. Cold energy travels along the liver meridian to reach the top of the head, which is the reason for the headache at the top of the head that is intensified by coldness.

Clinical Signs and Symptoms. Major signs: Pain and swelling in the chest and hypochondrium regions. Median signs: Abdominal rumbling, belching, chest discomfort, hiccups, pain at the top of the head or in the temple that is intensified by coldness. Minor signs: Irregular bowel movements, morning sickness, pain in the inner part of the stomach, vomiting of acid, vomiting of blood.

Applicable Western Diseases. Acute and chronic gastritis, acute and chronic hepatitis, chronic cholecystitis, chronic enteritis, erythema multiforme, gastric and duodenal bulbar ulcer, gastrointestinal neurosis, nervous vomiting, pyloric spasm and obstruction, stomach cancer, viral hepatitis (nonjaundice type).

Treatment Symptoms. Stomachache, vomiting, hiccups.

Clinical Cases. (1) A thirty-two-year-old female patient by the name of Yu had recurrent stomach discomfort and regurgitation of acid; other symptoms she exhibited included discomfort in the right hypochondrium region, insecure sleep, palpitations, and a bitter taste in the mouth, as well as being scared easily, all of which often showed up during her menstrual periods. She also had two to three bowel movements every day. A Chinese doctor diagnosed Yu's condition as Disharmony between the Liver and Stomach chiefly because of her stomach discomfort and the discomfort she felt in the right hypochondrium. (2) A female patient named Pan, age thirty-two, suffered from headaches on the right side of the head that would become more severe in the middle of the night. She also had these other symptoms: vomiting that would be triggered by severe headaches, palpitations, nervousness, a poor appetite, and a greasy coating on the tongue. A Chinese doctor diagnosed her condition as Disharmony between the Liver and Stomach mainly because of the headaches in her temple and the vomiting.

Treatment Principles. To disperse the liver and harmonize the stomach.

Foods Chosen Based on Y-Scores. Brown sugar (Liver 4, Stomach 4), celery (Liver -1, Stomach -1), Chinese chive (Liver 6, Stomach 6), chive (Chinese leek) (Liver 6, Stomach 6), hawthorn fruit (Liver 2, Stomach 2), perch (Liver 2, Stomach 2), vinegar (Liver -1, Stomach -1), whitefish (Liver 2, Stomach 2), wine (Liver 3, Stomach 3). Foods can also be chosen under the individual organs involved.

Generally Beneficial Foods and Other Foods to Be Chosen or Avoided. 1. Foods that are considered to be generally good for this syndrome are barley, brown sugar, carp, celery, chestnut, corn silk, date (red or black), kumquat, peanut, sweet orange, and white fungus. 2. Avoid these hot and spicy items: alcohol, chili pepper (cayenne pepper), chive (Chinese), cinnamon bark (cassia), cinnamon twig, clove, coffee, garlic, ginger (fresh or dried), green onion (leaf and white head), mustard seed, nutmeg, onion, pepper (black or white), tea, and wine. They force yin energy to excrete through perspiration, which is harmful to yin and energy. 3. Avoid these greasy and fatty foods: animal fats (including lamb fat and oil), butter, chicken egg (especially the yolk), creams, fatty meats, fish-liver oils, fried foods, and lard. They can generate heat and produce phlegm, which are bad for indigestion, poor appetite, jaundice, dysentery, and diarrhea. 4. Choose from these foods that can stop vomiting: areca nut (unripe), common button mushroom, fresh ginger, hyacinth-bean leaf, mandarin orange (sour), mango, mung-bean leaf, orange peel (sour), raspberry root, and sweet potato (vine and leaf).

Beneficial Herbs to Be Applied One Herb at a Time. Bai shao yao (Radix Paeoniae Alba), 11 g; ban xia (Rhizoma Pinelliae), 12 g;

chai hu (Radix Bupleuri), 16 g; chuan lian zi (Fructus Meliae Toosendan), 11 g; gan cao (Radix Glycyrrhizae), 11 g; huang lian (Rhizoma Coptidis), 12 g; wa leng zi (Concha Arcae), 11 g; wu zhu yu (Fructus Euodiae), 7 g; xiang fu (Rhizoma Cyperi), 11 g; zhi qiao (Fructus Aurantii), 11 g.

Beneficial Herbal Formulas to Be Applied One Formula at a Time. Bao He Wan, Jin Ling Zi San, Ping Wei San, Si Ni San.

15.10 Liver Fire Offending the Lungs

When you are in good health, your y-scores are Liver 4 and Lungs 3; when you are ill, your y-scores are Liver 8 and Lungs 7.

Definition of the Syndrome. Liver Fire Offending the Lungs refers to energy congestion in the liver that transforms into fire, burning up yin energy in the lungs, or to pathogenic heat that has accumulated in the liver meridian and that travels upward, offending the lungs.

Liver fire flames upward, burning up the yin energy in the lungs, and this accounts for the coughing up or vomiting of fresh blood. Liver fire burns up fluids, making them into sticky and yellowish phlegm. Liver fire travels along the liver meridian, which is the reason for the burning pain in the chest and hypochondrium as well as for the jumpiness and anger. Liver fire flames upward to the face and head, which leads to the dizziness, red eyes, and bitter taste in the mouth.

Clinical Signs and Symptoms. Major signs: Coughing up yellowish phlegm, burning pain in the chest and hypochondrium. Median signs: Meager and sticky phlegm, coughing up or vomiting fresh blood, jumpiness and being prone to anger, dizziness, red eyes, bitter taste in the mouth, reddish complexion. Minor signs: Rapid breath, phlegm with blood.

Applicable Western Diseases. Bronchiectasis, bronchitis, pneumonia, pulmonary tuberculosis.

Treatment Symptoms. Cough, discharge of blood from the mouth.

Clinical Cases. (1) For six months, a fifty-four-year-old male patient named Mu had been vomiting a mixture of phlegm and blood. Then a couple of weeks ago, he started vomiting profuse amounts of blood; this usually occurred around midnight and seemed to be triggered by an emotional disturbance, anger, or bad dreams. A Chinese doctor diagnosed his condition as Liver Fire Offending the Lungs, primarily because vomiting is a sign of a stomach disorder and vomiting that is triggered by an emotional disturbance points to a liver disease. (2) A thirty-five-year-old female patient named Wang had a history of chronic bronchitis, and over the past decade she frequently coughed up blood. Recently, she complained of coughing up phlegm containing huge amounts of blood, in addition to chest pain, hot sensations in the upper half of her body, dry stools, and a thin coating on her tongue. A Chinese doctor diagnosed her condition as Liver Fire Offending the Lungs, mainly because coughing up blood and chest pain are important signs of this syndrome.

Treatment Principles. To clear heat and sedate fire in the liver, to relieve cough.

Foods Chosen Based on Y-Scores. Foods can be chosen under the individual organs involved.

Generally Beneficial Foods and Other Foods to Be Chosen or Avoided. 1. Foods that are generally good for this syndrome are abalone, asparagus, black fungus, chestnut, chicken egg, duck egg, olive, pork, royal jelly, rye, shepherd's purse, soya milk, spinach, vinegar, and white fungus. 2. Choose from among these foods that can promote energy circulation: ambergris, beef, black-eyed pea, camphor mint, caraway seed, cardamom seed, carrot, chicken egg, chive (Chinese), chive (Chinese leek), chive root and bulb (Chinese), chufa rhizome, chufa stem and leaf (earth almond, nut grass), citron (fingered), clam (freshwater or saltwater), common button mushroom, dill seed, fennel seed, fingered citron (Buddha's hand), garlic, grapefruit, green onion (fibrous root and white head), hawthorn fruit, jasmine flower, kumquat, leaf or brown mustard, lemon leaf, lime (young trifoliate orange), litchi nut (including seed), longan seed, loquat seed, lotus stem, malt, mango leaf, marjoram, muskmelon seed, mussel, mustard seed, orange leaf, oregano (wild), radish leaf, rapeseed, red bean, rose, saffron, scallion bulb, shiitake mushroom, spearmint, star anise, string bean, sweet basil, sweet green, orange peel, tangerine (including peel), trifoliate orange, trifoliate orange (near ripe), turmeric, and vinegar. 3. Avoid these items that are likely to trigger a chronic fire syndrome or intensify an existing one: alcohol, chili pepper (cayenne pepper), ginger (fresh or dried), fried foods, garlic, pepper (black or white), and tobacco. 4. Choose from the following foods that are good for fire deficiency: asparagus, bamboo shoots, banana, bitter endive, black fungus, cattail, chicken egg, cucumber, duck egg, Job's tears, leaf beet, lily flower, liver, mung bean, oyster, peppermint, pork, purslane, salt, spinach, and strawberry. 5. Foods to be avoided in cases of fire deficiency are garlic, Japanese cassia bark, lichi nut, prickly ash, star anise, and walnut. 6. Foods to be avoided in cases of excess fire are apricot, chicken, long-tailed anchovy, pepper (black or white), and prickly ash.

Beneficial Herbs to Be Applied One Herb at a Time. Di gu pi (Cortex Lycii Radicis), 11 g; huang qin (Radix Scutellariae), 15 g; long dan (Radix Gentianae), 10 g; mu dan pi (Cortex Moutan Radicis), 11 g; sang bai pi (Cortex Mori Radicis), 11 g; zhi zi (Fructus Gardeniae), 16 g.

Beneficial Herbal Formulas to Be Applied One Formula at a Time. Ke Xue Fang, Long Dan Xie Gan Tang, Xie Bai San.

Part III

CHINESE FOOD CURES

16

An Overview of Chinese Food Cures

FUNDAMENTAL CONCEPTS OF CHINESE FOOD CURES

The practice of Chinese food cures is part of the system of traditional Chinese medicine, and it refers to curing diseases by consuming certain foods. It is a common belief that we consume foods to nourish the body so that the body can grow and stay in good health; in other words, foods provide the human body with nutrients. However, traditional Chinese physicians have long recognized that not only can foods provide the human body with nutrients but they can also cure diseases. Chinese food cures are based upon a theory that combines nourishment with therapy, and they have three distinct advantages.

First, the practice of food cures is derived from many thousands of years of experience. Countless numbers of recipes are recorded in Chinese classics of the past, and they have still been found to be very effective and easy to apply. In addition, many of these ancient recipes have been substantiated scientifically.

Second, food cures are an easy way to combat disease in everyday living, and the meals that you can prepare following the recipes are also delicious. For example, one recipe recorded in a Chinese classic on food cures that was published in the twelfth century is called "Deep-Pot Red Beans in Hen," and it says to do the following: Prepare a 500-g hen, remove the internal organs, squeeze 60 g of red beans into the hen's stomach, boil in water in a deep pot, and season to taste. Chicken acts on the spleen; it is a spleen tonic. Red beans can remove water from the body. Together, they can cure

223

ascites and edema due to the syndrome Spleen Energy Deficiency. This dish is somewhat sweet and very tasty. Another recipe, called "Honey Steamed with Lily," which was recorded in a classic of food cures that was published in 992, offers another typical example. This dish is easy to prepare. All you do is put 60 g of lily in a bowl and add 30 g of honey; then you place the bowl in a pot to steam, with the water reaching close to the top of the bowl. Lily can lubricate the lungs and stop coughing, and honey can strengthen the lungs and lubricate internal dryness. This recipe is used primarily to treat the syndrome Lungs Dryness, and it can cure a cough, a sore throat, constipation, coughing up blood as in tuberculosis, and chronic bronchitis with a dry cough that is often suffered by the elderly.

The third advantage of Chinese food cures is that the focus of the practice is the individual who is regarded as a whole person and the aim is to root out the cause of the disease; in other words, it is not a piecemeal approach to separate symptoms. For example, a person can display a variety of symptoms, such as being allergic to many things, being easily susceptible to the common cold, and sneezing frequently, all of which can be due to the syndrome Lungs Energy Deficiency. In this case, the approach of Chinese food cures is to strengthen the energy in the lungs in order to correct Lungs Energy Deficiency, which is a far cry from dealing with fragmented symptoms.

A BRIEF HISTORY OF CHINESE FOOD CURES

Chinese legend has it that a king in the prehistoric age tasted 100 plants and suffered seventy poisonings every day in his attempt to determine the effects of various plants on the human body. The plants included both herbs and foods, so the king was regarded by the Chinese people as a pioneer of Chinese herbal medicine and food cures.

During the period of the Shang dynasty (from the sixteenth to the eleventh century B.C.), a government official by the name of Yi Yin started using soups to cure disease, marking the beginning of Chinese food cures. During the years of the Western Zhou Dynasty (from the eleventh century to 771 B.C.), a food-cure specialist was established at the Imperial Palace to look after the emperor's diet.

The Yellow Emperor's Classics of Internal Medicine, published in the third century B.C., is the first Chinese medical classic. The following passage from this ancient text gives us a glimpse of the status of food cures in Chinese medicine at that time: "One should take toxic herbs to combat pathogens, consume five grains to nourish the five vital internal organs, reinforce them with five fruits, strengthen them with five animal meats, and supplement them with five vegetables. Energy and flavor should be balanced to produce vital energy in the body."

The first Chinese herbal classic was published during the Qin Dynasty (221-206 B.C.) and was called *The Agriculture Emperor's Materia Medica*. A total of 252 herbs are listed, but many of them are actually foods, such as rice, fruit, fish, and animals. However, it was not until the early years of the Tang Dynasty (618–907) that the system of Chinese food cures was established. This can be attributed to the publication in 652 of a celebrated Chinese medical classic entitled *The Thousand Gold Formulas*. In it, one whole chapter is devoted to the discussion of food cures, listing 154 foods that are divided into fruit, vegetables, grains, birds, and animals, with this emphatic statement at the beginning: "Good health basically relies on foods, because foods not only can destroy pathogens and secure the internal organs, but they can also please the spirits and activate will power for the production of energy and blood; those who can prescribe effective recipes to cure disease and relieve mental suffering are truly good physicians."

The first Chinese medical classic specifically dealing with food cures was published in 1330 and entitled *Proper Ways of Drinking and Eating*. In this classic, a total of 230 foods are listed with 168 illustrations and 238 recipes. The foods are divided into seven categories: rice, grains, animals, birds, fish, fruit, and vegetables. Foods are discussed in terms of their energies, flavors, actions, indications, and proper applications. Colorless spirit distilled from sorghum or maize, which had been widely used for cooking only among the Chinese minority nationalities, was introduced to the Chinese people for the first time through this classic; it has since become a very important ingredient in Chinese food cures. And when Li Shi-Zhen published his famous *Compendium of Materia Medica* in 1578, he included more than 500 foods, most of them accompanied by recipes. It is believed that more than 300 food-cure classics have been published over the course of Chinese history, but only sixteen of them are still available today.

PROPERTIES OF FOOD: ENERGIES AND FLAVORS

Energies of Foods

Foods have different properties, including energies and flavors. Energies of foods refer to their nature, which can be cold, cool, warm, hot, or neutral, as determined by their effects on the human body. For example, from many years of experience, the Chinese have come to know that watermelon has a cold energy. So, when we eat a slice of watermelon, we will probably get a cold feeling, which is good for us when we are hot but detrimental for us when we are already cold. Likewise, mutton has been found to have a hot energy. When we eat mutton, chances are we will get a hot or very warm feeling, and this is beneficial when we are cold but harmful when we are hot already.

Although certain foods can be cold or hot in nature, most of the foods we eat every day do not produce such a pronounced sensation, which is why many foods are further classified into warm or cool foods upon closer examination. The foods that do not produce a particular sensation (either hot or warm, or cold or cool) are classified as neutral foods, examples of which are rice and pineapple.

The energies of foods are reflected in their effects on the human body. When a food has a cold energy, it clears heat in the body; when a food has a hot energy, it warms the body; and when a food has a neutral energy, it is mild and does not produce any apparent energy reaction in the body. Knowing about the energy of foods is essential to the application of food cures.

Flavors of Foods

Flavors of foods refer to how they taste, which can be pungent, sweet, sour, bitter, or salty. These are the five major flavors, but there are also obstructive, light, and aromatic flavors, adding up to a total of eight flavors. One way of determining the flavor of a given food is to taste it directly; another way is to make an educated guess.

Pungent Flavor

Pungent foods can promote circulation and disperse substances. For example, they can promote energy circulation and perspiration, which is considered beneficial if you are under the attack of heat, as occurs with a common cold or the flu. Radish, onion, and fresh ginger are common pungent foods. It is important to realize that, because pungent foods can induce perspiration and deplete body energy, they should be avoided by weak people and by those who have excessive perspiration. According to modern research, pungent foods contain volatile oil, which is partially responsible for their effects.

Sweet Flavor

Sweet foods can nourish the body and slow down the progression of acute symptoms, and they are considered to be good for people with a deficient condition or for people who are under the attack of an acute disease. Sweet foods include yam, which can nourish the body's energy; red date, which can nourish the blood; and sugarcane, which can nourish yin energy. However, sweet foods can also cause an accumulation of dampness in the body; this is one important reason why people gain weight when they eat sweets. Modern research has shown that sweet foods contain carbohydrates and that this in part accounts for their effects.

Sour Flavor

Sour foods can constrict and solidify; therefore, they are good for diarrhea, seminal emission in men, and vaginal discharge in women. Lemon and vinegar are examples of sour foods. It is important to know that, if you are recuperating from an illness, you should avoid sour foods, because such foods can obstruct and slow down recovery.

Bitter Flavor

Bitter foods can excrete, so they are beneficial if you have constipation or excessive water retention in your body. Balsam pear is a typical bitter food. However, if you are skinny or have dry skin, you should avoid bitter foods, because such foods can drain off water from the body.

Salty Flavor

Salty foods can induce bowel movements and soften up hard symptoms, so they are considered to be good for constipation and hard symptoms such as a goiter. Seaweed is a typical salty food that is beneficial for a goiter. But salty foods should be avoided by those suffering from a falling symptom, such as falling of the uterus in women and falling of the stomach, because such foods can lubricate and intensify falling symptoms.

Obstructive or Constrictive Flavor

Some foods have an obstructive flavor, which means that they can constrict or restrict movements. Thus, they are considered good for diarrhea, seminal emission in men, excessive perspiration, and bleeding, as well as for many other symptoms of a sliding nature. Because foods with an obstructive effect are similar to sour foods in terms of effect, and because many sour foods also have an obstructive and constrictive flavor, the Chinese say, "Obstructive effects and sour flavor go hand in hand." Unripe guava is a typical obstructive food that can cause constipation.

Light or Bland Flavor

Some foods have little or no taste, so they are classified as having a light or bland flavor. Such foods can promote urination and are considered to be beneficial for edema and water retention. Job's tears are a typical light food.

Aromatic Flavor

Some foods are aromatic, particularly when they are fried. Foods with a strong aroma can reduce dampness in the body and open up blockages such as nasal congestion.

ORGAN Y-SCORES OF FOODS

The action of particular foods on certain internal organs has a wide application in Chinese food cures. The disease of a specific internal organ is best treated by consuming those foods that act upon that organ, although there are also other important factors to be taken into account. For example, if a person suffers from a disease of the gallbladder, naturally that disease should be treated with the foods that can affect the gallbladder. This is based on a concept called the "organ actions of foods" in traditional Chinese medicine, and, if we know about the organ actions of foods, we can apply them in treatment. After we have identified the y-scores of the internal organs, we need to identify the organ y-scores of foods, in order to know what specific foods will benefit particular internal organs.

ASSIGNING Y-SCORES FOR THE FIVE ENERGIES OF FOOD

	YANG		Neutral	YIN	
Five Food Energies	Hot	Warm		Cool	Cold
Y-Scores	+8	+4	0	-4	-8

ASSIGNING Y-SCORES FOR THE SIX FLAVORS OF FOOD

	YANG		Neutral	YIN		
Six Food Flavors	Pungent	Sweet	Light	Sour	Salty	Bitter
Y-Scores	+8	+4	0	-4	-6	-8

To determine the y-score for each food, follow this formula: (Y-Score of Energy + Y-Score of Flavor) ÷ 2 = Y-Score of Food. For example, here is how to figure out the y-score for beef, which has a sweet flavor and a neutral energy.

Y-SCORE FOR ENERGY OF BEEF

	YANG		Neutral	YIN	
Five Food Energies	Hot	Warm		Cool	Cold
Y-Scores	+8	+4	0	-4	-8

To determine the y-score for beef, follow this formula: $(4 + 0) \div 2 = 2$. Because beef acts on two internal organs (the spleen and the stomach), and because its y-score is 2, it follows that the organ y-score of beef is 2 for spleen and 2 for stomach, which can be indicated as Spleen 2 and Stomach 2.

What follows is a chart showing y-scores and organ y-scores of foods. But first look over these examples from the chart, so that you will know how to read the chart. We can see that the y-score of abalone is -1 and that its organ y-score is Liver -1; this means that the consumption of abalone can bring the y-score of your liver to -1. The y-score of apple is -2, and its organ y-score is Spleen -2, which means that eating an apple can bring the y-score of your spleen to -2. The y-score of banana is -2, and its organ y-scores are Spleen -2 and Stomach -2, so eating a banana can bring the y-score of your spleen and that of your stomach to -2.

CHART FIVE: Y-SCORES AND ORGAN Y-SCORES OF FOODS

Food	Y-Score	Lungs	L. Intestine	S. Intestine	Gallbladder	Bladder	Liver	Kidneys	Spleen	Heart	Stomach	Notes
Abalone	-1						-1					
Adzuki bean	0		0						0			
Agar	-5						-5					
Amaranth	0		0									
Ambergris	0											Heart tonic
Apple	-2								-2			Yin tonic
Apricot (sweet)	0	0	0									

FOOD	Y-Score	Lungs	L. Intestine	S. Intestine	Gallbladder	Bladder	Liver	Kidneys	Spleen	Heart	Stomach	NOTES
Apricot pit (bitter powder)	2											Toxic
Apricot pit (sweet powder)	1											
Areca nut	-2		-2								-2	
Arrowhead	-2						-2		-2			
Asparagus	1										1	Yin tonic
Autumn bottle gourd	2							2	2			
Azalea flower	2											Stomach tonic
Bamboo shoots	-2										-2	Glossy
Banana	-2								-2	-2		
Barley	-3								-3	-3		
Bean curd (tofu)	0		0						0		0	Energy tonic, yin tonic
Beef	2								2		2	Energy tonic, blood tonic, spleen-stomach tonic
Beetroot (sugar beet)	2											
Bird's nest	2							2			2	Energy tonic, yin tonic
Bitter gourd (balsam pear)	-8								-8	-8	-8	Yin tonic
Bitter-gourd seed	-2											Energy tonic
Black fungus	2		2								2	
Black pepper	8		8								8	
Black sesame seed	2						2	2				Liver tonic

Food	Y-Score	Lungs	L. Intestine	S. Intestine	Gallbladder	Bladder	Liver	Kidneys	Spleen	Heart	Stomach	Notes
Black soybean skin	0											Blood tonic
Blood clam	4								4		4	Blood tonic, stomach tonic
Bottle gourd (calabash)	-2			-2								
Broad bean (horse bean)	2								2		2	Spleen tonic
Brome seed	0									0	0	
Broomcorn	2		2						2		2	Blood tonic, spleen tonic
Brown sugar	4						4		4		4	Yin tonic
Buckwheat	0	0							0		0	
Butter	4											
Cabbage (Chinese)	2	2									2	
Caraway	6							6			6	
Carp (common)	2							2	2			
Carp (gold)	2								2		2	
Carp (grass)	4								4		4	
Carrot	2								2			Spleen tonic
Castor bean	3		3									
Catfish	4					4					4	
Celery	-1						-1				-1	
Cheeses	0											Yin tonic, lung tonic
Cherry	4						4		4			Energy tonic
Cherry seed	0											
Chestnut	4							4	4		4	Yang tonic, spleen-stomach tonic

Food	Y-Score	Lungs	L. Intestine	S. Intestine	Gallbladder	Bladder	Liver	Kidneys	Spleen	Heart	Stomach	Notes
Chicken	4								4		4	Energy tonic
Chicken egg	2											Blood tonic, yin tonic
Chicken egg white	-2	-2										
Chicken egg yolk	2							2		2		
Chicory	-6				-6		-6					Heart tonic
Chili pepper (cayenne)	8								8	8		
Chinese chive	6						6	6			6	Obstructive
Chinese toon leaf	-4		-4								-4	
Chinese wax gourd (winter melon)	0		0	0		0						
Chive (Chinese leek)	6						6	6			6	
Chive root (Chinese)	6											
Chive seed (Chinese)	3						3	3				Yang tonic
Cinnamon bark	7					7		7	7			Yang tonic, spleen tonic
Cinnamon twig	5					5				5		
Clam (freshwater)	-5						-5	-5				Stomach tonic
Clam (saltwater)	-7										-7	Stomach tonic
Clamshell (river)	-5						-5	-5				
Clamshell (sea)	-7										-7	
Clove	6							6	6		6	Yang tonic

FOOD	Y-Score	Lungs	L. Intestine	S. Intestine	Gallbladder	Bladder	Liver	Kidneys	Spleen	Heart	Stomach	NOTES
Clove oil	7							7	7		7	Yang tonic
Coconut meat	2		2						2		2	Obstructive, energy tonic
Coconut milk	4											Yin tonic
Coconut shell	0											
Coffee	1									1		Heart tonic
Common button mushroom	0		0	0							0	
Coriander (Chinese parsley)	6								6			
Corn cob	2		2								2	Spleen tonic
Corn silk	2				2		2					
Cottonseed	8											
Cottonseed oil	8		8									Slightly toxic
Crab	-7						-7				-7	Yin tonic
Crabapple	0						0			0		
Crane meat	-3											Energy tonic
Crown daisy	6								6		6	Stomach-spleen tonic
Cucumber	0		0						0		0	
Cuttlebone	-2						-2	-2				
Cuttlefish	-3						-3	-3				Blood tonic, yin tonic
Danggui	1						1		1	1		Blood tonic
Date (red or black)	4								4		4	Energy tonic, spleen-stomach tonic
Day lily	0						0	0	0			
Dill seed	6							6	6			Yang tonic, spleen tonic
Dry mandarin orange peel	2								2			Yin tonic

Food	Y-Score	Lungs	L. Intestine	S. Intestine	Gallbladder	Bladder	Liver	Kidneys	Spleen	Heart	Stomach	Notes
Duck	-1							-1				Yin tonic
Duck egg	0	0						0				Yin tonic
Eel blood	-3						-3	-3				
Eggplant	0								0		0	
Fennel	6					6		6			6	Yang tonic, stomach tonic
Fennel root	2							2				Yang tonic
Fenugreek seed (Oriental)	-2											Yang tonic
Fermented glutinous rice	5											Energy tonic
Fig	2		2						2			Yin tonic
Fishy vegetable	0	0										
Frog (forest)	-5							-5				Yin tonic, spleen tonic
Frog (pond)	-2											
Garlic	6								6		6	Lung tonic, spleen tonic
Ginger (dried)	8								8		8	
Ginger (fresh)	6								6		6	
Gingko leaf	-2									-2		Heart tonic
Ginkgo (cooked)	-2							-2				Energy tonic, lung tonic
Ginseng	1								1			Energy tonic, heart tonic
Goose egg	-8								-8			
Goose meat	2								2			Energy tonic
Gorgan fruit	2							2	2			
Grape	0							0	0			Energy tonic, blood tonic-
Grapefruit	-4							-4	-4			
Grapefruit peel	3					3		3	3			

FOOD	Y-Score	Lungs	L. Intestine	S. Intestine	Gallbladder	Bladder	Liver	Kidneys	Spleen	Heart	Stomach	NOTES
Green-onion leaf	6											
Green-onion seed	6							6				Yang tonic
Green-onion white head	6										6	
Green turtle	2						2					Yin tonic
Guava	4		4									Obstructive
Guava leaf	2											Obstructive
Hair vegetable	-2											
Hairtail	4						4		4			
Ham	-1								-1			Blood tonic
Hami melon	-2									-2	-2	
Hawthorn fruit	2						2		2		2	
Herring	2								2			Energy tonic
Honey	2		2						2			Energy tonic, yin tonic
Hops	-6					-6			-6			
Hyacinth bean	2								2		2	Spleen tonic
Hyacinth-bean flower	2								2		2	Spleen-stomach tonic
Jackfruit	0										0	Energy tonic
Japanese cassia bark	6						6	6	6	6		Spleen-stomach tonic
Japanese cassia fruit	5						5	5		5		Yang tonic, stomach tonic
Jellyfish	-3						-3	-3				
Jellyfish skin	-1						-1					
Job's tears	0							0	0			Lung tonic
Job's tears leaf	2										2	Stomach tonic
Job's tears root	-5					-5			-5			Spleen tonic

Food	Y-Score	Lungs	L. Intestine	S. Intestine	Gallbladder	Bladder	Liver	Kidneys	Spleen	Heart	Stomach	Notes
Kelp	-7						-7	-7			-7	
Kidney (beef)	2							2				Yang tonic, kidney tonic
Kidney (deer)	2						2	2				Yang tonic
Kidney (pork)	-3							-3				
Kidney (sheep or goat)	4							4				
Kidney bean	2											Yin tonic
Kiwifruit (Chinese gooseberry)	-4							-4			-4	
Kohlrabi (turnip cabbage)	1		1			1						
Kumquat	3											Yin tonic
Lard	0								0		0	Yin tonic
Laver	-5	-5										
Leaf or brown mustard	6	6									6	
Leek	6						6					
Lemon	2											Yin tonic
Lettuce (leaf and stalk)	-2		-2								-2	
Lettuce seed	-2		-2								-2	
Licorice	2								2		2	Energy tonic
Lily	-2									-2		
Lily flower	0											
Ling	0		0	0							0	
Litchi nut	2						2		2			Blood tonic, yin tonic
Liver (beef)	2						2					Energy tonic, liver tonic
Liver (chicken)	4						4	4				

Food	Y-Score	Lungs	L. Intestine	S. Intestine	Gallbladder	Bladder	Liver	Kidneys	Spleen	Heart	Stomach	Notes
Liver (pork)	1						1					Blood tonic, liver tonic
Liver (sheep or goat)	-3						-3					Blood tonic, liver tonic
Loach	2								2			
Lobster	1							1				
Longevity fruit	0								0			
Longan	4								4	4		Energy and blood, heart and spleen tonic
Long-kissing sturgeon	2					2			2		2	
Long-tailed anchovy	4						4		4			Energy tonic
Loquat	-2						-2		-2			Yin tonic
Lotus (fruit, seed, and root)	2							2	2	2		Obstructive, heart-spleen tonic
Lotus plumule	-8						-8			-8		Obstructive
Lotus-rhizome powder	-1								-1			Energy tonic
Mackerel	2								2		2	Energy tonic
Mackerel gall	-8						-8					
Malt	4								4		4	
Maltose	4								4		4	Yin tonic
Mandarin fish	2										2	Energy tonic, yin tonic
Mandarin orange	-2								-2		-2	Yin tonic
Mango	-2								-2		-2	Yin tonic
Marjoram	2		2			2					2	

Food	Y-Score	Lungs	L. Intestine	S. Intestine	Gallbladder	Bladder	Liver	Kidneys	Spleen	Heart	Stomach	Notes
Matrimony-vine fruit	2						2	2				Blood tonic
Matrimony-vine leaf	4							-4	-4	-4		Yin tonic
Milk (cow's)	2									2	2	Yin tonic, lung-stomach tonic
Milk (goat's)	4		4				4				4	
Milk (human)	-1									-1	-1	Blood tonic
Milk (mare's)	0								0			Blood tonic
Millet	2	2	2						2			
Mulberry	-2						-2	-2				Blood tonic
Mung bean	0									0	0	
Mung bean sprouts	-2								-2		-2	
Murrel (snakehead)	-2								-2		-2	Energy tonic
Muskmelon (cantaloupe)	-2									-2	-2	Yin tonic
Mussel	-1						-1	-1				Yin tonic, liver tonic
Mutton	4							4	4		4	
Nutmeg	6		6						6			
Octopus	-4								-4			Energy tonic, blood tonic
Olive (Chinese)	0										0	Obstructive
Onion	6								6		6	
Oxtail	1							1	1			Blood tonic, yang tonic
Oyster	-1									-1		Blood tonic, yin tonic
Oyster shell	-5						-5	-5				

FOOD	Y-Score	Lungs	L. Intestine	S. Intestine	Gallbladder	Bladder	Liver	Kidneys	Spleen	Heart	Stomach	NOTES
Palm seed	-4		-4									Blood tonic, constrictive
Papaya	2								2		2	
Pea	2								2		2	
Peach	2		2								2	
Peanut	2								2			
Pear	-2										-2	Yin tonic
Pearl sago	4								4		4	Spleen tonic
Peppermint	2						2					
Perch	2						2	2	2		2	Liver tonic, spleen-stomach tonic
Persimmon	-2		-2							-2		Obstructive
Pheasant	2								2	2	2	Spleen tonic
Pigeon egg	0							0				Energy tonic
Pigeon meat	-2							-2				Energy tonic, yin tonic
Pineapple	0								0		0	Yin tonic, spleen tonic
Pine-nut kernel	4		4				4					
Pistachio nut	7							7	7			Yang tonic, spleen tonic
Plum	0						0	0				
Polished rice	2								2		2	Energy-yin, spleen-stomach tonic
Pomegranate (sour fruit)	0											Constrictive
Pomegranate (sweet fruit)	2		2								2	Yin tonic
Pork	-1							-1	-1		-1	Yin tonic
Pork lung	2	2										Lung tonic

Food	Y-Score	Lungs	L. Intestine	S. Intestine	Gallbladder	Bladder	Liver	Kidneys	Spleen	Heart	Stomach	Notes
Pork marrow	-2							-2				Lung tonic, kidney tonic
Pork testes	4							4				Yang tonic
Pork trotter	-1										-1	Blood tonic
Potato (Irish)	2								2		2	Energy tonic
Prickly ash	6							6	6			
Prickly ash root	8							8				Yang tonic
Processed black-bean seed	-8										-8	
Pumpkin	0	0										
Purslane	-6		-6				-6		-6			
Rabbit	0		0				0					Energy tonic, yin tonic
Radish	1										1	
Radish leaf	0								0		0	
Rape	2						2		2			
Rape oil	6		6				6					
Raspberry	2						2	2				Yang tonic, liver tonic
Red bayberry	2										2	Yin tonic
Red or green pepper (chili pepper, cayenne pepper)	8								8	8		
Red-vine spinach	-4		-4	-4			-4		-4	-4		
Rice bran	3		3								3	
River snail	-5		-5	-5		-5					-5	
Rock sugar	2								2			Energy tonic, heart tonic
Rosemary	6	6									6	

FOOD	Y-Score	Lungs	L. Intestine	S. Intestine	Gallbladder	Bladder	Liver	Kidneys	Spleen	Heart	Stomach	NOTES
Royal jelly	2	2	2						2			Yin tonic, liver and spleen tonic
Saffron	2						2			2		
Salt	-7		-7	-7				-7			-7	
Scallion bulb	2		2						2			
Sea cucumber	-1							-1	-1			Blood tonic, yin tonic
Seaweed (marine alga)	-8						-8	-8			-8	
Sesame oil	0		0									
Shark air bladder	-1							-1	-1			Yin tonic, yang tonic, lung and heart tonic
Shark's fin	-1							-1	-1			Energy tonic
Sheep or goat blood	3								-3			Spleen tonic, energy tonic
Shepherd's purse	2						2					
Shiitake mushroom	2										2	Energy tonic, stomach tonic
Shrimp	4								4		4	
Silver carp	4								4		4	Energy tonic
Small white cabbage	2		2	2							2	
Small-eyed carp	4										4	
Sorghum	4		4						4		4	
Sour date	0				0		0		0	0		Liver tonic
Sour plum (prune)	-3						-3					

FOOD	Y-Score	Lungs	L. Intestine	S. Intestine	Gallbladder	Bladder	Liver	Kidneys	Spleen	Heart	Stomach	NOTES
Soybean (black)	2							2	2			
Soybean (yellow)	2		2						2			
Soybean oil	7		7									
Soybean sprouts (yellow)	4		4						4			
Soy sauce	-7							-7	-7		-7	
Spearmint	5	5					5					
Spinach	0		0	0								Glossy, blood tonic
Spiral-shelled snail	-2					-2						
Squash	4								4		4	Energy tonic
Star anise	5						5	5	5			Yang tonic
Star fruit (carambola)	-4								-4		-4	Yin tonic
Strawberry	-2	-2							-2			Liver tonic
String bean	2							2	2			Yin tonic, spleen tonic
Sugarcane	-2										-2	Yin tonic
Sunflower seeds	3		3									
Sweet basil	6		6						6		6	
Sweet potato	-2		-2						-2		-2	Energy tonic
Sweet rice (glutinous)	4										4	Energy tonic, lung tonic
Sword bean	4		4								4	Yang tonic
Tangerine	-2							-2			-2	
Taro	3		3								3	Glossy
Taro flower	0		0								0	Numbing taste

Food	Y-Score	Lungs	L. Intestine	S. Intestine	Gallbladder	Bladder	Liver	Kidneys	Spleen	Heart	Stomach	Notes
Taro leaf	2	2	2									
Tea	-6									-6	-6	Heart tonic
Tea melon	-2		-2	-2							-2	
Tobacco	6	6										
Tomato	-4						-4				-4	Yin tonic
Towel gourd	0						0				0	
Trifoliate orange	-2		-2						-2			Stomach tonic
Turnip flower	4						4					Liver tonic
Variegated carp	4					4					4	Yin tonic
Vinegar	-1						-1				-1	
Walnut	4							4				Yin tonic, lung tonic
Water chestnut	-2										-2	
Water spinach	-2		-2	-2			-2		-2			
Watermelon	-2					-2			-2			Yin tonic
Western ginseng	-3										-3	Lung tonic, energy tonic
Wheat	0							0	0	0		Heart tonic
Wheat bran	0										0	
White eel	2						2	2	2			
White fungus	2	2						2			2	Glossy, yin tonic, stomach tonic
White pepper	8		8								8	
White sugar	2								2			Yin tonic
Whitebait	2								2		2	Yin tonic, lung-stomach tonic, energy tonic
Whitefish	2						2				2	Spleen-stomach tonic, energy tonic

FOOD	Y-Score	Lungs	L. Intestine	S. Intestine	Gallbladder	Bladder	Liver	Kidneys	Spleen	Heart	Stomach	NOTES
Wild cabbage	2								2		2	
Wild rice gall	-2						-2		-2			
Wine	3						3				3	
Winter melon	-1	-1	-1	-1		-1						
Yam	2							2	2			Yin tonic, lung-spleen tonic
Yam bean	0										0	
Yellow croaker	-1										-1	

17

Six Classes of Foods and Their Effects

FRUIT AND NUTS

Fruit can be either fresh or dried. Fresh fruit such as pears and peaches contain juice; dried fruit like chestnuts and walnuts have a hard shell on the outside and virtually no juice. Fruit that have been left to dry in the sun are also called dried fruit. Persimmon cake is one example. When fresh persimmons are peeled and left to dry in the hot sun, they become persimmon cakes.

There is a wide variety of fresh and juicy fruit, most of which can tone deficiency, nourish yin energy, produce fluids, overcome mental depression, assist digestion, increase appetite, relieve hangover, lubricate the intestines, and promote bowel movements.

Modern research indicates that fruit and vegetables have similar nutritional components. Both contain vitamin C primarily, followed by inorganic salts, organic acid, and carbohydrates. Regular and moderate consumption of fruit increases the energy and vitality of the body, while also assisting the body in preventing hypertension, arteriosclerosis, coronal heart disease, and many other disorders. The pectin that is found in some dried fruit is capable of absorbing bacterial toxins and preventing the body from losing its immune power; for this reason, certain dried fruit are useful in preventing cancers.

Fruit can be cold or warm. If you have a cold disease, you should avoid cold fruit; if you have a hot disease, stay away from warm fruit. An excessive consumption of fruit should also be avoided.

What follows is a list of fruits and nuts with their organ y-scores and indications.

Apple   *Spleen -2*
Dry throat, thirst, dry cough, intoxication, chronic diarrhea.
Apricot (sweet)   *Lungs 0, L. intestine 0*
Cough, thirst, copious phlegm, asthma.The ripe fruit taste both
sweet and sour. The pits taste bitter and are ground into powder for
use as an herb. Apricot pit is an important powdered herb in Chi-
nese medicine for relieving a cough and expelling phlegm.
Areca nut   *L. intestine -2, Stomach -2*
Edema, beriberi, parasites (tapeworms, hookworms, roundworms,
fasciolopsis). Ripe, the nuts are used as food, unripe, as an herb.
Banana   *Spleen -2, Stomach -2*
Bleeding in hemorrhoids, dry cough, constipation with dry stools.
Cherry   *Liver 4, Spleen 4*
Measles before eruption, rheumatism, numbness, paralysis.
Chestnut   *Kidneys 4, Spleen 4, Stomach 4*
Diarrhea, vomiting of blood, nosebleed, weak bones or poor
growth of bones in children.
Coconut   *L. intestine 2, Spleen 2, Stomach 2*
Malnutrition in children, tapeworm.
Fig   *L. intestine 2, Spleen 2*
Dysentery, constipation, hemorrhoids, prolapse of anus..
Ginkgo   *Spleen 6, Stomach 6*
Cough with copious phlegm, whitish vaginal discharge, enuresis.
Before use, remove the shell and then crush the seeds and steam
them for consumption; ingest only 6 to 10 g each time, to prevent
poisoning that can arise from excessive dosages. The leaf of this tree
is also used as an herb for similar effects.
Gorgan fruit (water lily)   *Kidneys 2, Spleen 2*
Chronic diarrhea, frequent urination. Remove the seeds from the
fruit, and crack the seeds to obtain kernels to dry in the sun for con-
sumption. Gorgan fruit is also an important Chinese herb.
Grape   *Kidneys 0, Spleen 0*
Palpitations, fatigue, night sweats, hoarseness, urination difficulty,
dry throat.
Grapefruit   *Kidneys -4, Spleen -4*
Indigestion, coughing up copious phlegm, jaundice, bad breath
due to intoxication.
Guava   *L. intestine*
Diarrhea, pain, bleeding, inflammation. Unripe, the fruit of this
shrub is more obstructive than when ripe, but the ripe tastes better.

Hami melon   *Heart -2, Stomach -2*
Thirst, diminished urination, canker sore in the mouth. Hami melon is primarily cultivated in Hami, located in Xinjiang province in China. It is a variety of muskmelon.

Hawthorn fruit   *Liver 2, Spleen 2, Stomach 2*
Menstrual pain, abdominal pain, indigestion, diarrhea, dysentery, hypertension, coronary heart disease.

Kiwifruit (Chinese gooseberry)   *Kidneys -4, Stomach -4*
Thirst, poor appetite, indigestion, urinary stones, jaundice.

Lemon
Thirst, poor appetite among pregnant women, insecure fetus.

Ling   *L. intestine 0, S. intestine 0, Stomach 0*
Poor appetite, shortness of breath, diabetes, alcoholism.

Litchi nut   *Liver 2, Spleen 2*
Vaginal bleeding, hiccups, abdominal pain, palpitations, insomnia, forgetfulness.

Longan nut   *Spleen 4, Heart 4*
Palpitations, nervousness, anemia, neurasthenia, forgetfulness.

Longevity fruit   *Spleen 8*
Whooping cough, sore throat, constipation particularly among the elderly. Bake the fruit until dry, to become dried fruit, which produce noise on beating not unlike a drum. The dried fruit are consumed either having been boiled in water or having been ground into powder.

Loquat   *Liver -2, Spleen -2*
Coughing up blood, hoarseness, thirst, hiccups, vomiting.

Lotus seed   *Kidneys 2, Spleen 2, Heart 2*
Chronic diarrhea, fasting dysentery, seminal emission, premature ejaculation, palpitations, frequent urination.

Mandarin orange   *Spleen -2, Stomach -2*
Thirst, intoxication, urination difficulty.

Mango   *Spleen -2, Stomach -2*
Thirst, vomiting, motion sickness, dizziness, diminished urination.

Matrimony-vine fruit   *Liver 2, Kidneys 2*
Blurred vision, dizziness, weak loins, seminal emission, diabetes. Matrimony vine is cultivated for its berries. The dried berries are an important Chinese herb.

Mulberry   *Liver -2, Kidneys -2*
Dizziness, thirst, constipation with dry stools, blurred vision, premature gray hair.

Muskmelon (cantaloupe)   *Heart -2, Stomach -2*
Thirst, poor appetite, diminished urination, mental depression.
Olive (Chinese)   *Stomach 0*
Thirst, sore throat, cough, vomiting of blood, fish bone stuck in
the throat.
Papaya   *Spleen 2, Stomach 2*
Indigestion, stomachache, dysentery.
Peach   *l. intestine 2, Stomach 2*
Constipation with dry stools, thirst.
Peanut   *Spleen 2*
Dry cough, whooping cough, shortage of milk secretion in nurs-
ing mothers.
Pear   *Stomach -2*
Hot sensations in the body, thirst as in diabetes, diminished uri-
nation.
Persimmon   *L. intestine -2, Heart -2*
Dry cough or coughing up blood, bleeding in hemorrhoids. The
fruit is edible only when completely ripe and red and no longer
tastes obstructive. Green persimmons can be picked, but they are
edible only when the obstructive taste is gone.
Pineapple   *Spleen 0, Stomach 0*
Thirst due to summer heat, indigestion, diarrhea, heart disease.
Pine-nut kernel   *L. intestine 4, Liver 4*
Dry cough, dry constipation particularly in the elderly and
women after delivery.
Plum   *Liver 0, Kidneys 0*
Chronic cough, dysentery, blood in stool and urine, vaginal
bleeding, chronic diarrhea, abdominal pain caused by roundworms.
Pomegranate (sour fruit)   *Lungs 2, Stomach 2*
Thirst, chronic diarrhea, discharge of blood from the anus, vagi-
nal discharge.
Red bayberry   *Stomach 2*
Thirst, vomiting, diarrhea.
Red date   *Spleen 4, Stomach 4*
Fatigue, nervousness, hysteria in women, neurosis.
Star fruit (carambola)   *Spleen -4, Stomach -4*
Thirst, cough in the common cold, ulcers in the mouth and on the
tongue, sore throat, toothache, urination difficulty, pain on urination.
Sugarcane   *Stomach -2*
Dry cough, thirst, fever, measles before eruption, vomiting.

Sunflower seed   *l. intestine 3*
Enterobiasis (pinworm infestation), blood in stools.
Tangerine   *Kidneys -2, Stomach -2*
Hiccups, poor appetite, abdominal swelling, diabetes, coughing up copious phlegm.
Tomato   *Liver -4, Stomach -4*
Thirst, indigestion, hypertension, poor appetite.
Walnut   *Kidneys 4*
Impotence, seminal emission, frequent urination, premature aging, urinary stones, asthma.
Water chestnut   *Stomach -2*
Thirst, cough with copious phlegm, indigestion, vaginal bleeding.
Watermelon   *Bladder -2, Heart -2*
Thirst, diminished urination, mental depression.
Yam bean   *Stomach 0*
Thirst, chronic alcoholism.

VEGETABLES

Vegetables are plants that are cultivated for their edible roots, stems, leaves, or flowers. There are terrestrial plants, meaning plants that grow on land, and aquatic plants, meaning those growing in or on the water. Plants growing on land can be divided into garden and farm plants and wild plants. Generally, garden and farm plants, such as squash and hyacinth bean, tone the body's energy. Most wild plants can clear heat and detoxify.

The various kinds of vegetables and edible parts have different effects. In general, hot and pungent vegetables like cayenne pepper are warm, whereas most other types of vegetable are cold or cool.

Vegetables basically harmonize the middle region of the body and strengthen the spleen, as well as assist in digestion, wake up the appetite, clear heat, produce fluids, and promote urination and defecation. If you are experiencing a poor appetite, indigestion, abdominal distension, or fatigue due to disorders of the spleen and the stomach, it is likely you would benefit from eating vegetables.

Modern research indicates that vegetables are more than 70 percent juice. This is especially true of fresh vegetables, which also taste delicious and are the primary sources of vitamins, inorganic salts, pectin, and carbohydrates.

Fruit and vegetables contain salts of alkaline metals (calcium, magnesium, potassium, sodium). Such alkaline metals exert an alkaline effect in the body, neutralizing acids so as to maintain an acid-base balance. In general, fruit and vegetables are alkali-producing foods, and foods containing protein are acid-producing foods.

The acids and alkalis must be kept in a state of balance so that the normal pH range of systemic arterial blood can be maintained between 7.35 and 7.45. When it is below 7.35, it is called "acidosis," with the principal effect's being depression of the nervous system. When it is higher than 7.45, it is called "alkalosis," and in this case the primary effect is overexcitability in both the central nervous system and the peripheral nerves.

Now here is a list of vegetables with their organ y-scores and indications.

Agar   *Liver -5*

Coughing up phlegm, goiter, scrofula. Agar is a purplish-red or yellow-green food substance obtained from *Eucheuma gelatinae.*

Amaranth   *L. intestine 0*

Diminished urination, dysentery, constipation with dry stools.

Arrowhead   *Liver-2, Heart-2*

Coughing up phlegm containing blood, failure to expel placenta, urination difficulty. Arrowhead is an aquatic or marsh plant with arrowhead-shaped leaves and edible corn. The flowers and leaves of this plant are used as herbs.

Asparagus   *Stomach 1*

Diminished urination, urination difficulty, thirst.

Autumn bottle gourd   *Kidneys 2, Spleen 2*

Dry cough, thirst, diminished urination, edema, jaundice, urination disorders.

Bamboo shoots   *Stomach -2*

Dry mouth, constipation, indigestion, coughing up copious phlegm, measles with difficult eruption, difficult urination and defecation.

Bean curd (tofu)   *l. intestine 0, Spleen 0, Stomach 0*

Poor appetite, shortage of milk secretion in nursing mother, diminished urination, coughing up copious phlegm. Tofu is made of soybeans with gypsum as a coagulant.

Bitter gourd (balsam pear)   *Spleen -8, Heart -8, Stomach -8*

Sunstroke, dysentery. Balsam pear is a vine bearing a long, egg-shaped, edible melon. Because the melon tastes extremely bitter, it is commonly called "bitter gourd" by the Chinese people.

Black fungus   *L. intestine 2, Stomach 2*
Bleeding symptoms, including bloody dysentery, blood in urine, vaginal bleeding, and bleeding in hemorrhoids, prevention of cerebrovascular disease, coronary heart disease.

Bottle gourd (calabash)   *S. intestine -2*
Edema, diminished urination, abdominal swelling.

Carrot   *Spleen 2*
Poor appetite, constipation with dry stools.

Celery   *Liver -1, Stomach -1*
Dizziness, red complexion, pink eyes, hypertension, high cholesterol.

Chili pepper (cayenne pepper)   *Heart 8, Spleen 8*
Indigestion, vomiting, diarrhea, frostbite. The ground dried fruit and seeds of hot peppers.

Chinese cabbage   *L. intestine 2, Stomach 2*
Diminished urination, the common cold.

Chinese chive   *Liver 6, Kidneys 6*
Swallowing difficulty, vomiting, chest pain, stomachache, impotence, seminal emission, enuresis. Chinese chive, *Allium tuberosumis*, is different from the chive in the West, *Allium schoenoprasum*, which has hollow, grasslike leaves, as the leaves of Chinese chive are solid.

Chinese toon leaf   *L. intestine -4, Stomach -4*
Dysentery, boils, scabies, tinea capitis. Chinese toon is planted for its tender leaves that are used as food and for its bark, seeds, and juice that are used as herbs.

Common button mushroom   *L. intestine 0, S. intestine 0, Stomach 0*
Poor appetite, fatigue, shortage of milk secretion in nursing mothers, acute and chronic hepatitis.

Coriander (Chinese parsley)   *Spleen 6*
The common cold, measles before eruption, indigestion. Coriander *(Coriandrum sativumis)* is widely cultivated, and the entire plant, including the root, is edible. The dried ripe seeds are used as an herb, a condiment, and a corrective. Coriander bears a resemblance to parsley *(Petroselinum crispum)*, whose leaves are used for seasoning with similar therapeutic effects.

Crown daisy   *Spleen 8, Stomach 8*
Diminished urination, poor appetite, coughing up copious phlegm.

Cucumber *L. intestine 0, Spleen 0, Stomach 0*
Pink eyes, sore throat, thirst, edema.

Day lily *Liver 0, Kidneys 0, Spleen 0*
Dizziness, ringing in the ears, diminished urination, edema, urination disorders, vomiting of blood, nosebleed, discharge of blood from the anus.

Eggplant *Spleen 0, Stomach 0*
Blood in urine, bleeding in hemorrhoids.

Fishy vegetable *Lungs 0*
Cough, diminished urination, edema, dysentery, pulmonary abscess. Fishy vegetable *(Houttuynia cordatais)* is a plant that is edible in its entirety, including the root, and it can be consumed fresh or dried. It is called "fishy vegetable," because its leaves smell fishy.

Garlic *Spleen 6, Stomach 6*
Cold abdomen, diarrhea, high cholesterol, hypertension, pulmonary tuberculosis, flu, whooping cough.

Hair vegetable *Spleen -2*
Goiter, scrofula, tumor, diminished urination, edema, cardiovascular disease, obesity, cancers. Hair vegetable is a purplish-brown substance obtained from *Gracilaria verrucosa* for use as food.

Hyacinth bean *Spleen 2, Stomach 2*
Poor appetite, fatigue, edema in the lower limbs, chronic diarrhea. Hyacinth bean *(Dolichos lablabis)* is a twining vine bearing edible pods and seeds.

Kelp *Liver -7, Kidneys -7, Stomach -7*
Goiter, scrofula, swelling and pain in the testicle, skin itch.

Kidney bean
Edema, diminished urination, beriberi.

Kohlrabi (turnip cabbage) *L. intestine 1, Bladder 1*
Urination difficulty, swelling, blood in stools..

Laver *Lungs -5*
Goiter, tumor, beriberi, edema, urination disorders, chronic tracheitis, cough.

Leaf or brown mustard *Lungs 6, Stomach 6*
Cough, hiccups, chest congestion. Leaf or brown mustard *(Brassica juncea)* is widely cultivated in China for its edible stalks and leaves. The seeds are pungent and hot, with a y-score of Lungs 8, and are used to warm the lungs.

Lettuce   *L. intestine -2, Stomach -2*
Diminished urination, blood in urine, shortage of milk secretion in nursing mothers.

Lily (bulb and leaf)   *Heart -2*
Chronic cough, insomnia, discharge of blood from the mouth, insomnia.

Lotus   *Kidneys 2, Spleen 2, Heart 2*
Thirst, vomiting of blood, nosebleed, chronic diarrhea, poor appetite after a long illness. Lotus *(Nelumbo nuciferais)* is an aquatic plant with edible, fleshy rhizomes; it is dug out in autumn and winter.

Matrimony-vine leaf   *Kidneys -4, Spleen -4, Heart -4*
Fever, blurred vision, night blindness, pink eyes with pain, corneal opacity, thirst, loose teeth, toothache. See "Matrimony-vine fruit," described in the list above.

Mung bean sprouts   *Spleen -2, Stomach -2*
Thirst, mental depression, diminished urination, alcoholism.

Onion   *Spleen 6, Stomach 6*
Decreased appetite, abdominal swelling, diarrhea, hypertension, high cholesterol, vaginitis, ulcer, wounds..

Potato (Irish)   *Spleen 2, Stomach 2*
Stomachache, constipation, peptic ulcer, habitual constipation.

Processed black-bean seed   *Stomach -8*
The common cold, congested chest, insomnia, hypertension, cancers, aging. This food is fermented and salted soya beans; it is a mixture of three essential ingredients: black soybeans with mulberry leaf and southern wood.

Purslane   *L. intestine -6, Liver -6, Spleen -6*
Dysentery, diarrhea, acute enteritis. The whole plant is edible. The seed is used as an herb to cure dacryocystitis and glaucoma.

Radish   *Stomach 1*
Diabetes, dry mouth, nosebleed, coughing up blood, indigestion, phlegm, bacillary dysentery.

Rape   *Liver 2, Spleen 2*
Abdominal pain after delivery, blood in stools, acute mastitis. Rape *(Brassica campestris)* is a plant that is widely cultivated in China for its edible, tender stalks and leaves.

Red-vine spinach   *Heart -4, Liver -4, Spleen -4,*
                                      L. intestine -4, S. intestine -4
Constipation, urination difficulty, blood in stools, boils, cystitis.

Scallion bulb   *L. intestine 2, Heart 2*
Heart pain, shortness of breath, dysentery, tenesmus.
Seaweed (marine alga)   *Liver -8, Kidneys -8, Stomach -8*
Goiter, scrofula, edema, beriberi, swelling and pain in the testicle, chronic tracheitis.
Shepherd's purse   *Liver 2*
Bleeding, pink eyes, dizziness, diminished urination, swelling, chyluria.
Shiitake mushroom   *Stomach 2*
Decreased appetite, tumors, measles with poor eruption, cancers.
Small white cabbage   *l. intestine 2, S. intestine 2,*
                                                  Stomach 10
Cough, constipation, acute jaundice type of hepatitis.
Soybean sprouts   *l. intestine 4, Spleen 4*
Dry skin, verruca vulgaris, corns.
Spinach   *L. intestine 0, S. intestine 0*
Blood in stools, diabetes, blurred vision, constipation with dry stools, hemorrhoids.
Squash   *Spleen 4, Stomach 4*
Malnutrition in children, diabetes.
String bean   *Kidneys 2, Spleen 2*
Diarrhea, poor appetite, seminal emission, diminished urination.
Sweet potato   *L. intestine -2, Spleen -2, Stomach -2*
Fatigue, thirst, constipation, poor complexion.
Sword bean   *L. intestine 4, Stomach 4*
Hiccups, vomiting, chronic diarrhea, lumbago, suppression of menses.
Taro   *L. intestine 3, Stomach 3*
Scrofula, indigestion, chronic nephritis.
Tea melon   *L. intestine -2, S. intestine -2, Stomach -2*
Diminished urination, thirst, alcoholism.
Towel gourd   *Liver 0, Stomach 0*
Thirst, hemorrhoids, blood in urine, coughing up copious phlegm, shortage of milk secretion in nursing mothers.
Water spinach   *L. intestine -2, S. intestine -2,*
                                          Liver -2, Heart -2
Diminished urination, nosebleed, coughing up blood, vomiting of blood, blood in stools and urine, urination disorders.
White fungus   *Lungs 2, Kidneys 2, Stomach 2*
Dry cough, blood in phlegm, constipation, vomiting of blood,

discharge of blood from the mouth, blood in stools, vaginal bleeding, chronic bronchitis.

Wild cabbage   *Spleen 2, Stomach 2*

Pain in the upper abdomen, pain in peptic ulcer, cholescystitis.

Wild rice gall   *Liver -2, Spleen -2*

Thirst, intoxication, diminished urination, jaundice, constipation. Wild rice *(Zizania caduciflorais)* is a tall aquatic grass, and gall is a swelling of its flowering stem caused by the stimulation of *Ustilago esculenta*. Boil 30 to 60 g of fresh gall in water for consumption each time.

Winter melon (Chinese wax gourd)   *Lungs -1, L. intestine -1,*
S. intestine -1, Bladder -1

Edema, diminished urination, diabetes, asthma, coughing up copious phlegm, nephritis.

Yam   *Kidneys 2, Spleen 2*

Poor appetite, diarrhea, vaginal discharge, chronic cough, seminal emission, diabetes.

MEAT, POULTRY, AND EGGS

Meat is flesh used as food, as distinguished from fish or fowl. Meat is primarily warm in energy, so it can tone the body and is good for the spleen and the stomach; meat can also water and tone the liver, kidneys, and blood. Thus, meat is very important when it comes to combating a deficient disease and a weakness of the body, and it plays a significant role in promoting growth and strengthening the body's energy.

Foods in this category are beneficial to deficiency, poor spirits, fatigue, skinniness, and a yellowish complexion. Different foods are chosen to correct different kinds of deficiency. According to Traditional Chinese medicine, animal organs are beneficial for corresponding human organs. Eggs are primarily neutral in energy and mild in action; they are most suitable for infants and people with anemia and physical weakness.

Modern research indicates that meat is an important source of nutrition for the human body. The nutrients contained in meat (primarily proteins, fat, and carbohydrates) are very similar to those required by the human body. Various meats and vegetables can be mixed to supplement one another. Because meats are more essential than vegetables for correcting the deficient conditions of the human body, the Chinese customarily call meats "compassionate friends of flesh and blood." In addition, meats that contain proteins are acid-producing foods, whereas fruit and vegetables are alkali-producing foods. Therefore, when meats and vegetables are mixed, they keep the acids and alkalis in a state of balance, so that the normal pH range of systemic arterial blood can be maintained between 7.35 and 7.45, and so that we will be neither depressed nor overexcited.

Yet it should be noted that meats have a tendency to produce damp heat and generate phlegm, which may not be beneficial if you have Liver Yang Upsurging. And if you have a cold or cool physical constitution, you should avoid eating meats with a cold or cool energy, as such meats can easily cause harm to the spleen and induce diarrhea.

Here is a list of meats, poultry, and eggs with their organ y-scores and indications.

Beef   *Spleen 2, Stomach 2*
Skinniness and weakness, diabetes, edema, fatigue.

Beef liver   *Liver 2*
Blurred vision, night blindness, withered and yellowish complexion, skinniness and weakness, dizziness.

Bird's nest   *Kidneys 2, Stomach 2*
Cough, discharge of blood from the mouth, chronic diarrhea, swallowing difficulty, upset stomach. Bird's nest is the nest made by esculent swifts from regurgitated gelatinous substances, and it is available in most large Chinese food stores.

Chicken   *Spleen 4, Stomach 4*
Poor appetite, diarrhea, edema, vaginal discharge and bleeding, weakness after childbirth, shortage of milk secretion in nursing mothers, dizziness.

Chicken egg white   *Lungs -2*
Sore throat, pink eyes, cough, hiccups.

Chicken egg yolk   *Kidneys 2, Heart 2*
Insomnia, convulsion, vomiting of blood due to exhaustion.

Chicken liver   *Liver 4, Kidneys 4*
Blurred vision, night blindness, malnutrition in children, miscarriage, anemia after childbirth in women.

Cow's milk   *Heart 2, Stomach 2*
Upset stomach, swallowing difficulty, diabetes, constipation, high cholesterol, peptic ulcer, poor growth in children, weakness in the elderly, recuperating period after childbirth in women.

Duck   *Kidneys -1*
Hot sensation, night sweats, seminal emission, cough, coughing up blood, dry throat, thirst, meager menstrual flow, edema, ascites.

Duck egg   *Kidneys 0, Lungs 0*
Dry cough or coughing up a little phlegm, dry throat, sore throat, toothache, diarrhea, insomnia.

Goat's liver   *Liver -3*
Withered and yellowish complexion, skinniness, blurred vision.

Goat's milk   *l. intestine 4, Kidneys 4, Stomach 4*
Diabetes, dry mouth, hiccups, upset stomach, constipation with dry stools, weakness, skinniness.

Goose   *Spleen 2*
Fatigue, poor appetite, dry mouth, cough, shortness of breath, diabetes.

Goose egg   *Spleen -8*
Poor appetite, fatigue.

Mutton   *Kidneys 4, Spleen 4, Stomach 4*
Lack of energy, acute abdominal pain, pain in the hypochondrium, cold hernia pain, frequent urination, impotence.

Pork   *Kidneys -1, Spleen -1, Stomach -1*
Dry cough, sore throat, constipation with dry stools, hemorrhoids. Pork is not recommended if you have hypertension or high cholesterol, if you are obese, of if you have copious phlegm. Also, if you are under the attack of external atmosphere energies such as occurs with the common cold and flu, you should avoid pork.

Pork kidney   *Kidneys -3*
Lumbago, seminal emission, night sweats, deafness in the elderly.

Pork liver   *Liver 1*
Blurred vision, anemia, withered and yellowish complexion, dry eyes, night blindness.

Rabbit meat   *L. intestine 0, Liver 0*
Fatigue, poor appetite, diabetes, dry mouth.

AQUATIC FOOD

Aquatic food can be divided into animal food and plant food. Plant food has been discussed under the heading of "Vegetables" earlier, leaving animal food to be addressed here. This category includes edible fish and shellfish either from rivers, lakes, or streams (freshwater) or the sea (saltwater).

Aquatic animals are primarily warm in energy, having a toning effect, as they can strengthen the spleen and the kidneys and build up energy and blood. Some of them can promote urination and heal swelling. Aquatic foods are good for deficient body energy and for people who are recuperating from an illness. They are also beneficial following childbirth or for physical weakness due to spleen and stomach deficiencies, fatigue, poor appetite, edema, or ascites. The vast majority of foods in this category have a toning effect without causing energy stagnation.

According to modern research, edible fish contain abundant nutrients and are beneficial to the normal growth of the brain. Regular consumption of fish will bring about clear and quick thinking as well as a good night's sleep, prevent cardiovascular disease, and improve vitality. Yet aquatic animals have been known to trigger a recurrence of an old disease; they can also cause some carbuncles, boils, and skin diseases. So, if you tend to get allergic reactions or have a skin rash, scabies, or eczema, eat such foods with caution.

The following is a list of aquatic foods with their organ y-scores and indications.

Abalone   *Liver -1*
Shortage of milk secretion in nursing mothers, vaginal discharge, hot sensations, night sweats, glaucoma, blurred vision.

Blood clam   *Spleen 4, Stomach 4*
Anemia, cold stomachache, indigestion.

Catfish   *Bladder 4, Stomach 4*
Edema, diminished urination, poor appetite, shortage of milk secretion in nursing mothers, dizziness.

Clam   *Liver -5, Kidneys -5*
Pink eyes, eczema, boils, alcoholism, blurred vision, dizziness.

Common carp   *Kidneys 2, Spleen 2*
Poor appetite, edema, diminished urination, shortage of milk secretion in nursing mothers. It is also being used to treat edema due to chronic nephritis and hepatic ascites.

Crab   *Liver -7, Stomach -7*
Bone fracture, swelling and pain caused by blood coagulation, difficult labor, jaundice.

Cuttlefish   *Liver -3, Kidneys -3*
Shortage of milk secretion in nursing mothers, suppression of menses, meager menstrual flow, vaginal bleeding, ringing in the ears, dizziness, seminal emission, premature ejaculation.

Eel   *Liver 4, Kidneys 4, Spleen 4*
Fatigue, chronic diarrhea, bleeding in hemorrhoids, rheumatism.

Freshwater shrimp   *Spleen 4, Stomach 4*
Impotence, seminal emission, enuresis, insufficient sperm, shortage of milk secretion in nursing mothers.

Frog   *Kidneys -5*
Weakness while recuperating from an illness, malnutrition in children, dysentery, diarrhea after meals.

Gold carp   *Spleen 2, Stomach 2*
Poor appetite, shortage of milk secretion in nursing mothers, edema, diminished urination.

Grass carp   *Spleen 4, Stomach 4*
Cold stomachache, poor appetite, headache, bitter taste in the mouth, pink eyes, prone to anger.

Hairtail   *Liver 4, Spleen 4*
Fatigue, nausea, withered hair, shortage of milk secretion in nursing mothers. The oil is used to treat viral hepatitis.

Herring   *Spleen 2*
Poor growth in children, weakness in women after childbirth.

Jellyfish   *Liver -3, Kidneys -3*
Cough, asthma, scrofula, constipation.

Loach   *Spleen 2*
Diminished urination, jaundice, impotence, diarrhea, various kinds of hepatitis. Modern research indicates that loach can reduce jaundice and bring down the transaminase level.

Lobster   *Kidneys 1*
Impotence, weakness after childbirth, shortage of milk secretion in nursing mothers.

Long-kissing sturgeon   *Bladder 2, Spleen 2*
Edema in the lower limbs, poor appetite, diminished urination.

Long-tailed anchovy   *Liver 4, Spleen 4*
Poor appetite, abdominal swelling, fatigue.

Mackerel   *Spleen 2, Stomach 2*
Edema and weakness in the lower limbs, beriberi, diminished urination, dizziness, premature aging.

Mackerel gallbladder   *Liver -8*
The gallbladder of the mackerel is removed and placed in a drafty, cool room to dry; when dried, it is ground into powder. Good for pink eyes, pain in the eyes, corneal opacity, eczema, hemorrhoids, otitis media.

Mandarin fish   *Stomach 2*
Weakness, poor appetite, pulmonary tuberculosis.
Murrel (snakehead)   *Spleen -2, Stomach -2*
Edema, beriberi, diminished urination, scabies, carbuncle, leprosy.
Mussel   *Liver -1, Kidneys -1*
Dizziness, vaginal discharge, excessive menstrual flow, hypertension.
Oyster   *Heart -1*
Insomnia, night sweats, dizziness after intoxication. Modern research indicates that oysters can enhance male sexual capacity.
Perch   *Liver 2, Kidneys 2, Spleen 2, Stomach 2*
Edema, diminished urination, insecure fetus.
River clamshell   *Liver -5, Kidneys -5*
Coughing up copious phlegm, stomachache, hiccups, whitish vaginal discharge, eczema. River clamshell is used in powder form.
River snail   *L. intestine -5, S. intestine -5,*
                                         Bladder -5, Stomach -5
Pain on urination, edema, frequent urination, diabetes..
Sea cucumber   *Kidneys -1, Heart -1*
Impotence, seminal emission, sliding emission, frequent urination, lumbago, constipation with dry stools. Modern research indicates that sea cucumber is effective for spasmodic numbness in strokes and for chronic hepatitis.
Silver carp   *Spleen 4, Stomach 4*
Cold stomachache, decreased appetite.
Small-eyed carp   *Stomach 4*
Cold stomachache.
Spiral-shelled snail   *Bladder -2*
Diminished urination, pain in beriberi, pain on urination, pink eyes, blurred vision.
Variegated carp (bighead)   *Liver 4*
Cold abdominal pain, coughing up phlegm particularly in the elderly.
White eel   *Liver 2, Kidneys 2, Spleen 2*
Cough, rheumatism, carbuncle, hemorrhoids.
Whitebait   *Spleen 2, Stomach 2*
Poor appetite, indigestion, chronic diarrhea, dry cough, skinniness.
Yellow croaker   *Stomach -1*
Stomachache, poor appetite, vomiting of blood, dizziness, ringing in the ears, whitish vaginal discharge.

SUGARS, OILS, AND SPICES

Sugars, oils, and spices are additives frequently used in cooking. Such additives can wake up and increase the appetite, strengthen the spleen, and promote digestion. Some additives can also wake up the spirits. Additives can be divided into the following five categories: sweet foods, drinks, sour and salty condiments, spices, and oils.

Sweet foods, such as white sugar and honey, are foods that contain carbohydrates. They taste sweet and are neutral in energy, and most of them can tone the spleen and strengthen the stomach, slow down acute symptoms, and relieve pain. They are frequently used to treat symptoms arising from spleen and stomach deficiencies, including a poor appetite and abdominal pain. However, an excessive consumption of carbohydrates can cause abdominal swelling and a decreased appetite, because such foods are slow in movement; eating too many sweet foods can also contribute to an accumulation of dampness that generates phlegm.

The second category includes drinks such as tea and wine. Most drinks can strengthen the spleen and the stomach. They are also stimulating and can relieve fatigue and excite the spirits. But an excessive consumption can have a negative effect.

Sour and salty condiments include vinegar and soy sauce. Most of them can wake up the appetite and promote digestion. However, they have to be consumed in moderate quantities to be beneficial, as their primary function is to improve the taste of foods.

Most spices can wake up the appetite and improve digestion. But because they are pungent in flavor, they can waste energy and generate fire, which are harmful to yin energy. Thus, spices should not be consumed inadvertently.

Oils, such as sesame oil and soybean oil, are indispensable seasonings in cooking. Oils can be divided into vegetable oils and animal oils. Oils are very important nutrients for the human body; they are an indispensable driving force in maintaining the normal functions of the internal organs. The consumption of oils in adequate quantities can help maintain normal body temperature, moist and smooth skin, and shiny hair; however, an excessive consumption can cause harm to the body, as this increases the burden of the heart.

The following list shows organ y-scores and indications for sugars, oils, and spices.

Beer
Poor digestion, weak stomach, diminished urination, edema.

Black and white pepper   *L. intestine 8, Stomach 8*
Cold stomachache, vomiting of clear water, poor appetite, indigestion, chronic tracheitis.

Brown sugar   *Liver 4, Spleen 4, Stomach 4*
Lochia after childbirth that does not stop or abdominal pain due to blood coagulation, irregular menstruation, menstrual pain, meager menstrual flow.

Coffee   *Heart 1*
Sleepiness, low spirits due to intoxication, edema, diminished urination.

Cottonseed oil   *L. intestine 8*
Constipation with dry stools, scabies, cough.

Fresh ginger   *Spleen 6, Stomach 6*
The common cold, vomiting, food poisoning.

Green onion   *Seed: Kidneys 6; white head: Stomach 6*
The common cold, headache, nasal congestion, mastitis, chest pain.

Honey   *L. intestine 2, Spleen 2*
Fatigue, poor appetite, abdominal pain, cold limbs, dry cough, constipation.

Hops   *Spleen -6, Bladder -6*
Indigestion, abdominal swelling, edema, pulmonary tuberculosis, insomnia. Hops are used to bitter beer.

Japanese cassia bark   *Liver 5, Kidneys 5, Heart 5*
Cold abdominal pain, vomiting, hiccups, rheumatism.

Lard   *Spleen 0, Stomach 0*
Poor spirits and weakness, withered hair, excessive perspiration, dry cough, cracked skin.

Maltose (malt sugar)   *Spleen 4, Stomach 4*
Fatigue, shortness of breath, poor appetite, abdominal pain, dry cough, gastric ulcer, duodenal ulcer.

Monosodium glutamate
Poor appetite, malnutrition. A prolonged use can produce toxicity; it is not recommended for people with incomplete kidney function.

Prickly ash   *Kidneys 6, Spleen 6*
Cold abdominal pain, vomiting, diarrhea, indigestion in children.

Rape oil   *l. intestine 6, Liver 6*
Various disorders of the abdomen after childbirth, constipation
with dry stools, skin itch, eczema.
Rock sugar   *Spleen 2*
Fasting dysentery, coughing up phlegm, poor appetite in children.
Salt   *L. intestine -7, S. intestine -7, Kidneys -7, Stomach -7*
Sore throat, bleeding from gums, ulcers in the mouth and on the
tongue, habitual constipation.
Sesame oil   *L. intestine 0*
Constipation with dry stools, falling out of hair.
Soy sauce   *Kidneys -7, Spleen -7, Stomach -7*
Bleeding during pregnancy, blood in urine.
Soybean oil   *L. intestine 7*
Constipation, intestinal obstruction, arteriosclerosis, high choles-
terol.
Star anise   *Liver 5, Kidneys 5, Spleen 5*
Cold abdominal pain, falling of the testis on one side, vomiting,
poor appetite.
Tea   *Heart -6, Stomach -6*
Thirst, alcoholism, diarrhea, diminished urination, discharge of
blood from the anus, enteritis, dysentery, ulcers.
Vinegar   *Liver -1, Stomach -1*
Abdominal swelling due to blood coagulation, vomiting of blood,
nosebleed, discharge of blood from the anus.
White sugar   *Spleen 2*
Abdominal pain, dry cough or coughing up a little phlegm, dry
mouth, thirst.
Wine   *Liver 3, Stomach 3*
Cold rheumatism, spasms, chest pain, also used to speed the
action of certain herbs.

GRAINS

Grains primarily taste sweet and have a neutral energy. It is very
seldom that they are extremely cold or hot; for this reason, they
can be consumed on a regular basis for a long time without harmful effects. Grains can strengthen the spleen and the stomach, and
they can support the body's energy and cure symptoms arising
from spleen and stomach deficiencies, such as a poor appetite and

fatigue. Because grains have a moderate energy, they do not cause any harm to the body as long as they are consumed in moderate quantities.

Many people prefer the taste of polished grains and polished-grain products like flour, but they contain fewer nutrients. So, it is not wise to eat polished grains and polished-grain products for a prolonged period of time, in order to avoid vitamin deficiency and other physical disorders.

According to modern research, grains contribute to the growth and development of the human body, and they are primarily acid-producing foods, as opposed to fruit and vegetables, which are alkali-producing foods. When grains and vegetables are consumed together, they keep acids and alkalis in a state of balance, so that the normal pH range of systemic arterial blood can be maintained.

The following list shows the organ y-scores and indications for various grains.

Adzuki bean *S. intestine 0, Heart 0*
Edema, beriberi, diarrhea, mumps, hepatic ascites.

Barley *Spleen -3, Stomach -3*
Abdominal swelling, diminished urination, urination difficulty, indigestion.

Black sesame seed *Liver 2, Kidneys 2*
Premature gray hair, constipation with dry stools, dizziness.

Black soybean *Kidneys 2, Spleen 2*
Diabetes, dizziness, blurred vision, rheumatism, spasms of the four limbs, edema, beriberi. See "Yellow soybean" below.

Broad bean (horse bean, fava bean) *Spleen 2, Stomach 2*
Poor appetite, edema, diminished urination, beriberi

Brome seed *Heart 0, Stomach 0*
Poor appetite, difficult bowel movements.

Broomcorn (faxtail millet) *L. intestine 2, Spleen 2, Stomach 2*
Cough, diarrhea, thirst, stomachache, vomiting, hiccups.

Buckwheat *L. intestine 0, Spleen 0, Stomach 0*
Diarrhea, whitish vaginal discharge, abdominal pain.

Corn (Indian corn, maize) *L. intestine 2, Stomach 2*
Poor appetite, indigestion, edema, urination disorders, urinary stones, chronic nephritis.

Corn silk *Gallbladder 2, Liver 2*
Edema, diminished urination, burning sensation on urination, jaundice.

Job's tears (coix seed)   *Kidneys 0, Spleen 0*
Diarrhea, edema, rheumatism, urination difficulty, chronic enteritis. Modern research indicates that it can inhibit the growth of cancers, and it is most frequently used to treat cervical cancer. The seeds are used as an herb and a food. It is widely available in Chinese herb shops under the name Yi-Yi-Ren.

Millet   *Lungs 2, L. intestine 2, Spleen 2*
Upset stomach, vomiting, diarrhea and indigestion in children, diabetes, dry mouth.

Mung bean   *Heart 0, Stomach 0*
Diminished urination, red urine, diarrhea, dermatitis, enteritis, mumps, lead poisoning.

Pea   *Spleen 2, Stomach 2*
Shortage of milk secretion in nursing mothers, vomiting, hiccups, thirst, diarrhea.

Polished rice   *Spleen 2, Stomach 2*
Recuperating patients and women after childbirth, diarrhea, thirst, diminished urination.

Sorghum   *L. intestine 4, Spleen 4, Stomach 4*
Indigestion in children, diarrhea, vomiting, diminished urination.

Sweet rice (glutinous rice)   *Stomach 4*
Chronic diarrhea, thirst, poor appetite, nausea, excessive perspiration, peptic ulcer.

Wheat   *Kidneys 0, Spleen 0, Heart 0*
Hysteria in women, chronic diarrhea, nervousness, mastitis, burns, thirst, diminished urination, spitting of blood.

Yellow soybean   *L. intestine 2, Spleen 2*
Skinniness, indigestion, boils, withered and yellowish complexion. Soybean is yellow or black in color and widely cultivated for its nutritious, edible seeds and bean sprouts. Tofu, soybean oil, and soy sauce are made from yellow soybeans, whereas black soybeans are used to make fermented soya beans.

GUIDE TO APPROXIMATE EQUIVALENTS

CUSTOMARY				METRIC
			1/4 t.	1.25 g
			1/2 t.	2.5 g
			1 t.	5 g
			2 t.	10 g
1/2 oz.		1 T.	3 t.	15 g
1 oz.		2 T.	6 t.	30 g
2 oz.	1/4 c.	4 T.	12 t.	60 g
4 oz.	1/2 c.	8 T.	24 t.	120 g
8 oz.	1 c.	16 T.	48 t.	240 g
1 lb.	2 c.			480 g
2 lb.	4 c.			960 g
2.2 lb.				1 kg

Keep in mind that these are not an exact conversions, but generally may be used in measuring herbs.

Index

accumulation of phlegm, 19–20, 28
acid-base balance, 251, 257, 265
aquatic food
overview of, 258–259
list of, with organ y-scores and
indications, 259–261
atmospheric energies, 13–18. *See also*
cold, dampness, dryness, fire,
summer heat, wind

bladder syndromes
Bladder Cold and Deficiency,
176–178
Bladder Damp Heat, 174–176
bladder, functions of, 12
blood coagulation, 18
blood deficiency, 20, 28

Chart Five: Y-Scores and Organ Y-
Scores of Foods, 230–245
Chart Four: Western Diseases with
Their Possible Syndromes, 62–75
Chart One: Signs and Symptoms,
34–46
Chart Three: Recording and Calculating for Individuals Who Are
Ill, 58–61
Chart Two: Recording and Calculating for Healthy Individuals,
52–55
Chinese food cures
advantages of, 223–224
fundamental concepts of, 223–224
history of, 224–225
cold, 14–15, 28

dampness, 15–16, 28
diseases with possible syndromes, list
of, 62–75
dryness, 16–17, 28

eggs. *See* meat, poultry, and eggs
energy congestion, 19

energy deficiency, 20, 28

fire, 17–18, 28
fish. *See* aquatic food
food energies, 226
food flavors, 226
aromatic, 228
bitter, 227–228
light or bland, 228
obstructive or constrictive, 228
pungent, 227
salty, 228
sour, 227
sweet, 227
food, y-scores for the five energies of,
229
food, y-scores for the six flavors of,
229
foods, list of, with y-scores and organ
y-scores, 230–245
foods, properties of, 226–228
fruit and nuts
overview of, 246
list of, with organ y-scores and
indications, 247–250

gallbladder syndromes
Gallbladder Energy Deficiency,
158–159
Gallbladder Excessive Heat,
156–158
gallbladder, functions of, 12
grains
overview of, 264–265
list of, with organ y-scores and
indications, 265–266

heart syndromes
Heart Blood Deficiency, 185–187
Heart Energy Deficiency, 179–181
Heart Fire Flaming, 187–189
Heart Yang Deficiency, 181–183
Heart Yin Deficiency, 183–185

No Communication between the
Kidneys and Heart (Heart Fire
Flaming with Kidneys Yin Defi-
ciency), 197–199
Phlegm Fire Disturbing the Heart,
189–191
Simultaneous Deficiency of the
Heart and Spleen, 199–201
Yang Deficiency of the Heart and
Kidneys, 201–203
heart, functions of, 9
herbal formulas, 80–81
herbs, decoction of, 80

internal organs
concept of in traditional Chinese
medicine, 5
determining y-scores of, 28, 30, 31
external and internal influences on,
12–22
functions of, 9–12 (*See also specific
internal organs*)

kidney syndromes
Insufficient Kidneys Pure Essence
(Kidneys Yin Deficiency Affect-
ing Reproduction), 166–168
Kidneys Unable to Absorb Inspira-
tion (Kidneys Deficiency Affect-
ing the Lungs), 171–173
Kidneys Yang Deficiency, 160–163
Kidneys Yin Deficiency, 163–166
Loosening of Kidneys Energy (Kid-
neys Energy Deficiency Affect-
ing the Bladder), 168–171
No Communication between the
Kidneys and Heart (Heart Fire
Flaming with Kidneys Yin Defi-
ciency), 197–199
Yang Deficiency of the Heart and
Kidneys, 201–203
Yang Deficiency of the Spleen and
Kidneys, 205–208
Yin Deficiency of the Liver and
Kidneys, 211–213
Yin Deficiency of the Lungs and
Kidneys, 208–211

kidneys, functions of, 10–11

large intestine syndromes
Large Intestine Damp Heat, 97–99
Large Intestine Deficiency and
Slippery Diarrhea, 102–104
Large Intestine Fluid Exhaustion
(Dry Large Intestine), 100–102
large intestine, functions of, 11
liver syndromes
Cold Obstructing the Liver Merid-
ian, 151–153
Damp Heat Attacking the Liver
and Gallbladder, 153–155
Disharmony between the Liver and
Spleen (Liver Excess with
Spleen Deficiency), 214–215
Disharmony between the Liver and
Stomach (Liver Energy Conges-
tion with Stomach Deficiency),
216–218
Internal Liver Wind Blowing,
149–151
Liver Blood Deficiency, 142–144
Liver Energy Congestion, 137–139
Liver Fire Flaming Upward,
140–142
Liver Fire Offending the Lungs,
218–220
Liver Yang Upsurging (Yin Defi-
ciency of the Liver and the Kid-
neys Affecting Liver Yang),
146–149
Liver Yin Deficiency, 144–146
Yin Deficiency of the Liver and
Kidneys, 211–213
liver, functions of, 10
lung syndromes
Deficient and Cold Lungs (Lungs
Yang Deficiency), 87–89
Dry Lungs, 94–96
Energy Deficiency of the Spleen
and Lungs, 203–205
Hot Lungs (Lungs Fire), 93–94
Liver Fire Offending the Lungs,
218–220
Lungs Energy Deficiency, 81–83

Lungs under the Attack of Wind and Cold, 85–87
Lungs Yin Deficiency (Deficient and Hot Lungs), 83–85
Phlegm Dampness Obstructing the Lungs, 89–90
Wind and Heat Attacking the Lungs, 90–93
Yin Deficiency of the Lungs and Kidneys, 208–211
lungs, functions of, 9–10

meat, poultry, and eggs
   overview of, 256–257
   list of, with organ y-scores and indications, 257–258

numbers and sums, recording of, 31, 46–51, 52–55, 55–61
nuts. *See* fruit and nuts

oils. *See* sugars, oils, and spices
"organ actions of foods," 229

poultry. *See* meat, poultry, and eggs

recipes
   "Deep-Pot Red Beans in Hen," 223
   "Honey Steamed with Lily," 224
recording numbers and sums of signs and symptoms, 31, 46–51, 52–55, 55–61

shellfish. *See* aquatic food
signs and symptoms
   categories of, 31–32
   chart, 34–46
   of abdomen, 34–35
   of anus and genitals, 35
   of appetite, 35
   of back, 35
   of belching, 35
   of bleeding, 35–36
   of bowel movement, 36
   of chest, 36
   of children, 37
   of cold and hot sensations, 37
   of cough and phlegm, 37–38
   of ears, 38
   of emotions and mental states, 38–39
   of eyes, 39
   of face, 39–40
   of habits and preferences, 40
   of head and neck, 40
   of hiccups, 40
   of limbs, 40
   of men, 40
   of mouth and lips, 41
   of nose, 41
   of pain, 41–43
   of perspiration, 43
   of respiration, 43
   of skin, 43
   of sleep, 43–44
   of teeth, 44
   of throat, 44
   of tongue, 44
   of urination, 44–45
   of voice, 45
   of vomiting, 45
   of whole body, 45–46
   of women (menstruation), 46
   of women (miscellaneous), 46
   of women (pregnancy and child-birth), 46
   of women (vaginal discharge), 46
signs, clinical, 23–24. *See also* signs and symptoms
small intestine syndromes
   Excessive Heat in the Small Intestine, 192–194
   Small Intestine Energy Congestion (Small Intestine Energy Pain), 194–196
small intestine, functions of, 11
spices. *See* sugars, oils, and spices
spleen syndromes
   Cold Dampness Troubling the Spleen (Dampness Troubling Spleen Yang), 118–121
   Damp Heat Steaming the Spleen, 121–124

Disharmony between the Liver and Spleen (Liver Excess with Spleen Deficiency), 214–215

Energy Deficiency of the Spleen and Lungs, 203–205

Middle Energy Cave-in (Deficient Spleen with Cave-in of Its Energy), 111–114

Simultaneous Deficiency of the Heart and Spleen, 199–201

Spleen Energy Deficiency, 105–108

Spleen Unable to Govern Blood (Spleen Deficiency and Cold), 115–118

Spleen Yang Deficiency (Deficient and Cold Spleen), 108–111

Yang Deficiency of the Spleen and Kidneys, 205–208

spleen, functions of, 10

Step 1: identifying your signs and symptoms, 31–46

Step 2: recording numbers and sums of signs and symptoms for healthy people, 31, 46–51, 52–55

Step 3: recording numbers and sums of signs and symptoms for people who are ill, 31, 55–61

Step 4: identifying the syndrome responsible for your disease and the y-score of your internal organs, 31, 61–75

steps for determining the y-scores of the internal organs, overview of, 31

stomach syndromes
Cold Stomach, 130–133
Disharmony between the Liver and Stomach (Liver Energy Congestion with Stomach Deficiency), 216–218
Food Stagnation in the Stomach (Stomach Energy Congestion), 128–130
Hot Stomach, 133–136

Stomach Yin Deficiency (Stomach Deficient Heat), 125–128

stomach, functions of, 11–12

sugars, oils, and spices
overview of, 262
list of, with organ y-scores and indications, 263–264

summer heat, 15, 28

symptoms, common, 23. *See also* signs and symptoms

syndromes. *See also specific syndromes under* bladder syndromes, gall-bladder syndromes, heart syndromes, kidney syndromes, large intestine syndromes, liver syndromes, lung syndromes, small intestine syndromes, spleen syndromes, stomach syndromes
causes of, 13,
definition of, 6, 24
establishing y-scores for, 30
explanations of categories for, 79–81
list of, with y-scores, 25–27

vegetables
overview of, 250–251
list of, with organ y-scores and indications, 251–256

Western diseases, 23, 61–75
wind, 13–14, 28

yang deficiency, 21, 28
yang scores, 5, 29
yin deficiency, 21–22, 28
yin scores, 5, 29
y-scores of food
concept of, 5, 229
formula for, 229–230
y-scores of the internal organs
concept of, 5, 24
determination of, 28, 31
range of, 28
with list of syndromes, 25–27